VIBRIOS IN
THE ENVIRONMENT

VIBRIOS IN THE ENVIRONMENT

EDITED BY

RITA R. COLWELL
University of Maryland

ASSOCIATE EDITORS

HENRY B. BRADFORD, Jr.
Department of Health and
Human Services State of Louisiana

NELL C. ROBERTS
Department of Health and
Human Services State of Louisiana

MARY A. HOOD
University of West Florida

RAMON J. SEIDLER
Oregon State University

ALWORTH D. LARSON
Louisiana State University

RONALD J. SIEBELING
Louisiana State University

TECHNICAL EDITOR

MARY BETH HATEM
University of Maryland

A WILEY-INTERSCIENCE PUBLICATION

JOHN WILEY & SONS

New York ● Chichester ● Brisbane ● Toronto ● Singapore

Library of Congress Cataloging in Publication Data
Main entry under title:

Vibrios in the environment.

  (Environmental science and technology)
  "A Wiley-Interscience publication."
  Includes index.
    1. Vibrio. 2. Vibrio cholerae. I. Colwell, Rita
R., 1934—   . II. Series. [DNLM: 1. Vibrio.
2. Vibrio cholerae. 3. Vibrio infections—Prevention
and control. 4. Environment. QW 141 V626]
QR82.S6V53 1984   614.5'14   83-21720
ISBN 0-471-87343-8

Printed in the United States of America

10 9 8 7 6 5 4 3 2 1

SERIES PREFACE

Environmental Science and Technology

The Environmental Science and Technology Series of Monographs, Textbooks, and Advances is devoted to the study of the quality of the environment and to the technology of its conservation. Environmental science therefore relates to the chemical, physical, and biological changes in the environment through contamination or modification, to the physical nature and biological behavior of air, water, soil, food, and waste as they are affected by man's agricultural, industrial, and social activities, and to the application of science and technology to the control and improvement of environmental quality.

The deterioration of environmental quality, which began when man first collected into villages and utilized fire, has existed as a serious problem under the ever-increasing impacts of exponentially increasing population and of industrializing society. Environmental contamination of air, water, soil, and food has become a threat to the continued existence of many plant and animal communities of the ecosystem and may ultimately threaten the very survival of the human race.

It seems clear that if we are to preserve for future generations some semblance of the biological order of the world of the past and hope to improve on the deteriorating standards of urban public health, environmental science and technology must quickly come to play a dominant role in designing our social and industrial structure for tomorrow. Scientifically rigorous criteria of environmental quality must be developed. Based in part on these criteria, realistic standards must be established and our technological progress must be tailored to meet them. It is obvious that civilization will continue to require increasing amounts of fuel, transportation, industrial chemicals, fertilizers, pesticides, and countless other products; and that it will continue to produce waste products of all descriptions. What is urgently needed is a total systems approach to modern civilization through which the pooled talents of scientists and engineers, in cooperation with social scientists and the medical profession, can be focused on the development of order and equilibrium in the presently disparate segments of the human environment. Most of the skills and tools that are needed are already in existence. We surely have a right to hope a technology that has created such manifold environmental problems is also capable of solving them. It is our hope that this Series in Environmental Sciences and Technology will not only serve to make this challenge more explicit to the established professionals, but that it also will help to stimulate the student toward the career opportunities in this vital area.

Robert L. Metcalf
Werner Stumm

CONTENTS

IMPLICATIONS FOR THE SEAFOOD INDUSTRY

VIBRIOS IN THE ENVIRONMENT

Rita R. Colwell

The past decade has seen an extraordinary increase in interest in the Vibrionaceae. The taxonomy of the genera and species of this family of bacteria has been much improved, with a clarified distinction of Vibrio from Aeromonas, Photobacterium, and Plesiomonas and improved definition of species within the genus. New species, Vibrio fluvialis, Vibrio vulnificus, Vibrio hollisae, Vibrio damsela, Vibrio mimicus, and the redefined Vibrio cholerae and Vibrio metschnikovii, have been published (see West and Colwell, this volume).

Recognition of the pathogenic potential of vibrios, other than that of Vibrio cholerae, has also been much broadened. The first of the noncholera vibrios to be widely recognized as a serious human pathogen was Vibrio parahaemolyticus, an estuarine, halophilic bacterium common in shellfish. It has been known for nearly three decades as a frequent cause of foodborne infection in Japan and is now widely recognized as an etiologic agent of gastroenteritis following consumption of contaminated seafood. It may also cause sores on bathers swimming in salt water. The literature on Vibrio parahaemolyticus, as a human pathogen, has been reviewed by Joseph, Colwell, and Kaper (1982).

Vibrios that are biochemically very similar to the epidemic strains of Vibrio cholerae (V. cholerae serovar O1), but that do not agglutinate in V. cholerae O group 1 antiserum are referred to as non-O1 V. cholerae, and have been called noncholera vibrios and "nonagglutinable" vibrios in the past. V. cholerae non-O1 have been isolated from the environment in several countries around the world (Colwell et al., 1977; Juras et al. 1979; Lee et al. 1982; Desmarchelier and Reichelt 1981).

Outbreaks of diarrheal illness have been associated with non-O1 V. cholerae infection (Aldova et al. 1968; Dakin et al. 1974; World Health Organization 1980). Non-O1 V. cholerae infections have also been associated with severe cholera-like diarrhea in Bangladesh (McIntyre et al. 1965). Recently, Wilson et al. (1981) reported a non-O group 1 Vibrio cholerae gastroenteritis during November 1979 in Florida, associated with eating raw oysters. The non-O1 V. cholerae organisms were isolated from oysters and water samples taken from areas where ill persons had collected oysters. Interestingly, in at least one instance the same serovar was isolated from a patient's stool specimen and from the water where the patient had collected oysters. In their study, Wilson et al. (1981) traced the source of oysters to Oyster Bay and Apalachicola Bay locations. None of the clinical or environmental isolates were toxigenic in the Y-1 adrenal cell assay. The fact that the sites were as much as 80 km apart made the likelihood of a single source very small.

The potential severity of non-O1 V. cholerae infections is highlighted by the report of Guard et al. (1980) who described a case of fatal septicemia caused by V. cholerae which did not agglutinate with O group 1 V. cholerae antiserum. The illness occurred in an Australian Aboriginal woman and the organism was isolated from multiple blood cultures and urine while the patient was living and from a large hepatic abscess found post mortem.

Thus, it is now recognized that V. cholerae other than O1 serovar can be responsible for a wide range of diseases, including severe systemic infections (Hughes et al. 1978; Back et al. 1974). Furthermore, the association of V. cholerae non-O1 with diarrheal illness has been widely reported, both in cholera-endemic areas (Zafari et al. 1973) and in areas where cholera is not considered to be a health problem (Back et al. 1974; Dakin et al. 1974).

The isolation of V. cholerae from extra-intestinal disease is no longer a rarity (Fearrington et al. 1974; Goei and Karthigasu 1978), with reports of isolation of the organism from the ear, respiratory tract, cerebrospinal fluid, wound infections, and blood. In contrast to the typical behavior of V. cholerae O1, the non-O1 serovars have the capacity to invade the blood stream (Robins-Browne et al. 1977).

Vibrio vulnificus, the lactose-fermenting, halophilic vibrio, is a bacterium of unusual virulence (Hollis et al. 1976), capable of causing death in laboratory animals injected intraperitoneally in less than three hours (Poole and Oliver 1978). Unlike V. parahaemolyticus or V. cholerae, V. vulnificus can cause death when inoculated subcutaneously. The bacteria produce an extremely potent vascular permeability factor which leads to dramatic vascular fluid loss in laboratory animals. A significant correlation between ingestion of raw oysters and fatal infections has been shown (Blake et al. 1979). The vascular permeability changes occurring in V. vulnificus infections appear to require direct contact between host cells and viable Vibrio cells, rather than being diffusible toxin-induced (Bowdre et al. 1981). The rapidly progressive invasion associated with V. vulnificus infections in both forms--the fulminating septicemia in which V. vulnificus is isolated from blood cultures and sometimes also from secondary skin lesions and the other a rapidly progressive cellulitis resulting from infection of seawater-associated wounds, such as those sustained while cleaning crabs or digging clams--is unique among Vibrio spp. (Carpenter 1979). The latter occurs in apparently healthly people and is characterized by marked edema and necrosis. Heat-labile, antigenic, extracellular toxins produced by V. vulnificus have been described (Kreger and Lockwood 1981), but their role in the pathogenesis of disease is not clear. Erythrocyte hemolysis by strains of V. vulnificus were studied by Johnson and Calia (1981). All V. vulnificus strains, both environmental and clinical, produce a hemolysin that affects human erythrocytes, in contrast to V. parahaemolyticus, in which only clinical isolates are hemolytic. However, the evidence to date is convincing that iron plays a major role in the pathogenesis of V. vulnificus. Added iron was found to be required in an iron-limiting environment, as in human serum (Wright et al. 1981), and a high correlation of V. vulnificus septicemia in humans with hepatic disorders has been observed (Blake et al. 1980b).

Unlike V. parahaemolyticus, V. vulnificus showed a rapid and dramatic decrease in viability, not attributable to cold shock or to environmental factors, when suspended in oyster homogenates held at 4°C (Oliver 1981). V. vulnificus cells incubated on raw whole oysters held at 0.5°C exhibited a less dramatic decline in viability. Oysters kept on ice apparently are not a likely source of V. vulnificus infections.

V. alginolyticus has been found to occur in the aquatic environment, as well as in shellfish, in widely diverse geographic locations (Baross and Liston 1970; Kamplemacher et al. 1972). V. alginolyticus has also been isolated from wound infections (Rubin and Tilton 1975; Hollis et al. 1976; Pien et al. 1977). Eight cases of V. alginolyticus infections in Hawaii (Pien et al. 1977) were superficial, most often after coral or surfboard accidents. Three isolates were recovered from otitis externa cases related to swimming and were similar to English coastal cases (Ryan 1976).

U.S. travelers to Asia, Africa, the Middle East, and Oceania often have been concerned about the risk of acquiring cholera. However, only ten cases of cholera in U.S. travelers have been reported since the current cholera pandemic began in 1961. Nine of the ten were infected by Vibrio cholerae O1 El Tor, the strain responsible for the current pandemic, with no secondary cases involved. In fact, the chance of acquiring a reported case of cholera is less than one case per 500,000 returning travelers (Snyder and Blake 1982).

Domestically acquired cholera in the United States was reported in 1973, after more than 50 years without any known cases except for a few acquired in laboratories. In 1973, a case of cholera was reported in Port Lavaca, Texas, on the Gulf Coast (Weissman et al. 1974). No source of infection was found. In 1978, eight cases of cholera, and three persons asymptomatically infected with V. cholerae

O1, were found in southwestern Louisiana and were traced to eating insufficiently cooked crabs caught locally in Gulf Coast marshes (Blake et al. 1980a). The Texas and Louisiana strains were all biotype El Tor serotype Inaba, of the same unusual phage type, and hemolytic. The majority of V. cholerae O1 strains worldwide are now nonhemolytic (Barrett and Blake 1981), except for a recent outbreak of classical V. cholerae in Bangladesh in December 1982. V. cholerae El Tor Inaba was isolated from the stool of a woman in Florida with a diarrheal illness in 1980 (Centers for Disease Control 1980), but the strain ultimately proved to be nontoxigenic. Two cases of cholera--that is, gastro-intestinal disease caused by toxigenic Vibrio cholerae O-group--were reported in Texas in May and June 1981. In both cases, the organism isolated was a toxigenic, hemo-lytic, biotype El Tor, and serotype Inaba (Kelly et al. 1981).

In September 1981, toxigenic V. cholerae O-group 1, biotype El Tor, serotype Inaba was isolated in Louisiana from the stool of a man with diarrheal disease. The victim became ill five days after beginning a 7-day tour on an oil rig in the Intracoastal Waterway in Jefferson County, south of Port Arthur, Texas (Centers for Disease Control 1981).

The occurrence of Vibrio cholerae serovar O1 in Chesapeake Bay in Maryland and estuaries and sewers in Louisiana was reported by Colwell et al. (1977; 1981). The isolation of V. cholerae in both the Chesapeake Bay and Louisiana in areas relatively free of fecal contamination, using the presence of E. coli as an index, has led to the hypothesis that V. cholerae is indeed a component of the autochthonous flora of brackish water, estuaries, and salt marshes of coastal areas of the temperate zone (Colwell et al. 1981). Additional reports of the isolation of V. cholerae O1 from other Gulf Coast areas have been published (Hood et al. 1981; Twedt et al. 1981).

Recent observations strongly suggest an association of V. cholerae, and related vibrios, with invertebrate animals and zooplankton in the estuarine and marine environment (Huq et al. 1983). In addition, the most recent discovery that V. cholerae can survive in the estuarine and marine environment in a viable, but nonrecoverable, stage opens new opportunities for understanding the ecological role of this organism (Xu et al. 1983).

Interestingly, members of the genus Vibrio have been implicated in outbreaks of disease in larvae of Crassostrea virginica (Tubiash et al. 1970; Brown et al. 1981; Elston et al. 1981) and in lobsters (Bowser et al. 1981). The incidence of Vibrio spp. associated with blue crabs in Chesapeake Bay (Sizemore et al. 1975; Tubiash et al. 1975) and in Galveston Bay, Texas (Davis and Sizemore 1982) has been reported.

This volume brings together a series of papers dealing with the epidemiology, serology, pathogenesis, molecular genetic aspects, and ecology of pathogenic vibrios and related organisms as well as their isolation, enumeration, and identification, and implications for the seafood industry. Clearly, the role of vibrios in the environment and their implication in human disease are compelling. It is hoped that the information available in this volume will provide answers to some of the questions and pave the way for new ideas, ultimately leading to the solution of the enigma of the pandemic of cholera over the centuries.

REFERENCES

Aldova, E., K. Laznickova, E. Stepankova, and J. Lietava. 1968. Isolation of nonagglutinable vibrios from an enteritis outbreak in Czechoslovakia. J. Infect. Dis. 118:25-31.

Back, E., A. Ljunggren, and H. Smith. 1974. Non-cholera vibrios in Sweden. Lancet 1:723-724.

Baross, J., and J. Liston. 1970. Occurrence of Vibrio parahaemolyticus and related hemolytic vibrios in marine environments of Washington State. Appl. Microbiol. 20:179-186.

Barrett, T.J., and P.A. Blake. 1981. Epidemiological usefulness of changes in hemolytic activity of Vibrio cholerae biotype El Tor during the seventh pandemic. J. Clin. Microbiol. 13:126-129.

Blake, P.A., M. H. Merson, R.E. Weaver, D.G. Hollis, and P.C. Heublein. 1979. Disease caused by a marine vibrio--clinical characteristics and epidemiology. N. Engl. J. Med. 300:1-5.

Blake, P.A., D.T. Allegra, J.D. Snyder, T.J. Barrett, L. McFarland, C.T. Caraway, J.C. Feeley, J.P. Craig, J.V. Lee, N.D. Puhr, and R.A. Feldman. 1980a. Cholera--a possible endemic focus in the United States. N. Engl. J. Med. 302:305-309.

Blake, P.A., R.E. Weaver, and D.G. Hollis. 1980b. Disease of humans (other than cholera) caused by vibrios. Ann. Rev. Microbiol. 34:341-367.

Bowdre, J.H., M.D. Poole, and J.D. Oliver. 1981. Edema and hemoconcentration in mice experimentally infected with Vibrio vulnificus. Infect. Immun. 32:1193-1199.

Bowser, P.R., R. Rosemark, and C.R. Reiner. 1981. A preliminary report of vibriosis in cultured American lobsters, Homarus americanus. J. Invertebr. Pathol. 37:80-85.

Brown, C. 1981. A study of two shellfish-pathogenic Vibrio strains isolated from a Long Island hatchery during a recent outbreak of disease. J. Shellfish Res. 1:83-87.

Carpenter, C.C.J. 1979. More pathogenic vibrios. New Engl. J. Med. 300:39-41.

Centers for Disease Control. 1980. Cholera--Florida. Morbid. Mortal. Wkly. Rep. 29:601.

Centers for Disease Control. 1981. Cholera on a Gulf Coast oil rig--Texas. Morbid. Mortal. Wkly. Rep. 30:589-590.

Colwell, R.R., J. Kaper, and S.W. Joseph. 1977. Vibrio cholerae, Vibrio parahaemolyticus, and other vibrios: occurrence and distribution in Chesapeake Bay. Science 198:394-396.

Colwell, R.R., R.J. Seidler, J. Kaper, S.W. Joseph, S. Garges, H. Lockman, D. Maneval, H.B. Bradford, N. Roberts, E. Remmers, I. Huq, and A. Huq. 1981. Occurrence of Vibrio cholerae serotype O1 in Maryland and Louisiana estuaries. Appl. Environ. Microbiol. 41:555-558.

Dakin, W.P.H., D.J. Howell, R.G.A. Sutton, M.F. O'Keefe, and P. Thomas. 1974. Gastroenteritis due to non-agglutinable (non-cholera) vibrios. Med. J. Australia 2:487-490.

Davis, J.W. and R.K. Sizemore. 1982. Incidence of Vibrio species associated with blue crabs (Callinectes sapidus) from Galveston Bay, Texas. Appl. Environ. Microbiol. 43:1092-1097.

Desmarchelier, P.M., and J.L. Reichelt. 1981. Phenotypic characterization of clinical and environmental isolates of Vibrio cholerae from Australia. Curr. Microbiol. 5:123-129.

Elston, R., L. Leibovitz, D. Relyea, and J. Zatila. 1981. Diagnosis of vibriosis in a commercial oyster hatchery epizootic: diagnostic tools and management features. Aquaculture 24:53-62.

Fearrington, E.L., C.H. Rand, Jr., A. Mewborn, and J. Wilkerson. 1974. Non-cholera Vibrio septicemia and meningoencephalitis. Ann. Intern. Med. 81:401.

Goei, S.H. and K.T. Karthigasu. 1978. Systemic vibriosis due to non-cholera vibrio. Med. J. Aust. 5:286-288.

Guard, R.W., M. Brigden, and P. Desmarchelier. 1980. Fulminating systemic infection caused by Vibrio cholerae species which does not agglutinate with O-1 <u>V</u>. <u>cholerae</u> antiserum. Med. J. Aust. 1:659-661.

Hollis, D.G., R.E. Weaver, C.N. Baker, and C. Thornsberry. 1976. Halophilic <u>Vibrio</u> species isolated from blood cultures. J. Clin. Microbiol. 3:425-431.

Hood, M.A., G.E. Ness, and G.E. Rodrick. 1981. Isolation of Vibrio cholerae serotype O1 from the eastern oyster, <u>Crassostrea virginica</u>. Appl. Environ. Microbiol. 41:559-560.

Hughes, J.M., D.G. Hollis, E.J. Gangarosa, and R.E. Weaver. 1978. Non-cholera vibrio infections in the United States. Clinical, epidemiologic and laboratory features. Ann. Intern. Med. 88:602-606.

Huq, A., E.B. Small, P.A. West, M.I. Huq, R. Rahman, and R.R. Colwell. 1983. Ecological relationships between <u>Vibrio cholerae</u> with planktonic crustacaen copepods. Appl. Environ. Microbiol. 45:275-283.

Johnson, D.E., and F.M. Calia. 1981. Hemolytic reaction of clinical and environmental strains of <u>Vibrio vulnificus</u>. J. Clin. Microbiol. 14:457-459.

Juras, H., U. Futh, D. Winkler, J. Friedmann, and T. Hillig. 1979. Vorkommen von NAG-vibrionen in Berliner geswassern. Zeit. fur Allem. Mikrobiologie 19:403-409.

Joseph, S.W., R.R. Colwell, and J. Kaper. 1982. <u>Vibrio parahaemolyticus</u> and related halophic vibrios. CRC Crit. Rev. Microbiol. 10:77-124.

Kamplemacher, E.H., L.M. Van Noorlejansen, D.A.A. Mossel, and F.J. Groen. 1972. A survey of <u>Vibrio parahaemolyticus</u> and <u>Vibrio alginolyticus</u> on mussels and oysters and in estuarine waters in the Netherlands. J. Appl. Bacteriol. 35:431-438.

Kelly, M.T., J.W. Peterson, H.E. Sarles, Jr., M. Romanko, D. Martin, and B. Hafkin. 1982. Cholera on the Texas Gulf Coast. J. Am. Med. Assoc. 247:1598-1599.

Kreger, A., and D. Lockwood. 1981. Detection of extra-cellular toxin(s) produced by Vibrio vulnificus. Infect. Immun. 33:583-590.

Lee, J.V., D.J. Bashford, T.J. Donovan, A.L. Furniss, and P.A. West. 1982. The incidence of Vibrio cholerae in water, animals, and birds in Kent, England. J. Appl. Bacteriol. 52:281-291.

McIntyre, O.R., J.C. Feeley, W.B. Greenough III, A.S. Benenson, S.I. Hassan, and A. Saad. 1965. Diarrhea caused by non-cholera vibrios. Am. J. Trop. Med. Hyg. 14:412-418.

Oliver, J.D. 1981. Lethal cold stress of Vibrio vulnificus in oysters. Appl. Environ. Microbiol. 41:710-717.

Pien, R., K. Lee, and H. Higa. 1977. Vibrio alginolyticus infections in Hawaii. J. Clin. Microbiol. 5:670-672.

Poole, M.D., and J.D. Oliver. 1978. Experimental patho-genicity and mortality in ligated ileal loop studies of the newly reported halophilic lactose-positive Vibrio sp. Infect. Immun. 20:126-129.

Robins-Browne, R.M., C.S. Still, M. Isaacsoon, H.J. Koornhof, P.C. Appelbaum, and J.N. Scragg. 1977. Pathogenic mechanisms of a non-agglutinable Vibrio cholerae strain: demonstration of invasive and entero-toxigenic properties. Infect. Immun. 18:542-545.

Rubin, S.J., and R.C. Tilton. 1975. Isolation of Vibrio alginolyticus from wound infections. J. Clin. Microbiol. 2:556-558.

Ryan, W.J. 1976. Marine vibrios associated with superficial septic lesions. J. Clin. Pathol. 29:1014-1015.

Sizemore, R.K., R.R. Colwell, H.S. Tubiash, and T.E. Lovelace. 1975. Bacterial flora of the hemolymph of the blue crab, Callinectes sapidus: numerical taxonomy. Appl. Microbiol. 29:393-399.

Snyder, J.D., and P.A. Blake. 1982. Is cholera a problem for U.S. travelers? J. Am. Med. Assoc. 247:2268-2269.

Tubiash, H.S., R.R. Colwell, and R. Sakazaki. 1970. Marine vibrios associated with bacillary necrosis, a disease of larval and juvenile bivalve molluscs. J. Bacteriol. 103:272-273.

Tubiash, H.S., R.K. Sizemore, and R.R. Colwell. 1975. Bacterial flora of the hemolymph of the blue crab Callinectes sapidus: most probable number. Appl. Microbiol. 29:388-392.

Twedt, R.M., J.M. Madden, J.M. Hunt, D.W. Francis, J.T. Peeler, A.P. Duran, W.O. Herbert, S.G. McCay, C.N. Roderick, G.T. Spite, and T.J. Wazenski. 1981. Characterization of Vibrio cholerae isolated from oysters. Appl. Environ. Microbiol. 41:1475-1478.

Weissman, J.B., W.E. Dewitt, J. Thompson, C.N. Muchnick, B.L. Portnoy, J.C. Feeley, and E.J. Gangarosa. 1974. A case of cholera in Texas, 1973. Am. J. Epidemiol. 100:487-498.

Wilson, R., S. Lieb, A. Roberts, S. Stryker, H. Janowski, R. Gunn, B. Davis, C.F. Riddle, T. Barrett, J.G. Morris, Jr., and P.A. Blake. 1981. Non-O-group 1 Vibrio cholerae gastroenteritis associated with eating raw oysters. Am. J. Epidemiol. 114:293-298.

World Health Organization. 1980. Cholera and other vibrio-associated diarrhoeas. Bull. W.H.O. 58:353-374.

Wright, A.C., L.M. Simpson, and J.D. Oliver. 1981. Role of iron in the pathogenesis of Vibrio vulnificus infection. Infect. Immun. 34:503-507.

Xu, H-S., F.L. Singleton, N. Roberts, R.W. Attwell, D.J. Grimes, and R.R. Colwell. 1983. Survival and viability of non-culturable Escherichia coli and Vibrio cholerae in the estuarine and marine environment. Microb. Ecol.: in press.

Zafari, Y., A.Z. Zafifi, S. Rahmanzadeh, and N. Fakhar. 1973. Diarrhoea caused by non-agglutinable Vibrio cholerae (non-cholera vibrio). Lancet 2:429-430.

Edipemiology and Serology

Chapter 1

CHARACTERIZATION OF <u>VIBRIO CHOLERAE</u> STRAINS FROM INFECTIONS AND FROM THE ENVIRONMENT

Charlotte D. Parker

Since Koch's discovery that comma-shaped bacilli isolated from the human intestine caused cholera, bacteriologists have needed methods to differentiate typical epidemic strains of <u>Vibrio cholerae</u> from all other vibrios found in the gut and in the environment. Such a differentiation is important for two reasons. Vibrios and vibrio-like bacteria abound in natural environments such as water and sediment; moreover, epidemic cholera is devastating to society. Thus, detection of the vibrios which can cause epidemic cholera and differentiation of them from all other microorganisms is an important public health challenge.

Webster defines virulence as "the relative capacity of a pathogen to overcome body defences." Virulence is a quantitative value, and has two measurable components. As defined by Davis et al. (1981), "The term <u>virulence</u> (degree of pathogenicity) is used to encompass two features of a pathogenic organism: its <u>infectivity</u> (the ability to colonize a host), and the <u>severity</u> of the disease produced. Virulence varies not only among bacterial species, but among strains." We usually consider virulence to relate only to the severity of the disease. Determination of the median lethal dose of a pathogenic organism for animals provides a numerical estimate of severity. I will designate the infectivity component of virulence as <u>epidemic virulence</u>,

15

and the severity component of virulence as <u>tissue</u> <u>virulence</u>. Both <u>tissue</u> <u>virulence</u> and <u>epidemic</u> <u>virulence</u> are quantitative terms.

In assessing virulence, consideration must be given to parasite properties, to host properties, and to environmental properties. Most laboratory techniques to assess virulence emphasize estimates of tissue virulence. Tissue virulence is primarily dependent on properties of the parasite, such as toxins and ability to grow in the host. However, certain host factors and environmental factors also affect tissue virulence. Laboratory techniques to measure epidemic virulence are not generally available. Rather, one must use historical information regarding outbreaks of the disease or correlate environmental and host properties which allow outbreaks to occur. Dependence of epidemic virulence on parasite and host and environment is accepted. As an example, one can consider the transmission of <u>Neisseria meningitidis</u>. Parasite properties include possession of specific capsules--A, B, C, etc. Host properties include age and antibody status; environmental properties include air temperature and humidity.

A semiquantitative graph of virulence for several diseases is shown in Figure 1. Each disease is given a rating on the axis which shows the relative virulence properties of the pathogen for humans. For example, smallpox is high in tissue virulence because it causes a severe disease with a high death rate. Gangrene and typhoid fever are similarly severe diseases. However, gangrene is not transmissible from person to person, and thus lacks epidemic virulence. Typhoid is transmissible, but is not so contagious as smallpox, so that it is intermediate in epidemic virulence. Influenza and the common cold are also high in epidemic virulence, but are lower in tissue virulence.

Evaluation of tissue virulence is based on the severity of the disease and its mortality rate. We could all agree that rabies, with a 100% mortality in man, is as high as the scale goes for tissue virulence. Evaluation of epidemic virulence is less obvious. However, two patterns of disease induction are characteristic of parasites which are highly successful in spreading among humans. Such parasites may

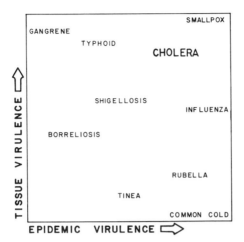

Figure 1. Relative virulence of several diseases for humans. Tissue virulence is a measure of severity of the disease, while epidemic virulence is a measure of the ability of the infectious agent to spread among humans.

either (1) cause epidemics and pandemics, or (2) infect all new susceptibles in the population so that the organism causes a childhood disease.

To apply this concept of virulence to cholera requires that we evaluate the history of the disease, and Figure 1 shows my evaluation. The cholera organisms have moderate or high epidemic and tissue virulence. This evaluation is based upon the ability of Vibrio cholerae to cause epidemic and pandemic disease, as well as upon the appreciable mortality caused by the disease.

Figure 2 compares the diseases caused by all Vibrio species. Only O1 strains of V. cholerae (made up of both classical and El Tor biotypes) can cause disease with high epidemic virulence. Other vibrios, including V. parahae-molyticus, V. vulnificus, and non-O1 V. cholerae, cause a variety of diseases of variable tissue virulence but very low epidemic virulence. El Tor strains of V. cholerae are as epidemically virulent as classical strains, but show lower tissue virulence (based on the incidence of mild versus severe disease; see Bart et al. 1970).

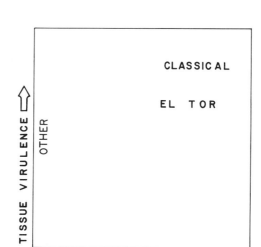

Figure 2. Relative virulence of Vibrio species diseases for humans. Classical refers to the classical biotype, O1 strains of V. cholerae, while El Tor refers to the El Tor biotype, O1 strains of V. cholerae. Together these strains make up the entry CHOLERA in Figure 1. OTHER refers to all other Vibrio species and strains, including V. parahaemolyticus, V. vulnificus, and non-O1 strains of V. cholerae.

Virulence prediction is based upon the correlation of properties parasites possess to the properties of parasites from previous disease outbreaks or cases. Koch originally evaluated the virulence of vibrios by microscopic examination of cell shape, motility, and arrangement of vibrios in the diarrheal fluid of cholera patients. He augmented the microscopic appearance evaluation with the necessity for a characteristic colonial appearance on gelatin medium (Pollitzer 1959). However, it was quickly discovered that vibrios with typical microscopic morphology and motility could be found in the gut of people who did not have choleraic diarrhea (Finkler and Prior 1884). Antibody tests, especially agglutination tests, became the method of choice to differentiate epidemiologically relevant strains of V. cholerae from all other vibrios (Gruber and Durham 1896; Gardner and Venkatraman 1935; Pollitzer 1959). The lesson learned from history is that agglutination to titer with specific O1 antiserum is the single best predictor of high tissue and epidemic virulence for vibrio strains.

Agglutination tests with O1 sera are not without problems, however. Technical problems and limitations of antiserum agglutination tests include the following: (1) Antisera may contain nonspecific antibody as well as specific antibody. The use of carefully absorbed sera, or monoclonal antiserum, and performance of titrations with antisera can help to minimize this difficulty. (2) Other gram-negative rods demonstrate antigens which cross-react with V. cholerae. Again, agglutination to titer will minimize difficulties with such organisms. (3) Rough strains of V. cholerae are not uncommonly found in diarrheal stool, although smooth strains are usually present also. Evaluation of such rough strains, whether from the gut or from the environment, is not possible with serotyping. (4) Serotyping may place a vibrio as a member of a particular group of known tissue and epidemic virulence, but serotyping cannot predict the virulence of the specific strain being tested. (5) A small, but disquieting, fraction of non-O1 strains of V. cholerae can make cholera toxin. Perhaps we should anticipate this observation, since vibrios can conjugate in the laboratory. Nevertheless, since the production of cholera toxin (CT) is such an important correlate of tissue virulence, the failure of O1 serotype tests to detect such strains is important.

Table 1 is a summary of techniques in current use which appear valuable in predicting tissue or epidemic virulence of V. cholerae. Many of these tests are suitable only for research laboratories, and cannot be used in the field. It may be possible to develop additional tests suited for field use, however, such as staphylococcal coagglutination tests to detect CT. Among enteropathogenic Escherichia coli strains, infectivity is associated with the presence of one of several adhesins (Evans et al. 1977; Evans and Evans 1978; Bergman et al. 1981). Finkelstein and Hanne have recently shown that V. cholerae strain CA401 has a highly specific adhesin. If this adhesin is highly correlated with infectivity, an additional easy test which predicts virulence may become available.

Table 1. Current Procedures Useful in Assessing the Virulence of _Vibrio cholerae_ Strains

Procedure	Advantages	Limitations
I. Serotyping (Ol versus non-Ol)	-Easy to do -Inexpensive -Proven predictive value for for both tissue virulence and epidemic virulence	-Antisera may contain antibodies to other bacteria -Cross-reacting antigens are found in Yersinia, Salmonella, Brucella and other organisms -Rough strains cannot be tested -Does not test for specific attributes of virulence
II. Toxicity Tests A. In vivo tests for CT production (ligated rabbit intestinal loop, infant rabbit oral challenge, etc.)	-Antibody blocking will show specificity for CT -Cells are incubated in vivo, so that they have maximum opportunity to make toxin	-Requires live animals -Requires research laboratory -NaCl, cytotoxins, etc., may induce fluid
B. Tests for biologically active CT produced in vitro (tests in II A, plus vascular permeability tests, adrenal and CHO cell tissue culture assays)	-Use fewer animals than tests in II A, or no animals -Highly sensitive -Specificity can be demonstrated by antibody blocking	-CT production is dependent on in vitro growth and toxin synthesis -Hemolysins, cytotoxins, and endotoxin may interfere
C. Detection of CT antigen (Enzyme Immunoassay and Radioimmunoassay, Passive Immune Hemolysis, etc.)	-Easy to perform -Specific for CT (no interference by cytotoxins, etc.) -Highly sensitive	-Dependent on culture conditions for expression of CT genes -Does not measure biological activity

20

Table 1. Continued

Procedure	Advantages	Limitations
D. DNA hybridization to detect toxin genes	-Highly specific -Does not depend on in vitro culture conditions for expression of CT -Very sensitive	-Technology to prepare the probe is not routinely available -May detect related DNA sequences which no longer code for CT
III. Infectivity Tests (Infant mouse oral infection, adult rabbit infection, chinchilla, primate, dog)	-Can evaluate both tissue virulence and some properties of epidemic virulence. -Can provide a rank order	-Difficult and expensive -Requires animals -Penetrating pathogens and organisms with cytolytic toxins may be difficult to assess

21

The single characteristic of V. cholerae, other than O serotype, which is routinely evaluated, is the ability to make CT or CT-like toxins. The various assay methods are given in Table 1. One major problem of the test, especially when examining non-O1 V. cholerae or other Vibrio species, is that the production of hemolysins and cytotoxins can significantly interfere with the test. A significant development in testing for toxin is the DNA hybridization technique which detects the genetic information for toxin synthesis (Kaper et al. 1981). Nevertheless, tests for CT suffer from the same limitation as tests for serotype--such tests may suggest that a strain can cause severe disease, but they do not predict that such a strain will cause severe disease.

Animal infection tests to assess the virulence of V. cholerae and related organisms show variable discrimination. Most animal tests, as listed in Table 1, are reasonably good assays for CT. However, only a few tests also appear to detect infectivity. The ligated adult rabbit loop test is primarily a test for in vivo toxin production, but can be altered by use of temporary ligatures. The altered test (Spira et al. 1981) appears useful for study of infectivity. The infant mouse oral challenge test was developed by Ujiiye and Kobari (1970) and has been extensively used in my laboratory. It can be used to measure some parameters of infectivity for strains of V. cholerae. It does not, however, possess predictive value for other vibrios. In addition, it suffers from the major flaw of all animal infection tests--one does not know which parameter of the parasite or host is being measured.

Animal infection tests are currently used to (1) evaluate the diarrheal response of the animal; (2) evaluate the in vivo multiplication of the parasite; (3) perform animal passage experiments to select for changes in the parasites; and; (4) perform in vivo competition experiments. In my discussion of these experiments, I will emphasize work with infant mice.

Evaluation of a diarrheal response in infant mice is dependent on the possession of cholera toxin genes by the parasite. However, more is required from the parasite than simply toxigenicity. In Figure 3, a dose response curve

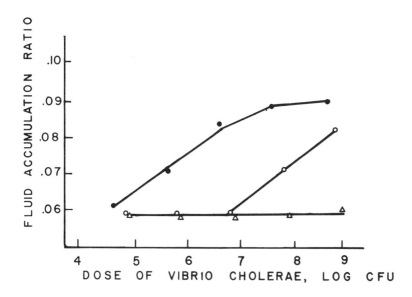

Figure 3. Dose response curves for <u>V. cholerae</u> strains CA401(O), and 569B(●), and VB12(△)--a rough derivative of strain CA401, selected by resistance to a smooth specific vibriophage. The graph shows the diarrheagenic response of orally inoculated infant mice to differing challenges of live vibrios. Sources of data: Baselski et al. 1977; V. Baselski, Ph.D. diss. University of Texas at Austin, 1978.

for fluid response is shown for several vibrio strains. Some strains which produce toxin cannot induce a fluid response. At high oral doses, strain 569B produces a fluid response, but at low doses it does not. CT given orally also causes a fluid response in doses greater than 0.25 micrograms/mouse.

Figure 3 also demonstrates that toxigenic strains which can multiply in vivo, such as CA 401 or CA 411, need a smaller inoculum to produce diarrhea than do rough strains (which do not multiply) or 569B, which multiplies only feebly. In mice, we developed a way to quantitate multiplicative ability of <u>V. cholerae</u> strains. Figure 4 shows the protocol and results for the strains shown in Figure 3. Note that in these tests for gut multiplication, we have

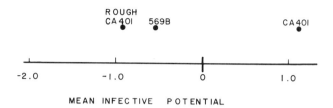

Figure 4. Mean infective potential for V. cholerae strains CA401, 569B, and VB12. The numbers represent the negative logarithm of the change in specific activity. Specific activity is cpm/cfu for time of inoculation (SA_0) and is cpm/cfu at 4 hours postinoculation (SA_4). A positive value indicates net multiplication, while a negative value indicates net death. Methods and calculations are described in Baselski et al. 1978.

examined only the upper bowel, only at 4 hours after oral infection. This limitation is due to the observation that nonmotile and nonchemotactic vibrios may multiply normally, but are washed quickly out of the upper intestine. Total counts of vibrios in the gut do not differ from motile strains, but the distribution of vibrios differs.

Figure 5 shows that ability to induce a fluid response correlates with the ability to multiply in vivo. For the strains shown, DNA hybridization experiments were done on the circled strains. These experiments correlate with the animal studies. Of seven strains tested by both techniques (see Sigel et al. 1980; Kaper et al. 1981), all were O1 serotype. Four, which multiplied in the gut and induced diarrheal fluid, were positive for the toxin gene, while three strains which were negative for the toxin gene were not able to multiply in infant mice or to induce diarrhea.

Strains of V. cholerae from a common source outbreak in Louisiana in 1978 were evaluated for ability to induce diarrhea, and for ability to multiply in infant mouse upper bowel. Figure 6 shows the results. The strain recovered from the crab vehicle was less diarrheagenic and less able to multiply in vivo than the isolates from stool or from the septic tank of patients. This finding suggests that passage through the human bowel selects for gut-adapted parasites. Figure 7 shows that passage through the mouse gut may, with some strains of V. cholerae, enhance the ability to

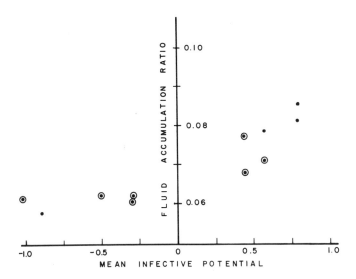

Figure 5. Mean infective potential (MIP) versus diarrheagenic potential for several V. cholerae O1 strains. Each circle represents a
single cholera strain, and is graphed for both MIP value and fluid
accumulation ratio. Circled dots represent strains tested by both Sigel
et al. 1980 and Kaper et al. 1981.

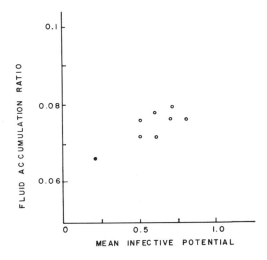

Figure 6. Mean infective potential versus diarrheagenic potential for
strains of V. cholerae from a common source outbreak in Louisiana in
1978. The filled circle represents the strain isolated from the crab
behicle, while open circles represent the strains isolated from infected
humans or their septic tanks. Source of data: Sigel et al. 1980.

produce a diarrheal response. Animal passage also selects for reversion to virulence among avirulent mutants (Finkelstein 1973) and for change in serotype (Sack and Miller 1969). Animal passage experiments have also been used to examine a mutant strain which does not produce the A subunit of cholera toxin (Honda and Finkelstein 1979). Passage of the mutant through mice did not restore diarrheagenic potential to the mutant strain. The animal-passaged strain was better able to multiply in the mouse intestine than the mutant strain, but was somewhat less able to multiply than the parent, toxigenic strain (Sigel et al. 1981; Sigel and Parker, unpublished results).

Competition experiments are animal infections in which two or more strains of microorganisms are used to coinfect animals. Then by determining the ratio of the strains at the time of infection, and during the infection, one can determine the relative ability of each strain to survive and multiply in the host. Table 2 shows some preliminary data on competition in infant mouse intestine, using various strains of V. cholerae. Such experiments may be a valuable method for determining virulence, especially if the results can be shown to correlate with virulence for man. However, this type of experiment is not suitable for use under field conditions, and its predictive value is unexamined to date.

Virulence prediction for vibrios other than O1 strains of V. cholerae is complicated and generally unsuccessful. No single toxin, or serologically detectible antigen, has been described for other vibrios which correlates with virulence. Certainly, the possession of CT is required for induction of choleraic diarrhea. But the ability to make CT is not sufficient for virulence. We can summarize by saying that only two tests, serotyping and CT detection, are of value in predicting virulence. (The Kanagawa hemolysin is of value for V. parahaemolyticus strains.) These tests need to be augmented with a test for adhesins and need to be available for field work. For the most effective analysis, it is likely that animal tests must be done. With all predictive tests, we must rely on the evidence of history. Thus it is unlikely that we can successfully predict the appearance of new and different pathogens. Should vibrios which are not

Table 2. Competition Experiments Using Various Vibrio cholerae Strains[a]

	Inoculum, cfu/mouse 0 Time			Recovery, cfu/mouse 16 Hours		
A	B		A/B Ratio	A	B	A/B Ratio
Texas Star 1×10^3	CA401 2.5×10^3		0.4	2.5×10^1	1×10^6	$\sim 10^{-4}$
CA411 1.2×10^6	CA401 2.2×10^6		0.55	5×10^6	4.5×10^7	0.11
2843-80A 5×10^5	CA401 1×10^6		0.5	2.5×10^3	6×10^7	$\sim 10^{-4}$

[a]In these experiments, a rifampin-resistant mutant of strain CA401 was inoculated simultaneously with a spectinomycin-resistant mutant of strain Texas Star, or a streptomycin-resistant mutant of strain CA411 and 2843-80A. Viable counts of the inoculum were performed on drug plates. Infant mice were retained for 16 hours after being inoculated orally. At 16 hours, the upper half of the intestine was removed, homogenized, and diluted for viable counts. The strains used include CA401 and CA411, classical cholera isolates from cholera cases; Texas Star, a mutant of an El Tor strain (3083) which does not produce the active subunit of cholera toxin; and 2843-80A, a nontoxin-producing O1 isolate from sewage in Carabella, Florida, 1980.

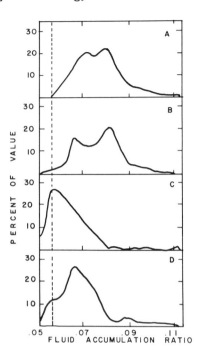

Figure 7. Effect of a single mouse passage on the diarrheagenic ability of V. cholerae strains CA 401 and Lou 14. Each panel represents the distribution of values of fluid accumulation ratios obtained for 50-100 single colonies of V. cholerae strains. a) Strain CA 401 prior to mouse passage; b) Strain CA 401 after mouse passage; c) Strain Lou 14, crab isolate from the Louisiana outbreak of 1978, before a single mouse passage; d) Strain Lou 14 after a single mouse passage. The dotted line indicates the area of shift after animal passage for strain Lou 14. Source of data: Sigel et al. 1980.

O-group 1 gain the ability to cause pandemic cholera, how could this be detected in the laboratory? I do not know, and I suspect that no one else knows.

Although not perfect, prediction of virulence is valuable. Continued study and characterization of the attributes of virulence may allow a more perfect prediction. For the present, we must use the tools we have, and make predictions based on correlations we have observed.

SUMMARY AND CONCLUSIONS

Tests to predict virulence for Vibrio species are necessary. The single best predictor for both tissue virulence and epidemic virulence is the possession of the O1 serotype antigen by V. cholerae. A second useful predictor is the ability to make cholera toxin. (Determination of the presence of a Kanagawa hemolysin also had predictive value for V. parahaemolyticus strains.) More specific tests for O serogroup are needed, as well as simpler tests for determination of cholera toxin production. Tests for adhesins need to be developed. Animal tests, while unsuitable for field work, can supplement simple tests as predictors. Animal models which are relevant for V. cholerae are not necessarily relevant for other vibrios.

ACKNOWLEDGMENTS

Much of the research described in this paper was supported by Public Health Service Grants AI 12819 and 17669.

REFERENCES

Bart, K.J., Z. Huq, M. Khan, and W.H. Moseley. 1970. Seroepidemiologic studies during a simultaneous epidemic of infection with El Tor Ogawa and classical Inaba Vibrio cholerae. J. Infect. Dis. (Suppl.) 121:S17.

Baselski, V., R. Briggs, and C. Parker. 1977. Intestinal fluid accumulation induced by oral challenge with Vibrio cholerae or cholera toxin in infant mice. Infect. Immun. 15:704-712.

Baselski, V., R. Medina, and C. Parker. 1978. Survival and multiplication of Vibrio cholerae in the upper bowel of infant mice. Infect. Immun. 22:435-440.

Bergman, M.J., W.S. Updike, S.J. Wood, S.E. Brown, and R.L. Guerrant. 1981. Attachment factors among enterotoxigenic Escherichia coli from patients with acute diarrhea from diverse geographic areas. Infect. Immun. 32:881-888.

Davis, B.D., R. Dulbecco, H. Eisen, and H.S. Ginsberg. 1980. Pages 552-553 in Microbiology, 3rd Edition. Harper and Row, Hagerstown.

Evans, D.G., and D.J. Evans. 1978. New surface-associated heat-labile colonization factor antigen (CFA II) produced by enterotoxigenic Escherichia coli of serogroups O6 and O8. Infect. Immun. 21:638-647.

Evans, D.G., D.J. Evans, and W. Tjoa. 1977. Hemagglutination of human group A erythrocyted by enterotoxigenic Escherichia coli isolated from adults with diarrhea. Infect. Immun. 18:330-337.

Finkelstein, R.A. 1973. Cholera. Crit. Rev. Microbiol. 2:553-623.

Finkler, D., and J. Prior. 1884. Untersuchungen uber Cholera nostras. Dtsch. Med. Wschr. 10:579.

Gardner, A.D. and K.V. Venkatraman. 1935. The antigens of the cholera group of vibrios. J. Hyg. 35:262.

Gruber, M., and H.E. Durham. 1896. Eine neue Methode zur raschen Erkennung des Choleravibrios und des Typhusbacillus. Munch. Med. Wschr. 43:285.

Honda, T., and R.A. Finkelstein. 1979. Selection and characteristics of a Vibrio cholerae mutant lacking the A (ADP-ribosylating) portion of the cholera enterotoxin. Proc. Nat. Acad. Sci. 76:2052-2056.

Kaper, J.B., S.L. Moseley, and S. Falkow. 1981. Molecular characterization of environmental and nontoxigenic strains of Vibrio cholerae. Infect. Immun. 32:661-667.

Pollitzer, R. 1959. Cholera. World Health Organization, Geneva, Switzerland.

Sack, R.B., and C.E. Miller. 1969. Progressive changes of vibrio serotypes in germ-free mice infected with Vibrio cholerae. J. Bacteriol. 99:688.

Sigel, S.P., R.A. Finkelstein, and C.D. Parker. 1981. Ability of an avirulent mutant of Vibrio cholerae to colonize in the infant mouse upper bowel. Infect. Immun. 32:474-479.

Sigel, S.P., S. Lanier, V.S. Baselski, and C.D. Parker. 1980. In vivo evaluation of pathogenicity of clinical and environmental isolates of Vibrio cholerae. Infect. Immun. 28:681-687.

Spira, W.M., R.B. Sack, and J.L. Froehlich. 1981. Simple adult rabbit model for Vibrio cholerae and enterotoxigenic Escherichia coli diarrhea. Infect. Immun. 32:739-747.

Ujiiye, A., and K. Kobari. 1970. Protective effect on infections with Vibrio cholerae in suckling mice caused by the passive immunization with milk of immune mothers. J. Infect. Dis. 121 (Suppl.):S50-S55.

Chapter 2

ANTIGENS AND SEROVAR--SPECIFIC ANTIGENS OF VIBRIO CHOLERAE

R.J. Siebeling, Linda B. Adams,
Zainal Yusof, and A.D. Larson

In addition to bacteriological surveillance for the presence of Vibrio species in the estuarine waters, sediments, and seafoods in Florida, Louisiana, Maryland, and Oregon, it was decided by investigators from institutions in each of these states to determine the spectrum of Vibrio cholerae serotypes/serovars present in the environmental specimens. We at Louisiana State University were charged with the responsibility of establishing a reliable system with which to serologically type the V. cholerae isolates collected from the four states.

The Two Existing Serological Typing Schemes

Gardner and Venkatraman (1935) divided V. cholerae into six serologically defined groups based on differences in heat-stable cell wall (O) antigens. The cholera vibrios, including the hemolytic El Tor strains, were included in O-subgroup I and non-cholera vibrios were placed into O subgroups II to VI inclusive (collectively referred to as non-O1). Some of the confusion in V. cholerae serology was eliminated when these investigators showed that all V. cholerae isolates O1 and non-O1 possess a species-specific H (flagellar) antigen and they cautioned their peers to refrain from using formalized cells for the production of "diagnostic serum" for identification of V. cholerae O1 (cholera vibrio) from among large numbers of isolates. Antiserum raised against "living" or formalized V. cholerae contains both anti-H activity which agglutinates all motile V. cholerae (O1 and non-O1) and anti-O activity which will discriminate from among the six O-subgroups only the O antigen present in the vaccine strain. Therefore, Gardner and Venkatraman recommended that "diagnostic serum" be raised in animals immunized with V. cholerae cells that have been "boiled or steamed for 2 hours to destroy the common H antigen," and that "suspensions of cultures under identification should be used in the unheated state, with or without formalin (0.2 %), since heated suspensions tend to show a common O cross agglutination with these sera." Sakazaki et al. (1970) extended the number of serologically distinguishable O-subgroups to 39. They suggested that the O-groups be referred to as serovars (a serological variety of a single serotype) because of the 405 non-O1 V. cholerae tested, 399 agglutinated in H antisera produced against V. cholerae 35A-3 and three non-O1 H vaccines, thereby confirming the observation of Gardner and Venkatraman that that non-O1 V. cholerae possess serologically identical H antigens with V. cholerae O1. By 1977 Sakazaki (1977a, 1977b) reported the existence of 60 serovars of V. cholerae.

In 1979 Smith reviewed the updated status of a sero-typing system he initiated in 1965 (Smith 1965) and reported the existence of 72 serotypes. The Smith or Vibrio Reference Laboratory (VRL) system starts numbering at 11, and with large gaps in the numbering nomenclature, ends at 350. Smith reported approximately 20% of vibrio strains tested either did not agglutinate (999) or spon-taneously agglutinated (998) in VRL typing serum. The difference between the Sakazaki system and the VRL is that Sakazaki followed the suggestions of Gardner and Venka-traman and raised typing serum in rabbits immunized with multiple injections of heat-killed organisms and serologically tests heat-killed cells by tube agglutination at 56°C. Smith immunizes rabbits with a single subcutaneous injection of live cells and serologically tests live isolates by slide agglutination.

The LSU Typing Serum

It was not our intention to add a third serological typing scheme, and its inherent nomenclature, to the two systems in use. Because the VRL system is based on serotyping isolates with serum produced in animals immunized with live vibrios, contrary to the advice offered by Gardner and Venkatraman, it would seem, as Gardner and Venkatraman stated in 1935, that such serum would lack specificity because of the potential presence of anti-H. We felt, as one of our primary goals, that the serological typing serum adopted to screen thousands of V. cholerae isolates should be dedicated to serological detection of a cell wall antigen that could ultimately be defined structurally. The Sakazaki system provides the first discriminating characteristic, heat stability, in defining the serovar-specific antigen.

The logistics and expense which would be incurred to send several thousand Vibrio isolates to Japan or England to be typed by the Sakazaki system was not practical. Therefore, there was impetus to establish a "local" serological typing serum. Typing serum was produced by rabbits immunized with multiple intravenous injections of heat-killed V. cholerae O1 and non-O1 vaccines. Vaccine preparation and immunization protocols were basically those reported by Sakazaki (1970). Table 1 shows the 54 different V. cholerae non-O1 vaccine strains used to produce typing serum. Each vaccine strain was assigned a temporary designation from the Roman alphabet (A through ZZ). There was an unfortunate lack of hindsight when the letters were assigned to the non-O1 vaccine strains in the temporary LSU system. The designations A, B, and C should not have been used because these letters were previously assigned to the antigens of Inaba (A,C) and Ogawa (A,B).

The vaccine strains were randomly chosen from among clinical isolates (H.B. Bradford, Department of Health and Human Resources, New Orleans), crab feces, hemolymph

Table 1. Non-O1 Vibrio cholerae Vaccine Strains[a] (LSU Systems)

Strain No.	Serovar Designation	Source	Sakazaki Serovar	VRL Serotype[b]
2022H	A	Human, LF	26	312
39	B	Crab homogenate		102
2026H	C	Human, LF	52/72	74
F8C	D	Crab feces	(14)[c]	33
F1A	E	Crab feces	(X66)[c,d]	38
H7C	F	Crab hemolymph		999
H10A	G	Crab hemolymph	(23)	19
F18B	H	Crab feces	(8)	25
N-37	Ia	Sewer, Lake Arthur	5	42
N-27	Id	Sewer, Lake Arthur	34	42
N-10	Ie	Sediment, Mud Lake	39	998
F46D	J	Crab feces	(6)	14
F50C	K	Crab feces	(19)	998
6391	L	Sewer, Lake Charles	(21)	44
2002H	M	Human, LA	(37)	23
2007H	N	Human, LA	41	106
N-38	O	Sewer, Lake Arthur	42	999
2019H	P	Human, LA	65	340
2012H	Q	Human, LA	2	17
N-24	R	Sewer, Lake Arthur	3	

N-83	S	Sewer, Cameron	12	33
2008H	T	Human, LA	18	25
N-13	U	Sediment, Mud Lake	36	
2015H	V	Human, LA	40	11
N-98	W	Sewer, Hackberry	51	40
2016H	X	Human, LA	57	999
N-128	Y	Sewer, Lake Charles	X64	350
2018H	Z	Human, LA	44	15
10-F2A	AA	Crab feces	27	37
10-F31A	BB	Crab feces		327
2009H	CC	Human, LA	20	999
2021H	DD	Human, LA	10	348
N-80	EE	Sewer, Cameron	X69	77
N-100	FF	Sewer, Welch	X82	999
N-69	GG	Sewer, Lake Arthur	16	344
N-11	HH	Sediment, Mud Lake	28	75
N-186	II	Sewer, West Lake	38	
N-157	JJ	Sewer, Sulphur	45	352
N-188	KK	Sewer, West Lake	32	325
N-125	LL	Sewer, Lake Charles	48	60
N-87	MM	Sewer, Cameron	56	999
N-46	NN	Sewer, Lake Arthur	X61	999
N-94	OO	Sewer, Hackberry	X64	998
N-104	PP	Sewer, Hackberry	46	76

Table 1. Continued

Strain No.	Serovar Designation	Source	Sakazaki Serovar	VRL Serotype[b]
N-1	QQ	Crab, homogenate	X64	360
N-96	RR	Sewer, Hackberry	X78	56
373	SS	Human, IL		29
1368	TT	Human, WI		12
2073	UU	Human, Dacca		21
2310	VV	Human, TX		59
TT3b	WW	Water, Vermilion Bay		
Fla-45	XX	Water, Florida		
Fla-106	YY	Water, Florida		
OSU-267	ZZ	Water, Oregon		

[a]Vaccine strains chosen from among V. cholerae non-O1 isolates typed by Sakazaki (Japan) or Lee/Donovan (Maidstone). Vaccine strains also typed by VRL (Jefferson Medical College, Philadelphia).

[b]VRL nomenclature: 998 = Spontaneous agglutination, 999 = Non-typeable.

[c]( ) = Probable Sakazaki serovar, not typed by either Sakazaki or Maidstone.

[d]X = Tentative Sakazaki serovar designation.

38

isolates (Susan Payne, LSU), and environmental isolates (Nell Roberts, Department of Health and Human Resources, Lake Charles). Most of the LSU vaccine strains were typed either in Japan or England by the Sakazaki systems (see Table 1, column 3) and by the VRL (Table 1, column 4). Vaccine strains C, G, L, M, N, CC, and KK are sucrose-negative, VP-negative and corn oil-negative which makes them candidates for inclusion in the newly proposed Vibrio mimicus (Fanning et al. 1981).

Correlation of Serological Nomenclature Between the Three Systems

An attempt was made to correlate the LSU nomenclature for Vibrio cholerae non-O1 (A through WW) with that of Sakazaki (2 through 82) and with that of Smith (11 through 350). Table 2 shows examples of agreement and disagreement among the three systems. Group I on Table 2 shows agreement among the three systems. The LSU vaccine strain F46D, assigned J in the temporary LSU nomenclature, was tentatively assigned Sakazaki serovar 6 and was typed by the VRL as 14. Environmental isolates N-53 and N-55 were typed by Sakazaki as serovar 6 and by the VRL as 14. Both isolates agglutinated in J antiserum in the LSU system.

Group II on Table 2 shows no correlation between the Sakazaki and VRL nomenclature. The LSU vaccine strain N-13 (U in the LSU nomenclature) was typed by Sakazaki as serovar 36 and by VRL as serotype 30. V. cholerae isolates N-52 and N-76 both agglutinated in anti-U serum and were typed by Sakazaki as 36, suggesting the LSU serovar U and Sakazaki 36 are the same. These three isolates--N-13, N-52, and N-76--were each recognized as a different serotype in the VRL system, therefore LSU serovar U cannot be translated into the VRL nomenclature. Similarly, LSU serovar O appears to be 42 in the Sakazaki serological nomenclature (Group II, Table 2); however, the five V. cholerae which agglutinated in anti-O serum (LSU) were each identified as a different serotype in the VRL system. Group III on Table 2 will be discussed below.

Table 2. Correlation of the LSU Serological Nomenclature with that of the Sakazaki and VRL System

LSU Vaccine Strain	V. cholerae Isolate	Serological Nomenclature of V. cholerae Isolates Typed by		
		LSU	Sakazaki	VRL
I. F46D		J	(6)[a]	14
	N-53	J	6	14
	N-55	J	6	14
II. N-13		U	36	30
	N-52	U	36	348
	N-76	U	36	31
N-38		O	42	347
	N-3	O	42	349
	N-40	O	42	348
	N-42		42	94
III. F8C		D	(14)[a]	33
N-83		S	12	33
	N-71	S	12	106

[a] ( ) = Probable Sakazaki serovar designation.

The above instances are examples of the difficulties encountered when attempts were made to correlate the serological nomenclature. Admittedly, our attempts to correlate the serological nomenclature were made through "third party" antiserum which could have prejudiced the findings and interpretations. It could be argued that if we had used antiserum produced by rabbits immunized with live vaccines, the LSU nomenclature might show closer agreement with that of the VRL system.

One reason for the apparent lack of correlation between the two serological nomenclatures originates with the disparity in the methods used to prepare the vaccines. Neither Sakazaki nor Smith attempt to define or identify the serovar or serotype-specific antigen(s) that each typing system purports to distinguish into VRL serological types or Sakazaki varieties. It would seem each system may be detecting different "classes" of antigens. Consider the array of potential antigens that the rabbit is confronted with when immunized with whole Vibrio cells, living or dead (Figure 1). The flagellar (H) antigen, eliminated in heat-killed vaccines, is identical in all V. cholerae isolates, O1 and non-O1 (Gardner and Venkatraman 1935; Sakazaki et al. 1970; Bhattacharyya and Mukerjee 1974; Bhattacharyya 1975; Bhattacharyya 1977). A capsular (K) antigen has not been identified as such; however, a mucoid (M) antigen has been described (Sakazaki et al. 1970) which is a poor immunogen and not present on most V. cholerae isolates. The M antigen is of importance since it inhibits agglutination by masking the cell wall (O) determinants. A sheath surrounds the flagellar core and appears to be contiguous with the outer cell membrane and may be serologically homogeneous among different serotypes (Hranitzky et al. 1981). Kabir (1980) characterized an outer membrane protein (OMP) common to both biotypes of V. cholerae O1 and to both serotypes, Inaba and Ogawa. The 48,000 MW OMP is immunogenic and antibody activity directed against the OMP will agglutinate V. cholerae O1. A single immunological variety of OMP shared by two serotypes, or more, would negate the production of serovar-specific antibody in rabbits immunized with live vaccines.

Antigens and Serovar-Specific Antigens of
Vibrio cholerae

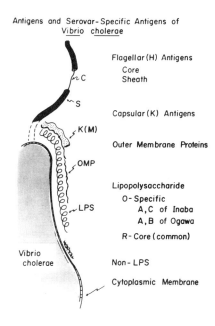

Figure 1. Antigens and serovar-specific antigens of Vibrio cholerae.

It is documented that, as in the Enterobacteriaceae, the O-antigen or serovar-specific antigen C in Inaba and B in Ogawa are constitutents of the polysaccharide portion of the lipopolysaccharide (LPS) which is associated with the outer membrane of the gram-negative cell wall (Redmond et al. 1973). Redmond (1979) reported that the O-antigen side chain of the LPS in V. cholerae Inaba 569B consists of a linear polymer, $\alpha(1 \to 2)$ D perosamine (4 amino,4,6 dideoxy D mannose) with the location of the antigenically important fructofuranosyl yet to be determined. Rough (R) determinants are poor immunogens and not serovar-specific (Shimada and Sakazaki 1973). They are serologically prominent and frequently encountered in V. cholerae isolates recovered from chronic carriers and at the tail end of epidemics.

There are reports which document the existence of nonserovar-specific heat-labile cell wall antigens (Ghosh and Mukerjee 1961) and heat-stable antigens of V. cholerae non-O1 which are identical with antigens on V. cholerae O1 (Ghosh and Mukerjee 1961) and a heat-stable protein antigen (Neoh and Rowley 1970).

LPS-Associated Antigens, the Serovar-Specific Antigen

From our vantage point it appears the serological nomenclature (serovar or serotype-specific antigen notations) of the two systems are irreconcilable. Whole cell vaccines, living or dead, present a diverse offering of antigens (serovar-specific and nonserovar-specific) to the antibody-producing facilities of the rabbit resulting in the potential production of a spectrum of antibodies possessing an array of serological specificities. In neither the Sakazaki nor the VRL system was an attempt made to define against what structure (antigen) on the Vibrio cell the "serovar or serotype-specific antibody" was directed, which makes it difficult to defend the specificity of either system. To us it makes good sense to dedicate or commit the serological typing of V. cholerae to the detection of LPS-associated antigens. As previously mentioned, there is precedent for such a commitment since the A, B, and C antigens in the O1 serogroup are LPS associated. This approach would lead to a standardized serological nomenclature with a defined serovar-specific antigen. In order to achieve the above, LPS must serve in some form as the immunogen, rather than whole cells, in order to provoke in the rabbit antiserum which is serologically active, specific, and of high titer.

LPS was extracted by the phenol-water procedure of Westphal and Jann (1965), from V. cholerae Inaba (LA 5875), Ogawa (CA 411) and from 14 of the LSU V. cholerae non-O1 vaccine strains. The LPS preparations were used as (1) antigen in serology to detect anti-LPS activity in the typing sera produced by the methods of Sakazaki, (2) antigen in serology to determine whether multiple determinants exist in the LPS of V. cholerae non-O1 serovars as they do in O1 serovars (i.e., A and B in Ogawa), (3) as an immunogen to provoke LPS-specific antibody, and (4) as antigen coupled to Sepharose beads to serve as an immunoabsorbent to facilitate removal of anti-LPS activity from whole anti-serum and thus separate anti-LPS activity from antibody activity directed against non-LPS nonserovar-specific determinants.

Serology

V. cholerae Ol and non-Ol LPS preparations were detoxified by the method of Auzins (1968) and diluted to give 50 μg LPS per ml. The detoxified LPS was coated into washed rabbit red blood cells (RRBC) and added to dilutions of the antiserum to be tested (Auzins 1968). Table 3 shows the serovar-specific anti-LPS activity present in each of 15 antisera produced in rabbits immunized with heat-killed whole cell vaccines prepared from 14 of the V. cholerae non-Ol LSU vaccine strains and V. cholerae Inaba (LS 5875). Each antiserum prior to serology was percolated through a cellulose R-antigen column (Bhattacharyya 1974) to remove antibody activity to the rough core antigen, a structure common to all V. cholerae. From the checker-board passive hemagglutination (PHA) titration (Table 3), it can be seen that each of the 15 antisera tested showed elevated antiserovar-specific antibody titers against the homologous LPS antigen. With the exception of anti-D and anti-S, there was no evidence of cross-reactivity. LPS serves well as the antigen in PHA serology to detect serovar-specific antigen(s). The results of the checker-board titration suggest that some V. cholerae non-Ol strains may present two or more antigenic determinants in the LPS (strain D and S).

Multiple Determinants

LSU vaccine strains H and T were typed as serotype 25 and vaccine strains D and S were both typed as serotype 33 in the VRL system (Table 1). The results of the PHA checkerboard titration (Table 3) show that anti-H did not agglutinate, by PHA, red cells coated with T-LPS, nor did the reciprocal titration show significant cross reactivity.

Table 3. Passive Hemagglutination Assay: Checkerboard Titration of 15 Anti-Vibrio Serum versus LPS-Coated Rabbit Red Cells

LPS Extracted From		Antiserum to the LSU-Serovar[a]													
		A	B	C	D	E	F	G	H	K	Q	S	T	Y	NN	O1
2022H	A	2560														
39	B		512													
2026H	C			1024												
F8C	D				10,240							40				
F1A	E					2560										
H7C	F						1024									
H10A	G							10,240								
F18B	H								2560				5			
F50C	K									10,240						
2012H	Q										10,240					
N-83	S											5120				
2008H	T												512			
N-128	Y													5120		
N-46	NN														10,240	
Inaba	O1															5120

[a]All antisera R-absorbed.

45

This would imply the VRL typing system detected an antigen shared by the H and T vaccine strains that was not of LPS origin. Serological evidence does suggest that multiple determinants in the LPS of non-O1 V. cholerae do exist. Anti-D serum agglutinated red cells coated with D- (homologous) LPS and S- (heterologous) LPS, which suggests vaccine strains D and S are antigenically identical or that they each may possess a serovar-specific LPS antigen and a second "public" antigen present in the LPS of both strains. To resolve this question, reciprocal absorption studies were done within the D versus S set.

Absorption Studies

Table 4 reviews the serological relationship of D-LPS to S-LPS. Absorption of anti-R activity from anti-D and anti-S sera did little to eliminate the reactivity in either serum to the heterologous antigen (middle columns, Table 4). Next, anti-D serum was percolated through a cellulose S-antigen column to remove anti-S activity. The absorbed anti-D reacted with D-LPS (titer of 5120) and failed to agglutinate S-LPS coated RRBC. This finding implies the presence of an antigenic determinant on the LPS of D which is unique to D (serovar-specific antigen) and not present on S-LPS. When anti-S serum was passed through a cellulose D-antigenic column, to remove anti-D activity, the absorbed serum would no longer react with either D or S-LPS by the PHA assay. This latter finding suggests that the vaccine strain D exhibits at least two LPS antigens: a D serovar-specific antigen (unique to D) and a public antigen which is also detectable on the LPS of the S vaccine strain. A second interpretation would suggest the D and S serovar are identical since they both express a common antigen and in addition the D strain expresses a second LPS antigen, which may be public.

Table 4. The Presence of Multiple Determinants in the LPS of LSU Vaccine Strain F8C (Serovar D)

	Passive Hemagglutination Titer					
	Whole Serum anti		Anti-R Absorbed anti		Reciprocal Absorption[a]	
LSU Vaccine Strain	D	S	D	S	D	S
D (F8C)	10,240	40	5120	40	5120	0
S (N-83)	2560	5120	640	5120	0	0

[a]Anti-D, absorbed with S-cells; anti-S, absorbed with D-cells.

Interference by Non-LPS Antibody

Rabbits from our colony immunized with heat-killed suspensions of whole Vibrio cells do not produce only anti-LPS-specific antibody, a fact which descended on us in the midst of typing large numbers of environmental V. cholerae non-O1 isolates. By way of example we received 66 isolates from the University of Maryland which were typed with our antisera. Twenty-six of these isolates agglutinated strongly in two, three, or four different typing serum. The top panel on Table 5 shows that isolate SGM-61 agglutinated by slide agglutination in anti-G, K, Y, and NN, which suggested this isolate possibly carried multiple determinants. The agglutination patterns for four additional isolates are also included in this table to show examples of multiple or single reactions. Next, SGM isolates 61 and 92 were selected for further serological testing and were tested against each of the five antisera by the tube agglutination test (Bhattacharyya 1977). Live and heated (100°C/10 min) cell suspensions of isolate 61 showed

Table 5. Presence of Antibody Activity to Heat-Stable Non-LPS Antigens in Typing Serum Produced in Rabbits Immunized with Heat-Killed Whole Cell Vaccines

Slide Agglutination

Maryland Isolates	Anti-serum to				
	G	K	Q	Y	NN
SGM-61	+++	+++	0	+++	+++
64	0	0	++	+++	+++
73	0	0	0	+++	+++
92	+++	0	0	+++	+++
108	0	+++	0	0	0

Tube Agglutination

	G	K	Q	Y	NN
Live 61	8	2048	8	512	512
Heated 61[a]	4	1024	8	512	512
Live 92	16	16	16	512	512
Heated 92[a]	8	16	4	16	16

Passive Hemagglutination

LPS Extract From					
SGM-61	0	1024	0	0	0
64	0	0	0	256	256
73	0	0	0	256	256
92	0	0	0	0	0
108	0	512	0	0	0

[a]Heated, 100°C, 10 minutes.

elevated titers in anti-K (2048), Y (512), and NN (512) while anti-G activity was negligible (middle panel, Table 5). The bacterial tube agglutination test is used in the Sakazaki system to type V. cholerae non-Ol. The results suggest SGM-61 is a multiple serovar K, Y, and NN, while SGM-92 appears to be Y and NN. Heated SGM-92 cells failed to show a significant agglutination pattern in either the anti-Y or anti-NN. The heating process may have, through some yet to be explained event, masked the O-determinants making them inaccessible to the agglutinating antibody. Gardner and Venkatraman (1935) cautioned their peers to "use the suspensions of cultures under identification in the unheated state, with formalin (0.2%) since heated suspensions tend to show a common O cross agglutination."

The LPS moiety was shown by PHA titrations to carry the serovar-specific antigen; therefore LPS was extracted from each of the five Maryland isolates, coated on to RRBC and tested by PHA against anti-G, K, Q, Y, and NN. The results of the passive agglutination assay are shown in the bottom panel on Table 5. SGM-61 tested by slide agglutination appeared to be serovar G, K, Y, and NN, a finding which was partially endorsed (except for G) by the tube agglutination test, but not confirmed by testing the LPS of this isolate by PHA. In the PHA assay SGM-61 was agglutinated by anti-K only, suggesting anti-G, Y, and NN reacted with non-LPS antigenic determinants on the SGM-61 cell. The heat-stable non-LPS determinant, it appears, is present on several of the LSU vaccine strains, most notably G, K, Y, and NN. Typing sera with a variety of specificities when used, will produce erroneous conclusions with respect to serotype and, as a result, confuse the serological interpretations.

The presence of high titer nonserovar-specific antibody activity in typing serum produced by rabbits immunized by Smith's (1979) or Sakazaki's (1970) methodology is shown in Table 6. The LSU vaccine strain NN was used to prepare three different vaccines. One group of rabbits were immunized with a subcutaneous injection of 10^7 live NN cells (Smith 1979). A second group of rabbits were immunized with several intravenous injections of a heat-killed suspensions of NN cells (Sakazaki et al. 1970) and a third

Table 6. Absence of Antibody Activity to Non-LPS Heat-Stable Antigens in Typing Serum Produced by Rabbits Immunized with LPS Preparations

Anti-NN raised in rabbits immunized with	NN (N-46)		SGM-61		SGM-92	
	cells	LPS	cells	LPS	cells	LPS
1. Live Vaccine	2048	1024	512	0	1024	0
2. Heat-Killed	1024	8192	512	0	512	0
3. LPS SRBC (iv)	512	8192	0	0	0	0
saline (ip)	2048	4096	5	0	5	0
Anti-NN (No. 2 above) through Sepharose 4B armed with NN-LPS						
4. Eluate	512	0	256	0	128	0

group of animals were immunized with LPS extracted from NN cells (Westphal and Jann 1965). The NN vaccine strain was chosen because NN antiserum (in the LSU system) agglutinated V. cholerae non-O1 isolates SGM-61 and 92 by slide and tube agglutination but not the LPS extracted from these two isolates in the PHA (Table 5). Both the live and heat-killed vaccines provoke agglutinating antibody activity against non-LPS determinants (line 1 and 2, Table 6). In both cases the anti-NN typing sera agglutinated the "live" cell suspensions of the vaccine strain (NN) and also SGM-61 and SGM-92. The same antisera agglutinated only RRBC coated with NN-LPS, but not LPS extracted from isolates 61 and 92. In vibrio serology live whole cells are tested, which presents the opportunity for nonspecific agglutination by antibody produced against non-LPS determinants.

To show the presence of high titer antibody to a heat-stable non-LPS determinant in anti-NN produced by rabbits immunized with heat-killed vaccines, anti-NN was passed through a column packed with Sepharose 4B beads armed with NN-LPS. The eluate (freed of anti-LPS activity) showed elevated agglutination titers against whole cells of the vaccine strain (serovar NN) SGM-61 (serovar K, Table 5) and SGM-92 (serovar unknown; Table 6, line 4). No anti-NN-LPS activity could be detected in the eluate when tested in the passive hemagglutination assay. At this time nothing is known about the location of the non-LPS antigen or of its chemical properties. The important finding is that the non-LPS antigen(s) is heat-stable and is shared across serovar lines.

LPS as an Immunogen

If the serological typing system used to distinguish V. cholerae serovars is committed to the detection of the serovar-specific antigen (LPS), then the background noise--the non-specific antibody activity present in typing sera raised in rabbits immunized with whole cell vaccines-- must be eliminated. One way to circumvent this problem is to use LPS in some form as the immunogen.

After a number of preliminary probes, we adopted two immunization protocols based on the work of Staub (1964). LPS was extracted from the vaccine strains G, K, Q, Y, and NN, and groups of rabbits were immunized with increasing doses of LPS-coated sheep red blood cell suspensions (Figure 2). A second group of rabbits were immunized with three intraperitoneal injections of whole LPS.

Figure 2 shows the immunization schedule along with the PHA titer for each of five representative rabbits immunized with LPS-SRBC suspensions. The anti-LPS responses to K, NN, and G were in the range (the gray area on Figure 2) of the anti-LPS titers seen in sera from rabbits immunized with heat-killed vaccines (Table 3). Anti-Y and Q responses were marginal.

The anti-NN LPS serum produced a PHA titer of 8192 with NN-LPS coated RRBC and a tube agglutination titer of 512 with live NN cells (line 3, Table 6). NN antiserum did not agglutinate live cells or the LPS extract from SGM-61 or 92, a finding which shows the specificity required of typing sera.

Table 7 shows the checkerboard titrations done by PHA of the five anti-LPS sera titrated against each of the five LPS preparations both before (top panel) and after (bottom panel) absorption of anti-R activity. Each antiserum shows low level activity against the four heterologous LPS preparations (anti-R). The anti-R was effectively removed by percolating each antiserum through a cellulose R-antigen column.

These latter experiments show that rabbits immunized with LPS extracted from the vaccine strain will produce serovar-specific antibody (Table 6) that will agglutinate live cells, by the slide or tube agglutination method, which bear the serovar-specific antigen. At the moment we are modifying LPS preparations and immunization protocols in an effort to provoke in the rabbit consistent levels of high titer antiserovar antibody.

Table 7. PHA Activity in Sera in Five Selected Rabbits Immunized with LPS Extracted from Five LSU Vaccine Strains

I Anti-LPS Titers Produced in Rabbits Immunized Intravenously with LPS-Coated Sheep Erythrocytes

Tested Against	Antiserum to				
	G	K	Q	Y	NN
H10A, G	2056	5	5	5	0
F50C, K	10	21,000	5	5	5
2012H, Q	20	5	640	5	5
N-128 Y	160	5	5	40	0
N-46 NN	10	20	20	20	10,240

II Absorption of Anti-R from Anti-LPS Serum by the Cellulose-R Antigen Column Method

	G	K	Q	Y	NN
G	320	0	0	0	0
K	0	1,280	0	0	0
Q	0	0	160	0	0
Y	0	0	0	20	0
N	0	0	0	0	640

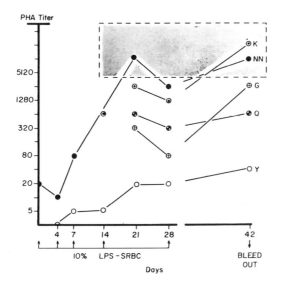

Figure 2. Anti-LPS response in rabbits immunized intravenously with LPS-coated SRBC.

ACKNOWLEDGMENTS

This research was supported by grants from the Louisiana Department of Health and Human Resources and National Oceanic and Atmospheric Administration Office of Sea Grant, Department of Commerce, under Grant NA79AA-D-00128.

REFERENCES

Auzins, H. 1968. A comparative assay of O-somatic antigen 5 of Salmonellae. Aust. J. Exp. Biol. Sci. 46:93-105.

Bhattacharyya, F.K., and S. Mukerjee. 1963. The use of starch gel filtration for the absorption of anti-cholera sera. Ann. Biochem. Exp. Med. 23:633-636.

Bhattacharyya, F.K., and S. Mukerjee. 1974. Serological analysis of the flagellar of H agglutinating antigens of cholera and NAG vibrios. Ann. Microbiol. 125A:167-181.

Bhattacharyya, F.K. 1975. Vibrio cholerae flagellar antigens: A serodiagnostic test, functional implications of H-reactivity and taxonomic importance of cross-reactions within the Vibrio genus. Med. Microbiol. Immunol. 162:29-41.

Bhattacharyya, F.K. 1977. The agglutination reactions of cholera vibrios. Jap. J. Med. Sci. Biol. 30:259-268.

Fanning, G.R., B. R. Davis, J.M. Madden, H.D. Bradford, A.G. Steigerwalt, and D.J. Brenner. 1981. Vibrio mimicus: A newly recognized cholera-like organism. Abstr. Am. Soc. Microbiol. Page 50.

Gardner, A.D., and K.V. Venkatraman. 1935. The antigens of the cholera group of vibrios. J. Hyg. 35:262-282.

Ghosh, S.N., and S. Mukerjee. 1961. Ann. Biochem. Exp. Med. 21:151-156.

Hranitzky, K.W., A. Mulholland, A.D. Larson, E.R. Eubanks, and L.T. Hart. 1980. Characterization of a flagellar sheath protein in Vibrio cholerae. Infect. Immun. 27:597-603.

Kabir, S. 1981. Composition and immunochemical properties of outer membrane proteins of Vibrio cholerae. J. Bacteriol. 144:382-389.

Neoh, S.H., and D. Rowley. 1971. Quantative assay of protein antigens of Vibrio cholerae involved in the vibriolytic action of antibody and complement. Aust. J. Exp. Biol. Med. Sci. 49:605-610.

Redmond, J.W., M.J. Korsch, and G.D.F. Jackson. 1973. Immunochemical studies of the O-antigens of Vibrio cholerae. Partial characterization of an acid-labile antigenic determinant. Aust. J. Exp. Biol. Med. Sci. 51:229-235.

Redmond, J.W. 1979. The structure of the O-antigenic side chain of the lipopolysaccharide of Vibrio cholerae 569B (Inaba). Biochem. Biophys. Acta. 584:346-352.

Sakazaki, R., K. Tamura, C.Z. Gomez, and R. Sen. 1970. Serological studies on the cholera group of vibrios. Jap. J. Med. Sci. Biol. 23:13-20.

Sakazaki, R., and T. Shimada. 1977. Serovars of Vibrio cholerae. Jap. J. Med. Sci. Biol. 30:279-282.

Shimada, T., and R. Sakazaki. 1973. R antigen of Vibrio cholerae. Jap. J. Med. Sci. Biol. 26:155-160.

Shimada, T., and R. Sakazaki. 1977. Additional serovars and inter-O-antigenic relationships of Vibrio cholerae. Jap. J. Med. Sci. Biol. 30:275-277.

Smith, H.L., Jr., and K. Goodner. 1965. On the classification of vibrios. Pages 408 in O.A. Bushnell and C.S. Brookhyser (Eds.), Proceedings of the Cholera Research Symposium, Honolulu, Hawaii.

Smith, H.L., Jr. 1979. Serotyping of non-cholera vibrios. J. Clin. Microbiol. 10:85-90.

Staub, A.M. 1964. The role of the polysaccharide moiety in determining the specificity and immunological activity of the O-antigen complex of Salmonellae. Pages 38-48 in M. Landy and W. Braun (Eds.), Bacterial endotoxins.

Westphal, O., and K. Jann. 1965. Bacterial lipopoly-
    saccharides. Extraction with phenol-water and further
    applications of the procedure. Pages 83-91 in R.L.
    Whistler (Ed.), Methods in carbohydrate chemistry,
    Vol. V.

Chapter 3

AN EPIDEMIOLOGICAL STUDY OF V. CHOLERAE IN LOUISIANA

Henry B. Bradford Jr.

Until recently, health professionals and scientists in the United States have had a false sense of security regarding the possibility of infections by toxigenic Vibrio cholerae. The first hint of a cholera problem to come arose in 1973 when a Port Lavaca, Texas man was diagnosed as having cholera. In 1978, national and international attention focused on Louisiana as the site of this country's first cholera outbreak since 1911. A medical technician at Abbeville General Hospital persisted in attempts to identify an unknown isolate recovered from an Abbeville man. The Centers for Disease Control (CDC) later identified the isolate as toxigenic Vibrio cholerae Ol Inaba.

In order to delineate the extent of the outbreak, the CDC and the Louisiana State Health Department launched an extensive investigation. Eleven cases of cholera were identified during the two-month investigation. Eight were symptomatic, and three cases were asymptomatic. All were associated with the consumption of home cooked crabs, either boiled or steamed. The incubation period ranged from 34 to 112 hours after consumption of crabs.

The contaminated crabs were caught in a variety of places--from Mud Lake, Louisiana in the extreme western portion of the state to Redfish Point 125 miles east in Vermilion Bay. Apparently no single point of contamination was responsible for the contaminated crabs. A large number of environmental samples were taken in order to delineate the extent of contamination by V. cholerae O1. Of the 1055 samples consisting of fresh shrimp, raw oysters, live crabs, crab meat, and estuarial waters, only three cultures yielded V. cholerae O1, suggesting that this organism was endemic in the area--but in very low numbers (Blake et al. 1980).

To determine whether the strains isolated from the 11 patients were identical, phage typing studies were initiated. It was determined that all the strains from Louisiana were identical and that they were also identical to the Port Lavaca strain of 1973 (Blake et al. 1980), thus suggesting that this particular strain of organism had become endemic in the states of Louisiana and Texas. When no additional cases had been discovered by the end of September, the CDC terminated its intensive epidemiological investigation. The state of Louisiana, however, continued surveillance for additional cases.

In 1978, the Division of Laboratory Services of the Office of Health Services and Environmental Quality isolated four strains of V. cholerae O1 from small communities throughout the southern part of the state. Isolation procedures are those described by Roberts and Seidler in this volume. No additional clinical cases of cholera were reported during this time, indicating that although V. cholerae O1 was still active in the state, the cases were at the subclinical level. With the onset of cold weather in the latter part of November, the isolation of V. cholerae O1 ceased.

Only four Vibrio cholerae O1 isolates were reported from Louisiana in 1979. The initial isolate of the year was made from the environment. An unusual observation was made in May of that year when a nontoxigenic Vibrio cholerae O1 was isolated from a gentleman presenting a history of a leg wound. The patient had broken a leg in an automobile accident and his recovery was unremarkable until the latter part of the convalescence period. At that time, a lesion on his lower leg was noticed and a culture was subsequently taken. Prior to receipt of the wound isolate, Vibrio cholerae O1 was isolated from a sewer in New Orleans. Epidemiological investigation revealed that the patient with the leg lesion was debreeding his lesion and placing the bandages in the commode, which was subsequently discharged into the sewage system. This isolate was shown to be nontoxigenic by Y-1 adrenal cells and ELISA toxigenicity studies. Later in the year two isolates were recovered in October from Lafayette. These isolates were not associated with any cholera case and were nontoxigenic. In 1980, a total of eight strains of <u>Vibrio cholerae</u> O1 were isolated from the western part of Louisiana. All isolates were nontoxigenic with the exception of the September isolate from Lake Charles, suggesting that at least one additional case was present in Louisiana, but was not severe enough to seek medical treatment. There were no further <u>V. cholerae</u> O1 isolations until June 1981 when another toxigenic O1 Inaba was isolated from the sewer system of Lake Charles. This isolate was made approximately the same time that two <u>Vibrio cholerae</u> O1 Inaba isolations were reported in the state of Texas. It is not known at this time whether the <u>V. cholerae</u> O1 from Lake Charles was identical to the Texas isolates. Additionally, an O1 Ogawa was isolated at the same time from the Lake Charles sewer system. In October 1981, <u>V. cholerae</u> O1 Inaba was again associated with a case of acute diarrhea. Investigations are ensuing and it is not known at this time as to the exact source of the infection.

The biochemical characteristics of the <u>Vibrio cholerae</u> strains isolated from Louisiana were studied. These assays included gelatinase detection, oxidase production, sensitivity to 0/129, reactivity on Kliglers iron agar, production of H_2S, indole production; and metabolism of lysine, arginine, ornithine, sucrose, arabinose, and mannitol. All isolates produced gelatinase and oxidase and were sensitive to 0/129. The organisms produced an alkaline slant and acid butt on the Kliglers iron agar, but did not produce hydrogen sulfide. Positive reactions in tryptophane broth, lysine, ornithine, sucrose, and mannitol were observed. The organisms did not metabolize arginine or arabinose. All isolates were agglutinated by <u>Vibrio cholerae</u>, polyvalent antisera--an O1 Inaba or O1 Ogawa monospecific antisera provided by the CDC.

In an attempt to further define the relatedness of all these Vibrio cholerae O1 Inaba isolates, phage pattern analysis was conducted (Table 1). It is easily seen that the isolates made in 1978 are all identical and these isolates were identical to the phage susceptibility patterns of the V. cholerae isolates associated with the 1978 outbreak (Blake et al. 1980). Furthermore, the strains cultured from Lake Charles in September 1980 and June 1981 were also identical to the 1978 strains with one exception, phage type 57 from June 1981. All of these strains were toxigenic. It is also interesting to note that the two isolates made in 1979, one environmental from Hopedale and the other from the leg lesion (Camp Plauche), were identical in phage reaction patterns, classical phage patterns III and IV. It is debatable at this time whether the environmental strains possessed the necessary virulence factors to initiate infection. Additionally, the appearance of the same phage pattern from the Cocodrie estuaries and the Houma sewers gives rise to some interesting speculation. These data suggest that the Houma isolate may be the result of some disease or disease process, and that the organism originated in the environment. However, there is no conclusive evidence that the Houma isolates were responsible for any type of disease. The fact that three different phage patterns were cultured from one sample station employing one sample suggests that this area has an unusually high number of different strains of Vibrio cholerae O1 Inaba in the environment. These organisms may play some role in the mediation of some infections. An important question to be raised is the relationship of the nontoxigenic V. cholerae O1 strains to the toxigenic. The toxigenic strains appear to be all of the same phage type; whereas the nontoxigenic strains have a wide variety of phage patterns.

With the increased awareness of the cholera problem, both the physician and the hospitals referred to the Division of Laboratory Services a number of non-O1 V. cholerae isolates. Table 2 provides a summation of the clinical symptoms that the patients presented in association with positive cultures; 96% of the patients had diarrhea, 75% experienced weakness; 34%, dizziness; 65%, nausea; 44%, vomiting; 62% had abdominal cramps; 72%, fever; and 55%,

Table 1. Phage Patterns of _Vibrio cholerae_ O1

Location	Date	Classical				El Tor								Experimental				
		I	II	III	IV	1	2	32	4	5	B	51	57	D	13	14	16	24
Franklin	Oct. 78					+	+			+	+	+		+	+		+	+
Guedan	Oct. 78					+	+			+	+	+		+	+		+	+
Pecan Island	Oct. 78					+	+			+	+	+		+	+		+	+
Lake Arthur	Nov. 78					+	+			+	+	+		+	+		+	+
Hopedale	Mar. 79			+	+													
Camp Plauche	May 79			+	+													
Lafayette	Oct. 79													+				
Lafayette	Oct. 79					+	+			+		+		+				
Cocodrie	Apr. 80			+	+													
Houma	Apr. 80			+	+													
Houma	May 80				+													
Houma	May 80															+		
Houma	May 80			+	+											+		
Bayou Teche	May 80					+	+			+	+	+						
Mud Lake	June 80																	
Lake Charles	Sept. 80					+	+			+	+	+		+	+		+	+
Lake Charles	June 81					+	+			+	+	+	+	+	+		+	+
Lake Charles	June 81						±			+	+	±						

Table 2. Symptoms of V. cholerae Non-O1 Infections

Patient	Strain	Diarrhea	Weakness	Dizziness	Nausea	Vomiting	Abdominal Cramps	Fever	Chills	Hospitalized	Seafood Eaten
	2022										
7	2026	X					X			No	Potatoes, Crabs
8	2024	X					X	X		No	Oysters
9	2025	X			X		X	X	X	Yes	Oysters, Shrimp
10	2027	X			X	X	X	X	X	No	Oysters
11	2000	X	X		X		X	X	X	Yes	Oysters
12	2023	X					X			No	Oysters
13	2002	X	X	X	X	X		X	X	Yes	Crabs
14	2001	X	X	X	X	X	X	X	X	No	Crabs, Crawfish
15	2004	X	X				X	X	X	Yes	None
16	2003	X	X		X		X	X		No	Crawfish
17	2008	X	X	X	X	X				Yes	Oysters, Crabmeat
18	2007	X	X				X			No	Shrimp
19	2005										
	2006	X	X	X	X	X	X	X	X	No	Crabs, Crawfish
20	2011	X	X		X	X				Yes	Shrimp, Crab Gumbo
21	2012	X	X	X			X	X	X	Yes	Crabs
22	2009	X	X	X			X	X	X	Yes	Crawfish
23	2010	X	X					X	X	Yes	None
24	2013	X								Yes	Raw Oysters
25	2014	X	X	X	X		X	X	X	Yes	Raw Oysters

No.	Year	C1	C2	C3	C4	C5	C6	C7	Response	Item
26	2015	X	X			X	X	X	No	Raw Oysters
27	2017	X	X	X	X	X		X	Yes	Raw Oysters
28	2018	X	X	X	X	X	X	X	Yes	Raw Oysters
29	2016	X	X	X			X	X	Yes	Raw Oysters
30	2019	X	X			X		X	Yes	Raw Osyters
31	2020	X	X	X			X		Yes	Raw Oysters
32	2021	X	X	X	X	X	X	X	Yes	Raw Oysters
33	2036	X	X	X	X	X	X	X	No	Raw Oysters
34	2034	X	X	X	X	X	X	X	Yes	Raw Oysters
35	2028	X	X	X	X	X	X	X	Yes	Raw Oysters
36	2035	X	X	X	X	X	X	X	Yes	Shrimp, Crab
	2030						X		No	
37	2031	X	X	X	X	X		X	No	Crawfish
38	2032	NA	NA	NA	X	X	X	NA	No	Crawfish
39	2033	NA	NA	NA	NA	NA	NA	NA	No	Crawfish

chills. It might also be noted that over 60% of the patients had such severe diarrhea that hospitalization was required. When the patients were questioned as to the foods they consumed, it was learned that 60% ate raw oysters, 13% ate shrimp or crawfish, 23% ate crabs, and 10% gave no history of seafood consumption. These data obviously suggest that persons consuming seafood, either raw or improperly prepared, placed themselves at greatest risk.

Table 3 provides data relevant to the biochemical characteristics of the non-O1 V. cholerae that the Division of Laboratory Services has studied over the past several years. This table also provides data regarding the serotypes of the respective organisms. The methodology for the preparation of antisera employed and the relationship of the Sakazaki to the LSU typing scheme are topics presented in this volume. The homogeneity of the biochemical characteristics of these organisms should be noted with one exception: the ability to ferment sucrose. Of the 37 strains, 20 could not ferment sucrose. Davis et al. (in press) will be publishing data to document that these sucrose-negative non-O1 V. cholerae are sufficiently different from the sucrose-positive V. cholerae non-O1's, that a special species name, V. mimicus, is in order. The serotype of these organisms is also very interesting in the respect that there is great antigenic diversity associated with disease. It is also noted that a number of organisms were nontypeable in the serotyping scheme of Sakasaki. All organisms were nontoxigenic with the exception of strains 2002 and 2011. Radioactive toxin gene probe studies were conducted and it was clearly shown that strains 2002 and 2011 did possess the toxgene. Restriction enzyme and electrophoretic migration studies were conducted on the labeled nuclear acid and it was clearly shown that the toxin genes were different from the genes of the organisms of the 1978 outbreak, suggesting that there are two distinct pools of cholera toxin gene in Louisiana.

Because of the impact of the environment on V. cholerae and the possible relationship to the mediation of cholera, a number of studies were undertaken in an attempt to elucidate the exact role the environment plays. Our data show that cholera organisms are present in large numbers

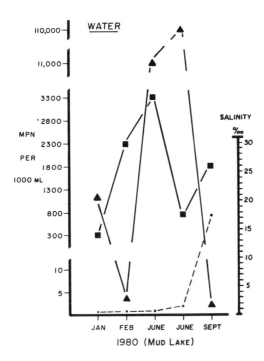

Figure 1. The relationship of V. cholerae (■) and fecal coliforms (▲) in Mud Lake to water salinity (●).

throughout the warm months. However, the numbers are greatly influenced by both salinity and temperature (Figure 1). It should also be noted that V. cholerae non-O1 will vary independently of the level of fecal coliforms. As might be expected, the seafood in such waters will reflect the amount of Vibrio cholerae non-O1 present. Figure 2 shows the colonization of Vibrio cholerae in crabs in waters that have relatively high numbers of V. cholerae non-O1.

Because of the high numbers of V. cholerae in the estuaries of Louisiana, it was decided to monitor sewers of several cities in south Louisiana for the presence of V. cholerae, both O1 and non-O1. It was discovered that a large number of serotypes could be cultured on any given day during the warm months. Figure 3 shows the relative

Table 3. Biochemical Characteristics of V. cholerae Non-O1

Strain	Gelatin	Oxidase	Urea	Indole	Lysine	Arginnine	Ornithine	Sucrose	Arabinose	Mannitol	Sakazaki Serotype
2022	+	+	-	+	+	-	+	-	-	+	26
2026	+	+	-	+	+	-	+	+	-	+	UK
2024	+	+	-	+	+	-	+	+	-	+	2
2025	+	+	-	+	+	-	+	-	-	+	X71
2027	+	+	-	+	+	-	+	-	-	+	20
2000	+	+	-	+	+	-	+	+	-	+	6
2023	+	+	-	+	+	-	+	-	-	+	51
2002	+	+	-	+	+	-	+	-	-	+	UK
2001	+	+	-	+	+	-	+	-	-	+	41
2004	+	+	-	+	+	-	+	+	-	+	41
2003	+	+	-	+	+	-	+	-	-	+	41
2008	+	+	-	+	+	-	+	+	-	+	18
2007	+	+	-	+	+	-	+	-	-	+	41
2005	+	+	-	+	+	-	+	-	-	+	6
2006	+	+	-	+	+	-	+	-	-	+	41
2011	+	+	-	+	+	-	+	+	-	+	UK
2012	+	+	-	+	+	-	+	-	-	+	2
2009	+	+	-	+	+	-	+	+	-	+	20
2010	+	+	-	+	+	-	+	-	-	+	8
2013	+	+	-	+	+	-	+	+	-	+	24
2014	+	+	-	+	+	-	+	+	-	+	24
2015	+	+	-	+	+	-	+	-	-	+	40
2017	+	+	-	+	+	-	+	-	-	+	8
2018	+	+	-	+	+	-	+	+	-	+	44
2016	+	+	-	+	+	-	+	+	-	+	58
2019	+	+	-	+	+	-	+	+	-	+	X65

Table 3. Continued

strain	Gelatin	Oxidase	Urea	Indole	Lysine	Arginnine	Ornithine	Sucrose	Arabinose	Mannitol	Sakazaki Serotype
2020	+	+	-	+	+	-	+	-	-	+	44
2021	+	+	-	+	+	-	+	-	-	+	10
2036	+	+	-	+	+	-	+	+	-	+	UK
2034	+	+	-	+	+	-	+	+	-	+	37
2028	+	+	-	+	+	-	+	-	-	+	8(52)
2035	+	+	-	+	+	-	+	+	-	+	UK
2030	+	+	-	+	+	-	+	+	-	+	UK
2031	+	+	-	+	+	-	+	-	-	+	20
2032	+	+	-	+	+	-	+	-	-	+	20
2033	+	+	-	+	+	-	+	-	-	+	20

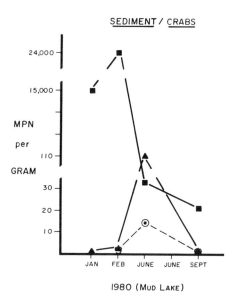

Figure 2. Occurrence of fecal coliforms (■) and V. cholerae in sediment (▲) in comparison to V. cholerae in crabs (◎).

distribution of serotypes of Vibrio cholerae in the environment, in the sewers, and in human cases. This preliminary data is very difficult to interpret; however, it can be said that there are no clear patterns as to which serotypes can be found in which of the three locations.

SUMMARY

Epidemiological studies of cases and environmental surveillance suggest that V. cholerae is endemic in Louisiana coastal waters. The coastal waters harbor a large number of different phage types of V. cholerae O1, and the relationship of these phage types to the mediation of cholera is not clear.

People consuming seafood that has been improperly cooked or handled are at increased risks of acquiring

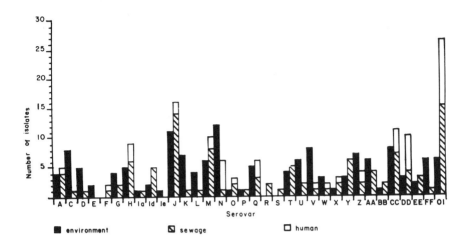

Figure 3. Vibrio cholerae serovar distribution from the environment, from sewage, and from human sources.

infection due to either O1 or non-O1 V. cholerae. Sucrose-positive and sucrose-negative non-O1 V. cholerae are as potentially serious to the individual patient as O1 V. cholerae. Environmental factors influence the colonization of seafood by V. cholerae, and these foods play a vital role in the distribution and morbidity of V. cholerae. All states with warm coastal waters should be concerned about cholera. I would like to challenge investigators to develop better assays to assess the pathogenicity of the Vibrio group.

ACKNOWLEDGMENTS

I gratefully acknowledge the assistance of Dr. Don Brenner of the Centers for Disease Control for toxin determination, and Dr. John Lee of the Public Health Laboratories in Kent, England, and Dr. Jim Kaper of the University of Maryland for genetic probe studies. I would like to thank Nell Roberts, Joan Barbay, Betty Planchard, and James Gillespie of my staff for technical assistance.

REFERENCES

Baser, S., and S. Mukeyie. 1968. Bacteriophage typing of _Vibrio_ el tor. Experientia. 1968:299-300.

Blake, P.A., D.T. Allegra, J.D. Snyder, T.J. Barrett, L. McFarland, C.T., Caraway, J.C. Feely, J.P. Craig, J.V. Lee, N.D. Puhr, and R.A. Feldman. 1980. Cholerae--a possible endemic focus in the United States. N. Engl. J. Med. 302:305-309.

David, B.R., A.R. Fanning, J.M. Madden, A.G. Steiger-wolt, H.B. Bradford, H.L. Smith, Jr., D.J. Brenner. 1982. Characterization of biochemically atypical strains of _Vibrio cholerae_ and designation of a new pathogenic species, _Vibrio mimicus_. J. Clin. Microbiol. In press.

Weissman, J.B., W.E., Dewitt, and J. Thompson. 1974. A case of cholera in Texas, 1973. Am. J. Epidemiol. 100:487-498.

Chapter 4

H ANTIGEN RELATIONSHIPS AMONG SEVERAL VIBRIO SPECIES

Mariela Tassin Stein, R.J. Siebeling
and A.D. Larson

Mukerjee in 1978 stated that "the heat-sensitive flagellar antigens of V. cholerae and possibly of all vibrios differ from those of other genera in that they are now known to be serologically uniform and definitive of the species. They may usefully be applied to identification at the species level. Contrary to common opinion, the flagella are good antigens and H agglutination under suitable conditions is sensitive, reactions occurring at high serum dilutions (1/40,000 and above). Interestingly, the H antigens are not involved in the immune immobilization reaction. This reaction involves the type-specific O determinants which may also be situated on the complex flagellar structure of vibrios. Relationships of possible phylogenetic importance between minor H determinants of V. cholerae and V. anguillarum, V. metschnikovii and V. proteus have been demonstrated. Recent studies suggest that this list be expanded to include isolates of Vibrio fluvialis, the tentative species name given to those organisms previously designated Group F or EF-6." Evidence for this suggestion will be presented.

Flagellar antisera were prepared by the method outlined by Bhattacharyya and Mukerjee (1974). Motile strains of desired Vibrio species were selected by serial passage through Craigie tubes containing Difco Motility GI medium supplemented with 1% NaCl. Smooth, motile strains were inoculated into Tryptic Soy Broth and incubated at 37°C for 18 hours. The broth culture was swabbed onto dry Tryptic Soy Agar in Kolle flasks, and incubated at 37°C for 48 hours. Bacterial growth was harvested in 20 ml of 0.3% formalized saline and stored at 4°C for 48 hours. The dense formalized whole cell suspension was standardized to 380 units at 540 nanometers in a Klett-Summerson Colorimeter. New Zealand White rabbits were injected intravenously in the marginal ear vein with the standardized suspension in 9 to 12 graded doses from 0.2 ml to 1.0 ml at 1- to 2- day intervals. Test bleeds showed anti-OH titers usually approached 20,000 or greater on the 21st day post immunization. The rabbits were exsanguinated on or about day 30 by cardiac puncture.

Unwanted anti-O activity was removed by cellulose-column absorption (Bhattacharyya and Mukerjee 1974). Homologous cells were heated for 20 minutes at 121°C and dispersed in a matrix of 16 grams (wet weight) of washed cellulose powder. The cellulose-O-cell suspension was delivered to a chromatography column and was washed with several volumes of saline until no obvious particulate material was seen in the wash. The bed volume was determined using hemoglobin as a tracer. A 1:10 dilution of flagellar (OH) antiserum in a volume equal to the bed volume was allowed to enter the bed and eluted with either saline or more antiserum. The antiserum was cycled over the column until anti-O activity was no longer detectable.

The cellulose-column method of absorption was chosen over the conventional absorption procedure because of its efficiency in removing anti-O activity without diminishing anti-H activity, thus avoiding the five- to tenfold "nonspecific" removal of anti-H activity by conventional absorption (Figure 1). This "nonspecific" loss of anti-H activity probably occurs as the result of the change in surface charge of the antibody-antigen complex, thus as it agglutinates, the H agglutinins are absorbed by electrostatic attraction or physically entrapped in the sedimenting agglutination particles. Agglutination complexes or particles are not formed in the column; therefore, anti-H antibody molecules are not physically entrapped.

Table 1. Serological Assay of Vibrio Species and Assorted Gram-Negative Bacilli Against OH Serum Raised Versus Vibrio cholerae Inaba (LA 5875) and Vibrio fluvialis (10-50D)

| Motile Isolate Tested | No. | H-Agglutination | |
		Anti-Vibrio cholerae	Anti-Vibrio fluvialis
V. cholerae 5875	1	20480	160
V. cholerae non-O1	24	1280-10240	80-320
V. parahaemolyticus	2	0	0
V. alginolyticus	2	0	0
V. anguillarum	1	1280	320
V. fluvialis 10-50D	1	2560	10240
V. fluvialis	41	640-2560	320-5120
V. metschnikovii	4	160	80
V. vulnificus	2	0	0
A. hydrophila	1	0	0
A. fecalis	1	0	0
A. hinshawii	1	0	0
E. coli	1	0	0
E. tarda	1	0	0
P. morgani	1	0	0
P. vulgaris	1	0	0
S. paratyphi A	1	0	0
S. typhimurium	1	0	0

Anti-Vibrio cholerae El Tor Inaba (LA 5875) OH serum was tested for species specificity by the tube H-agglutination test against motile Vibrio parahaemolyticus Vibrio alginolyticus, Vibrio anguillarum, Vibrio metschnikovii, Vibrio vulnificus, Vibrio fluvialis, representative genera in the families Enterobacteriaceae (Escherichia, Proteus, Edwardsiella, Arizona, and Salmonella),

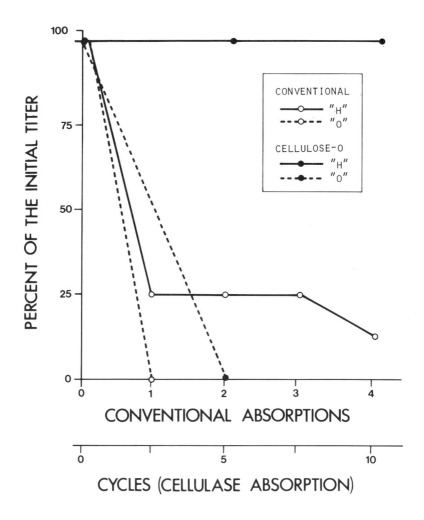

Figure 1. Cellulose "O" column absorption versus conventional absorption to remove anti-O activity.

Pseudomonadaceae (Alcaligenes), and the genus Aeromonas (Vibrionaceae). H-tube agglutinations were performed following the procedure outlined by Bhattacharyya and Mukerjee (1974) using a dense formalized suspension and a high reaction temperature. The antiserum agglutinated to a titer of 1280 against the environmental Vibrio fluvialis 10-50D (Table 1). An additional 41 motile isolates were tested and all were agglutinated in the anti-V. cholerae OH serum. Previously, Bhattacharyya (1975) reported that anti-V. cholerae OH sera agglutinated V. anguillarum and V. metschnikovii which was also seen in this assay (Table 1), whereas the remaining Vibrio species and assorted gram-negative bacilli showed no agglutination.

The same organisms were also screened with anti-flagellar antibody produced against a V. fluvialis crab isolate 10-50D (Table 1). Anti-V. fluvialis OH agglutinated the homologous antigen V. fluvialis and heterologous preparations of V. cholerae, V. anguillarum, and V. metschnikovii. H-agglutination titers against 25 V. cholerae isolates ranged from 80 to 320. These results suggest that an H-antigen relationship exists between V. fluvialis and the three cross-reacting species. Anti-V. fluvialis OH did not agglutinate motile V. parahaemolyticus, V. alginolyticus, V. vulnificus, nor the assortment of gram-negative organisms.

Next it was necessary to show that the antigenic relationships which exist between V. cholerae, V. fluvialis, V. anguillarum, and V. metschnikovii are restricted to shared H and not common "O" determinants. Anti-O activity was assayed by passive hemagglutination (PHA). Anti-V. cholerae 5875 OH serum showed no PHA activity to the LPS of V. fluvialis 10-50D or V. cholerae non-O1 2026H nor did anti-V. fluvialis 10-50D OH serum agglutinate 5875 or 2026H LPS (Table 2). This suggests that anti-O activity is not responsible for the cross-reactivity seen in the anti-OH serum.

In an attempt to produce "mono-specific H antisera" O agglutinins were first absorbed followed by subsequent removal of "cross-reacting" H agglutinins. Anti-H serum to V. cholerae 5875 and V. fluvialis 10-50D (O absorbed by the cellulose column) were titered against 41 isolates of V.

Table 2. Passive Hemagglutination (PHA) Titers: For Anti-O Activity in Anti-OH Serum Raised Against Vibrio cholerae O1 (LA 5875), non-O1 (LA 2026H), and Vibrio fluvialis 10-50D Formalized Vaccines

	PHA Titers[b]		
LSP Source[a] Coated onto RRBC	Anti- V. cholerae	Anti- Non-O1	Anti- V. fluvialis
V. cholerae O1	1024	32	4
V. cholerae non-O1	2	64	4
V. fluvialis 10-50D	2	2	128

[a]LPS extracted by Hot-Phenol (Westphal).
[b]Auzin.

fluvialis acquired from three different sources and included both biotypes: aerogenic and anaerogenic. Absorption of the anti-O activity from each antiserum did not eliminate the capacity of anti-V. cholerae 5875 serum to agglutinate V. fluvialis isolates (Table 3). H-agglutination titers of anti-V. cholerae 5875 "H" against the V. fluvialis isolates ranged from 640 to 2560, which confirmed the cross-reactivity observed with V. cholerae 5875 OH antiserum as being associated with anti-H activity. Activity of anti-V. fluvialis 10-50D antibody serologically titrated against the V. fluvialis isolates ranged from 320 to 10240 (Table 3).

Absorption of the anti-O activity from anti-V. cholerae OH, anti-V. fluvialis OH, anti-V. metschnikovii OH, and anti-V. anguillarum OH serum did not remove their capacities to agglutinate homologous antigen nor the three cross-reacting heterologous species. Anti-H produced against each of the four Vibrio species reacted with the H-antigen preparations of each of the three other species.

Table 3. The Agglutination of Vibrio fluvialis by "O" Absorbed Anti-Vibrio cholerae "H" Serum and Anti-Vibrio fluvialis "H" Serum

Motile Isolates Tested	Source	No. Tested	Anti-H Agglutination Titers	
			Anti- V. cholerae (5875)	Anti- V. fluvialis (10-50D)
V. fluvialis	Crabs (Louisiana)	20/Aerogenic	640-2560	1280-5120
	Water (Maryland)	12/Anaerogenic	640-2560	1280-10,240
		6/Anaerogenic	1280-2560	320-2560
	Human	3/Anaerogenic	1280-2560	2560-5120
V. fluvialis	Crab (10-50D)	1/Aerogenic	2560	10,240
V. cholerae	(LA 5875)	1/Anaerogenic	20,480	160

79

The H-agglutination titers to the heterologous antigens ranged from 80 to 1280 (Table 4).

Cross-absorption studies were done in which the cross-reacting anti-H activity of both anti-V. cholerae and anti-V. fluvialis was absorbed with a formalized heterologous cell suspension in a cellulose column. The heterologous H-titers for the absorbed sera are presented in Table 4. When anti-V. cholerae H was absorbed with V. fluvialis, the capacity to agglutinate V. cholerae and V. anguillarum remained unchanged, while the H activity to V. fluvialis and V. metschnikovii was removed. When anti-V. fluvialis was absorbed with V. cholerae, the absorbed serum agglutinated V. fluvialis and V. anguillarum to the same level as preabsorbed sera, while the H activity to V. cholerae and V. metschnikovii decreased significantly. This suggests that V. cholerae, V. fluvialis, and V. metschnikovii possess a common, possibly minor, H determinant(s).

The serological relationships between species of Vibrio become very important if flagellar antisera is to be used for the rapid screening of vibrios, most importantly, Vibrio cholerae. If anti-V. cholerae H is to be used to initially screen for V. cholerae isolates, strains of Vibrio fluvialis, Vibrio metschnikovii and Vibrio anguillarum could be tentatively and eroneously identified as Vibrio cholerae because they will agglutinate in nonabsorbed anti-V. cholerae H serum. To avoid this problem, cross-reacting antibody should be absorbed to render the H antiserum species-specific, or the investigator must be made aware of the interspecies H relationships.

Kauffman (1971) believes the principal basis for any system of bacterial classification or species recognition is serological relatedness between strains. The evidence presented and discussed confirms the relationship among three species of Vibrio, namely Vibrio cholerae, Vibrio metschnikovii and Vibrio anguillarum previously reported (Bhattacharyya 1975) and established an additional relationship between Vibrio fluvialis and the three above named species at the flagellar level. Serological H-typing for the genus Vibrio should thus provide an excellent means for presumptively identifying species of Vibrio, and together

Table 4. Cross-Absorption Analysis of the Four Cross-Reacting Vibrio Species

H Antisera	Absorbing Antigen	H-Agglutination Titers			
		V. cholerae	V. fluvialis	V. metschnikovii	V. anguillarum
Anti-V. cholerae (LA 5875)	none	5120	1280	160	1280
	10-50D	5120	0	10	640
Anti-V. fluvialis (10-50D)	none	160	5120	80	640
	5875	0	2560	20	640
Anti-V. metschnikovii	none	160	1280	20480	1280
Anti-V. anguillarum	none	640	1280	80	10240

with biochemical characterization, all probable Vibrio isolates could be rapidly and definitively identified.

REFERENCES

Bhattacharyya, F.K., and S. Mukerjee. 1971. Serological analysis of the flagellar or H agglutinating antigens of cholera and NAG Vibrios. Annals Microbiol. (Institute of Pasteur). 125:167-181.

Bhattacharyya, F.K. 1975. Vibrio cholerae flagellar antigens: a serodiagnostic test, functional implications of H-reactivity and taxonomic importance of cross-reactions with the Vibrio genus. Med. Microbiol. Immun. 162:20-41.

Furniss, A.L., J.V. Lee, and T.J. Donovan. 1977. Group F, a new Vibrio? Lancet 2. 565-566.

Jensen, M.J., P. Baumann, M. Mandel, and J.V. Lee. 1980. Characterization of facultatively anaerobic marine bacteria belonging to Group F of Lee, Donovan and Furniss. Curr. Microbiol. 3:373-376.

Kauffman, F. 1971. Klassifikation and Nomenklatur der Bacterien. Curr. Topics Microb. Immun. 56:1-12.

Mukerjee, S. 1978. Principles and practices of typing Vibrio cholerae. Pages 51-115 in Methods in microbiology, Vol. 12. Academic, New York.

Seidler, R.J., D.A. Allen, R.R. Colwell, S.W. Joseph, and O.P. Daily. 1981. Biochemical characteristics and virulence of environmental Group F bacteria isolated in the United States. Appl. Environ. Microbiol. 40:715-720.

CHAPTER 5

SEROLOGY AND SEROTYPING OF VIBRIO CHOLERAE

Terence Donovan

The serological classification of Vibrio cholerae was established by Gardner and Venkatraman in 1935. This was based on a common heat-labile H antigen and division into six subgroups with different heat-stable O antigens. The majority of isolates from cases of clinical cholera from several countries were found to have an identical O antigen and were designated subgroup 1. Other vibrios with similar biochemical reactions were found to have different O antigens and five other subgroups were recognized. The recognition of subgroup O1 for cholera vibrios led to the use of the following terms, nonagglutinating vibrio (NAG) or noncholera vibrio (NCV) for vibrios having the same biochemical characters as cholera vibrios, but not possessing the O1 antigen. In 1965 Smith and Goodner reported on the presence of 197 different serotypes but did not give information regarding the identification of species or the nature of the antigens used in their system. In 1970 Sakazaki et al. published a scheme of O typing Vibrio cholerae recognizing 39 O groups. They followed the nomenclature of Gardner and Venkatraman (1935) in designating cholera vibrios as O1 as had Smith and Goodner (1965). Some of the original Gardner and Venkatraman (1935) strains were still available and were included in their scheme. The relationship of some strains of V. cholerae included in the different schemes is given in Table 1. In 1977 Shimada and

83

Table 1. V. cholerae Non-O1 Type According to Scheme

Sakazaki et al. Groups 1-60		Gardner and Venkatraman Subgroups I-VI		Smith Serotypes 1-349 (72)
1	=	I	=	1
2	=	III	=	17
3	=	V	=	62
4	=	VI	=	20
5	=	--	=	12a
6	=	--	=	14
7	=	II	=	13

[a]Unconfirmed.

Sakazaki added a further 21 O groups to their scheme to give 60 O groups. In 1979 Harry Smith published a serotyping scheme recognizing now only 72 serotypes; he did not number his types sequentially but did retain the designation O1 for cholera vibrios. In 1978 Sakazaki added types 61-75 to his scheme; in 1980 types 76-83 were added (Sakazaki, personal communication). These types were mainly derived from Smith types (Smith 1979) and designated as provisional serotypes.

Interest in non-O1 V. cholerae has been stimulated by their potential pathogenicity for man (Blake et al. 1980) and by ecological surveys (Kaper et al. 1979). Several papers (Sakazaki and Shimada 1977; Nacescu and Ciufecu 1978; Szita et al. 1979; Smith 1979) have reported on the incidence of different serotypes; most workers have reported on the high incidence of Sakazaki O serotypes 5, 2, 7, and 37. These types also predominate in our own series of human isolates. The number of isolates of non-O1 V. cholerae in the United Kingdom for 1980 from cases of human diarrheal disease was 40; in 1979 the number was 32, and 1978, 12.

The specificity of a common H antigen for Vibrio cholerae has been questioned by Bhattacharyya (1975) and Shinoda et al. (1976). Smith (1974) found no evidence of H antigens. Most bacterial flagella are composed of a basal body, the flagellar hook, and flagellar core or filament (Silvermar and Simon 1977). The polar flagellum of Vibrio cholerae has, in addition, a sheath which encloses the filament (Follett and Gordon 1963). It has been suggested (Glauert et al. 1963) that the sheath is a continuation of the outer cell membrane. However, Hranitzky et al. (1980) suggested that the flagellar sheath of V. cholerae is a protein and is present on the outer membrane, but is not a simple extension of membrane lipopolysaccharide. The demonstration of an H filament or core antigen is difficult and the development of a simple slide agglutination test using phenol to remove the sheath has led to further interest in this field (Sil and Bhattacharyya 1978, Pastoris et al. 1980).

The presence of other common antigens found within the species V. cholerae has been reported by several workers. A common heat-stable R antigen was described by Gardner and Venkatraman in 1935 and Shimada and Sakazaki (1973). The presence of common heat-labile antigens has been noted by Gallut (1965) and White (1940).

MATERIALS AND METHODS

Non-Ol V. cholerae cultures were received from several sources. The main sources of environmental isolates were cultures isolated at Maidstone Public Health Laboratory, England; Hull Public Health Laboratory, England; Lake Charles Regional Laboratory, Louisiana; and the Microbiology Department, University of Maryland. The main sources of human isolates, almost all from patients showing symptoms of gastroenteritis, were Public Health laboratories in England; the Division of Laboratory Services in New Orleans, Louisiana; and the Cholera Research Laboratory, Dacca, Bangladesh.

V. cholerae antisera were raised in rabbits, using heated whole-cell suspensions for O sera, and unheated formalin-killed cells and flagellar suspensions for H sera as immunizing antigens.

The Phenol H Slide Agglutination Method of Sil and Bhattacharyya (1979) was modified for use by suspending the growth from an overnight culture in nutrient agar at 30°C in approximately 1 ml of Formal Phosphate-Buffered Saline (FPBS)--phosphate-buffered saline with 0.3% formalin. This suspension was lightly vortexed and allowed to stand for 20 minutes. Two separate loopfuls of the suspension were placed on a slide; one loopful of 3% Phenol in PBS was added to each suspension, and allowed to stand one minute. One loopful of H serum was then added to the first suspension and one loopful of FPBS to the second suspension. Each suspension was mixed by rocking. The H reaction took up to 2 minutes to develop and appeared finely granular, stringy or floccular; observation with a hand lens is recommended. The controls should remain stable (negative).

A tube H agglutination test was also used. The stock antigen as prepared for slide agglutination was diluted to McFarland Standard No. 5 (approximately 1.5×10^9 organisms/ml). Dilutions of H antisera were prepared in PBS with 0.01% Thiomersalate. Volumes of 0.3 ml of both antigen suspension and serum dilutions were added to glass serology tubes and incubated at 50°C in a water bath for 18 hours. Readings were made using a hand lens, examining both the button of cells and the suspension after gently resuspending the button. True H agglutination appears significantly different from O agglutination in its "stringy, floccular" appearance.

Before O serotyping, all cultures of V. cholerae were examined for viability and purity, and their identity was checked using the biochemical criteria given by Furniss et al. (1978). Strains were subcultured through Craigie tubes before plating on to nutrient agar plates and incubating at 30°C overnight. The growth was removed by means of a sterile swab into 1-2 ml of FPBS. Rugose or rough cultures were subcultured through further Craigie tubes to select smooth colony forms. All cultures were tested for the presence of the common H antigen using the modified Phenol slide test or preferably the tube agglutination method. V. cholerae O1 strains were eliminated by testing all strains with V. cholerae O1 antisera using slide agglutination.

From the stock antigen suspension, a diluted suspension was prepared (approximately 5×10^8 per ml) in 5 ml FPBS. Approximately 2 ml is retained as an unheated suspension (designated UH); the remainder (designated 5F) is removed and heated in a 100°C waterbath for 5 minutes and then cooled to room temperature.

Sera are used in 14 pools, each pool containing between 4-6 sera at dilutions to give good agglutination with their homologous O antigen. The O typing set of antisera used is given in Table 2. The method used is based on a method for serotyping salmonella used by Shipp and Rowe (1980). Volumes of 25 µl are used for both suspension UH and 5F · for separate rows in a U-well microtiter tray. Added to each row are 25 µl volumes of the 14 pools of sera. The sera are dispensed by 25 µl Microdel Reagent Bottles (Dynatech Laboratories) when small numbers of strains are being serotyped or by a Dynadrop MultiReagent Dispenser (Dynatech Laboratories) when large numbers of strains are being serotyped. The trays are gently mixed and incubated at 37°C overnight in a sealed, moist container. Results are read the following day using a hand lens and a mirror to aid observation of agglutination patterns in the wells. Strains are tested with single sera contained in pools which show agglutination. Strains reacting with one serum are reported as that type. Strains which react with more than one serum are investigated by titration of reacting sera and the use of absorbed sera to elucidate the extent of these reactions. Absorbed sera have been found to be required for the following pairs of related O types: 2 and 9, 13 and 29, 65 and 80, 34 and 75.

Biological Activity

Investigations of the biological activity of 75 cultures of non-O1 V. cholerae were performed by Richard Daniel of

Table 2.   Present O Typing Set Used at Maidstone

Sera	Prepared from Cultures
1–39	Supplied and Published, R. Sakazaki (1970)
40–60	Supplied and Published, R. Sakazaki (1977)
6–81, 83[a]	Supplied R. Sakazaki (1978/80)
LEN	Maidstone environmental type
Total	83

[a]Provisional type 82 was excluded from the set as it was found to be identical with type 62.

Surrey University, England, using methods published by Spira et al. (1979) and Daniel (1981).

Electron Microscopy

Formvar-carbon coated copper grids were used for electron microscopy and the grids were examined by A. Porter at the Electron Microscope Unit of the Virus Reference Laboratory, Central Public Health Laboratory, London, England.

RESULTS

O Typing

A total of 1116 cultures of non-O1 V. cholerae strains were serotyped at Maidstone Public Health Laboratory using the methods previously described. A summary of results is given in Tables 3 and 4.

Table 3. Serotyping of Non-Ol V. cholerae Strain (Maidstone)

	Human Isolates	Environmental Isolates	Human and Environmental Isolates
Total	288	828	1116
Not Typeable	50 (17.4%)[a]	293 (35.4%)	343 (30.7%)
Predominating	37 (30)[b]	4 (151)	4 (155)
O Types	5 (20)	34 (31)	34 (39)
	7 (18)	41 (27)	41 (39)
	40 (16)	3 (20)	37 (35)
	2 (15)	6 (20)	7 (32)
	41 (12)	49 (19)	6 (30)
	24 (12)	7 (14)	5 (25)
	6 (10)	62 (12)	2 (23)
	8 (9)	64 (11)	3 (21)
	34 (8)	12 (10)	49 (19)

[a]Percentage of strains not typeable.
[b]Number of strains.

Biological Activity

A total of 75 cultures of non-Ol V. cholerae were sero-typed and their biological activity evaluated by Richard Daniel of Surrey University, England (Daniel 1981). Represented were 25 different O types. More than one strain was found within eight different O types and of these types the following showed differences of biological activity.

Table 4. Serotyping of Human Isolates By Year

Year	Number	Different Types	Not Typeable	Predominating Types[a]
1973	12	8	2	5, 37
1974	3	2	1	
1975	7	6	0	24
1976	15	8	1	7, 19, 2
1977	16	8	3	5, 6
1978	12	8	2	2, 8
1979	33	18	8	5, 7, 34, 37
1980	40	20	7	2, 8, 24, 34, 37
	138		24 (17.4%)	

[a]Incidence of predominating types: 5 (12), 7 (11), 24 (11), 2 (9), 34 (8), 40 (8), 37 (6), 8 (6).

H Antigens

All strains of V. cholerae examined were agglutinated by V. cholerae anti-H sera using either the modified phenol slide or tube method. Some strains required subculture through Craigie tubes to select highly motile cells before the H agglutination test was positive.

The V. cholerae anti-H sera produced from both whole cells and flagellar preparations agglutinated V. cholerae suspensions of various O types to high titres (1:10,000). These sera did contain homologous O agglutinins at lower titres which could be removed by absorption with O homologous heated suspensions without removing H agglutinins. The H sera also agglutinated unheated suspensions of V. metschnikovii (1:3200), V. fluvialis (1:3200), and V. anguillarum (1:100) but did not agglutinate unheated suspensions of V. parahaemolyticus or V. alginolyticus. The

Table 5.   Biological Activity of Non-O1 V. cholerae Types

Numbers	Serotype	Cholera-like Toxin	Enteritis Activity	Inactivity
6	5	2	3	1
4	12	0	3	1
2	26	1	1	0
18	37	11	7	0
2	63	1	1	0
2	81	1	1	0

V. cholerae anti-H sera could be made species-specific for V. cholerae by absorption with V. metschnikovii and V. fluvialis suspensions.

Heating Experiments with
V. cholerae antigens

The results of heating experiments with suspensions of Vibrio cholerae demonstrated differences in the heat stability of the O antigens, as detected by agglutination techniques. Three patterns were found after heating at 100°C for 5 minutes: thermostable, themolabile, and thermoenhanced agglutination. These results were not serotype-related. Where the O antigen suspension appeared to have lost agglutinability after heat treatment, it was still capable of absorbing the homologous O antibody. Prolonged heating at 100°C allowed the detection of the nonspecific R antigen. The common H antigen of V. cholerae was destroyed after heating at 100°C. Suspending cultures in FPBS retarded the production of the R antigen and allowed detection of specific O antigens and the common H antigen.

Immobilization by Antisera

Immobilization experiments using V. cholerae H sera showed no immobilization in liquid or semi-solid media that could be attributed to a common anti-H or flagella component in the sera used. Immobilization that occurred appeared to be due to homologous O antigen-antibody reaction.

Electron Microscopy

Electron microscopy demonstrated sheathed polar single flagella in the cultures of V. cholerae examined. Examination of a preparation of V. cholerae O45 showed the presence of a partially detached structure resembling a microcapsule.

DISCUSSION

The results of O typing strains of non-O1 V. cholerae during this study demonstrated the presence of 64 different O types. The percentage of typeable cultures was 70%-- within the human isolate collection, 82% but only 65% of the environmental collection were typeable.

The predominating types found within the human isolate collection were O types 37, 5, 7, 40, and 2. These findings were similar to other workers' findings (Sakazaki and Shimada 1977; Nacescu and Ciufecu 1978; Szita et al. 1979; Smith 1979) as shown in Table 6.

O Type 5 was, in retrospect, responsible for an outbreak of diarrheal disease in Czechoslovakia in 1965 (Aldova et al. 1968) and type 37 for a large outbreak in the Sudan in 1968 (Kamal and Zinnaka 1971), probably due to fecal contamination of water. These conclusions were reached after the examination of strains supplied from other workers and from the reexamination of strains in the Maidstone Vibrio Collection which were deposited from these two sources. Both types 5 and 37 from these outbreaks produced a cholera-like toxin. However, other strains of

Table 6. Predominating Types of Non-O1 <u>V. cholerae</u>

Typing Done by	Total	Predominating Types
Sakazaki (1977)	1073	5, 3, 2, 6, 37, 40
Nacescu (1978)	30	5, 39, 2
Szita[a] (1979)	182	10, 6, 34, 11, 21, 30
Smith[a] (1979)	2608	5, 7, 37, 6, 18, 40
Maidstone Human	288	37, 5, 7, 40, 2, 41
Maidstone Environmental	828	4, 34, 41, 3, 6, 49

[a]Smith System used in the publications; given in the table as Sakazaki equivalent.

type 5 from Bangladesh did not produce a cholera-like toxin nor did some type 37 strains from Bangladesh. Eight strains of type 37 isolated in Bangladesh in 1977/78 produced a cholera-like toxin but were sucrose-negative, compared with the strains from the Sudan outbreak (Kamal and Zinnaka 1971) which were sucrose-positive. Both Davis et al. (1981) and Furniss et al. (1978) have suggested that sucrose-negative strains are distinguishable from sucrose-positive using additional tests such as Voges-Proskauer and starch hydrolysis. Davis et al. (1981) have suggested the species name <u>Vibrio mimicus</u> for these vibrios on the basis of only 30-50% DNA-relatedness to <u>Vibrio cholerae</u>. On this basis, the strains isolated from the Sudan outbreak and the Bangladesh strains are distinguishable.

There appeared to be no clear-cut relationship between serotype and toxin production as toxigenic and nontoxigenic strains are found within the same serotype. Strains within the same serotype may be distinguished by toxin testing and biochemical tests.

In addition to the epidemiological information on O types 5 and 37, there was epidemiological information linking seven isolates of O type 64 from Algeria, some evidence linking five environmental isolates of O type 41 with five isolations of this type with human diarrheal disease in Louisiana. O type 24 was high in our series of isolates from patients returning to the United Kingdom after holiday in Tunisia. In general amongst human isolates without strong epidemiological links, a variety of O serotypes were found; in one incident with a strong epidemiological link, two patients excreted three different O types.

The results of O typing strains of V. cholerae isolated from the environment showed O4 as the predominating type. The majority of the isolates were from the River Humber estuary in the Hull area in England. V. cholerae O4 has been isolated by the Hull Public Health Laboratory from the River Humber since 1979. Among human isolates, O4 strains are low in incidence. The predominating types among human isolates, O37 and O5, are low in incidence among environmental isolates. It is not possible to make valid comparisons between the human and environmental isolates as, apart from some isolates from Louisiana, the geographical origin of the collections are significantly different.

The results of heating suspensions of V. cholerae at 100°C demonstrated three patterns of stability of the suspensions when subsequently tested for O agglutination. There were marked reductions in heated suspensions' ability to be agglutinated by homologous O antisera compared with unheated suspensions (thermolabile), no reduction after 5 minutes heating suspensions at 100°C (thermostable), and an increase in agglutination after heating (thermoenhanced). These patterns appeared to be strain-dependent and were not related to serotype. The results of the heating experiments appear to be similar if not identical to the phenomenon of thermovariable inhibition of agglutination (TIA) in Pseudomonas aeruginosa described in a series of papers by Muller (Muller et al. 1973a; Muller et al. 1973b; Muller et al. 1973c; Muller et al. 1976a; Muller et al. 1976b) who concluded that a glyco-proteinaceous complex was formed during heating of suspensions of P. aeruginosa. This complex was inhibitory to O agglutination by obscuring the LPS sites in the outer cell membrane. Further details of this topic will be described by Donovan (1983).

Sera with high anti-H agglutinating titers were raised using both whole cell and flagella suspensions as immunizing agents. The H sera can be made species-specific for V. cholerae H antigen by absorption to remove type-specific anti-O and anti-H agglutinins which reacted with V. metschnikovii, V. fluvialis, and V. anguillarum. In this study modifying Sil and Bhattacharyya's (1979) slide agglutination method produced improved results: fewer strains showed autoagglutination. The tube agglutination method described gave reproducible results, proved useful in testing large numbers of isolates, gave a quantitative result, and would be the recommended method from this study. Despite lack of agreement on the existence (Smith 1974) and specificity (Bhattacharyya 1975; Shinoda et al. 1976) of the H antigen in Vibrio cholerae, which are probably due to significant differences in techniques used by the various workers, it would appear that V. cholerae anti-H sera could be of value in the identification of the species if sufficient detail is applied to the test conditions used.

Immobilization experiments with anti-H sera using two different techniques could not demonstrate immobilization due to anti-H sera. Immobilization occurred with sera containing a homologous O agglutinin, a finding in agreement with Bhattacharyya (1975) who found V. cholerae refractive to immobilization by H sera. The validity of the apparent immobilization by homologous O sera must be questioned in view of the suggestion of Hranitzky et al. (1980) that the flagella sheath is a protein and not a simple extension of the membrane lipopolysaccharide. Immobilization by homologous O sera may be due to agglutination of the cells and, therefore, a restriction of growth or motility rather than attachment to the flagellum. The presence of sheathed flagella may prevent specific attachment of anti-H sera to the flagellum core as it is known that antisera do not agglutinate suspensions of vibrios with an intact sheathed flagellum and only show agglutination with treated suspensions (Bhattacharyya 1975).

Electron microscopy confirmed the presence of single polar, mainly sheathed flagellum of V. cholerae (Follett and Gordon 1963). Some strains showed the presence of relatively more unsheathed flagella than other strains, and suspensions of these strains showed quicker reactions in H agglutination tests. H agglutination could be demonstrated without the addition of phenol (Sil and Bhattacharyya 1979); whereas other strains examined required treatment with phenol to remove the flagellum sheath to give H agglutination by a slide agglutination method. The presence of a partially detached structure, probably an envelope or microcapsule, was seen with strain 3396 (V. cholerae O45). This strain also showed thermaloenhanced O agglutination, which could be similar to the masking of O antigens with K antigens as found in Escherichia coli (Deb and Harry 1977).

CONCLUSIONS

O serotyping of V. cholerae offers a typing method which is discriminating and should be of value in distinguishing different sources of V. cholerae. If O serotyping of V. cholerae is to be used for further environmental studies it would be of value to increase the type-ability rate by adding additional types, but it would be prudent to await the final conclusions of the comparison of the Sakazaki et al. (1970) and Smith (1979) systems before attempting this.

ACKNOWLEDGMENTS

I would like to thank Dr. A.L. Furniss for his guidance and encouragement and Dr. R. Sakazaki for supplying the standard O antigen cultures and other help. To Dr. R. Daniel, I am grateful for collaborating on the study of the relationship of O types and their biological activity. I am also grateful to Mr. A.A. Porter for his help and guidance with the electron microscopy.

REFERENCES

Aldova, E., K. Laznickova, E. Stepankova, and J. Lietava. 1968. Isolation of non-agglutinable vibrios from an enteritis outbreak in Czechoslovakia. Infect. Dis. 118:25-31.

Bhattacharyya, F. 1975. Vibrio cholerae flagellar antigens; a serodiagnostic test, functional implications of H-reactivity and taxonomic importance of cross-reactions within the Vibrio genus. Med. Microbiol. Immun. 162:29-41.

Blake, P., R.E. Weaver, and D. Hollis. 1980. Diseases of humans (other than cholera) caused by vibrios. Ann. Rev. Microbiol. 341-367.

Daniel, R.R. 1981. The taxonomy and pathogenicity of human diarrhoeagenic vibrios. Ph.D. thesis, University of Surrey.

Davis, B.R., G.R. Fanning, J.M. Madden, A.G. Steigerwalt, H.B. Bradford, Jr., H.L. Smith, Jr., and D.J. Brenner. 1981. Characterization of biochemically atypical strains of Vibrio cholerae and designation of a new pathogenic species Vibrio mimicus, J. Clin. Microbiol. 14:631-639.

Deb, J.R., and E.G. Harry. 1977. Evaluation of methods for the determination of O and K antigens of an 02:K1(L) strain of Escherichia coli. J. Med. Microbiol. 10:77-85.

Donovan, T.J. 1983. Thermovariable inhibition of agglutination reactions with Vibrio cholerae. In press.

Follett, E.A.C., and J. Gordon. 1963. An electron microscopy study of vibrio flagella. J. Gen. Microbiol. 32:235-239.

Gallut, J. 1965. Antigenic structure of vibrios. Pages 235-243 in Proc. Cholera Research Symposium Honolulu, Hawaii. U.S. Government Printing Office, Washington, D.C.

Gardner, A.D., and K.V. Venkatraman. 1935. The antigens of the cholera group of vibrios. J. Hyg. 35:262-282.

Glauert, M., D. Kerridge, and R.W. Horne. 1963. The fine structure and mode of attachment of the sheathed flagellum of Vibrio metschnikovii. J. Cell. Biol. 18:327-336.

Hranitzky, K.W., A. Mulholland, A.D. Larson, E.R. Eubanks, and L.T. Hart. 1980. Characterization of a flagellar sheath protein of Vibrio cholerae. Infect. Immun. 27:597-603.

Kamal, A.M., and Y. Zinnaka. 1971. Outbreak of gastroenteritis by non-agglutinable (NAG) vibrios in the Republic of the Sudan. Egyptian Public Health Assoc. 46:125-173.

Kaper, J., H. Lockman, R.R. Colwell, and S.W. Joseph. 1979. Ecology, serology and enterotoxin production of Vibrio cholerae in Chesapeake Bay. Appl. Environ. Microbiol. 37:91-103.

Keilich, G., R. Brossmer, H. Muller, H. Pech, W.W. Franke, and H. Spring. 1976. Release by agitation of constituents from cell walls of Pseudomonas aeruginosa. II. Communication: Biochemistry of released components. Zentralbl. Bakteriol. Parasitenkd. Infektionskr. Hyg. Abt. 1 Orig. 234:317-326.

Lowry, O.H., N.H. Rosebrough, A.L. Farr, and R.J. Randall. 1951. Chemical analysis of microbial cells. J. Biol. Chem. 193:265-275.

Muller, H., Kleinmailer, and H. Pech. 1973a. Serological examinations for the envelope structure of Pseudomonas aeruginosa. I. Communication. Zentralbl. Bakteriol. Parasitenkd. Infektionskr. Hyg. Abt. 1 Orig. 225:487-503.

Muller, H., Kleinmailer, and H. Pech. 1973b. Serological examinations for the envelope structure of Pseudomonas aeruginosa. II. Communication. Zentralbl. Bakteriol. Parasitenkd. Infektionskr. Hyg. Abt. 1 Orig. 225:504-517.

Muller H., Kleinmailer, and H. Pech. 1973c. Serological examinations for the envelope structure of Pseudomonas aeruginosa. III. Communication. Zentralbl. Bakteriol. Parasitenkd. Infektionskr. Hyg. Abt. 1 Orig. 225:518-527.

Muller, H., H. Pech, G. Keilich, R. Brossmer, W.W. Franke, and H. Spring. 1976a. Release by agitation of constituents from cell walls of Pseudomonas aeruginosa. I. Communication: Serology. Zentralbl. Bakteriol. Parasitenkd. Infektionskr. Hyg. Abt. 1 Orig. 234:305-316.

Muller, H., H. Spring, W.W. Franke, H. Pech, G. Keilich, and R. Brossmer. 1976b. Release by agitation of constituents from cell walls of Pseudomonas aeruginosa. III. Communication: Electron microscopy. Zentralbl. Bakteriol. Parasitenkd. Infektionskr. Hyg. Abt. 1 Orig. 234:327-345.

Nacescu, N., and C. Ciufecu. 1978. Serotypes of NAG vibrios isolated from clinical and environmental sources. Zentralbl. Bakteriol. Parasitenkd. Infektionskr. Hyg. Abt. 1 Orig. 240:334-338.

Pastoris, M., Castellani, F. Bhattacharyya, and J. Sil. 1980. Evaluation of the phenol-induced flagellar agglutination test for the identification of the cholera group of vibrios. J. Med. Microbiol. 13:363-367.

Sakazaki, R., K. Tamura, C.Z. Gomez, and R. Sen. 1970. Serological studies on the cholera group of vibrios. Jap. J. Med. Sci. Biol. 23:13-20.

Sakazaki, R., and T. Shimada. 1977. Serovars of Vibrio cholerae identified during 1970-1975. Jap. J. Med. Sci. Biol. 30:279-282.

Shimada, T., and R. Sakazaki. 1977. Additional serovars and inter-O antigenic relationships of Vibrio cholerae. Jap. J. Med. Sci. Biol. 30:275-277.

Shimada, T., and R. Sakazaki. 1973. R antigens of Vibrio cholerae. Jap. J. Med. Sci. Biol. 26:155-160.

Shinoda, S., R. Kariyama, M. Ogawa, Y. Takeda, and T. Miwatani. 1976. Flagellar antigens of various species of the genus Vibrio and related genera. Int. J. System. Bact. 26:97-101.

Shipp, C.R., and B. Rowe. 1980. A mechanized micro-technique for salmonella serotyping. J. Clin. Pathol. 33:595-597.

Sil, J., and F. Bhattacharyya. 1979. A rapid test for the identification of all serotypes of Vibrio cholerae (including "non-agglutinating" vibrios). J. Med. Microbiol. 19:63-70.

Silvermar, M., and M.I. Simon. 1977. Bacterial flagella. Ann. Rev. Microbiol. 31:397-419.

Smith, H.L., Jr., and K. Goodner. 1965. On the classification of vibrio. Pages 4-8 in Proc. Cholera Research Symposium Honolulu, Hawaii, 1965. U.S. Government Printing Office, Washington, D.C.

Smith, H.L., Jr. 1979. Serotyping of non-cholera vibrios. J. Clin. Microbiol. 10:85-90.

Smith, H.L., Jr. 1974. Antibody responses in rabbits to injections of whole cell flagella, flagellin preparation of cholera and non-cholera vibrios. Appl. Microbiol. 27:375-378.

Spira, W.M., R.R. Daniel, Q.S. Ahmed, A. Huq, A. Yusuf, and D.A. Sack. 1979. Clinical features and pathogenicity of O group I non-agglutinating Vibrio cholerae and other vibrios isolated from cases of diarrhea in Dacca, Bangladesh. Pages 137-153 in Proc. 14th Joint Cholera Research Conference Karatsu 1978. U.S. Government Printing Office, Washington, D.C.

Szita, J., A. Svidro, H. Smith, E. Czirok, and K. Solt. 1979. Incidence of non-cholera vibrios in Hungary. Acta Microbiologica Academiae Scientuarum Hungaricae 26:71-83.

White, P.B. 1970. A heat-labile somatic protein antigen (HLSP) of vibrios. J. Path. Bacteriol. 50:165.

Chapter 6

PURIFIED H ANTIGENS OF VIBRIO CHOLERAE

A.D. Larson, K.W. Hranitzky, Sharon Norris,
Susan L. Payne, and R.J. Siebeling

Vibrio cholerae has a sheathed flagellum. The flagellar core
has a diameter of 150-170 nm and the sheath a thickness of
75 nm; the total diameter of the flagellum is about 300 nm
(Das and Chatterjee 1966). V. cholerae possess at least
one common H-antigenic determinant (Hranitzky et al. 1980;
Subcommittee on Taxonomy 1972). The flagellar core
protein (Yang et al. 1977) and flagellar sheath protein
(Hranitzky et al. 1980) represent H-antigenic determinants
which have been isolated and characterized. Therefore, we
prepared antiserum against flagellar cores and sheath
protein of V. cholerae O1 Inaba (CA 401) and surveyed
cultures of V. cholerae isolated from the hemolymph and
feces of Louisiana blue crabs (Callinectes sapidus) for the
sheath and core which would react with antisera prepared
against the respective antigens of O1 Inaba. We wished to
determine whether both sheath and core were common
antigens in V. cholerae.
Flagellar cores were purified as described by Yang et
al. (1977) and injected subcutaneously into rabbits at
intervals until significant agglutination titers were obtained.
Antibodies against flagellar sheath were raised as previously
described (Hranitzky et al. 1980). There was no demonstrable cross-reaction between the antisera and the antigens.
Both sheath and core antisera agglutinated Inaba and Ogawa

103

strains of V. cholerae. Thus, agglutination was employed to survey isolates of V. cholerae from blue crabs for the presence of core and sheath antigens which would react with the Inaba antisera.

Tube agglutinations were performed on 200 V. cholerae non-O1 isolates from blue crabs. The agglutinations were performed using cells standardized to 200 Klett units (blue filter). The cells were 18-hours-old and were grown on brain heart infusion slants at 37°C. In 100 x 13 mm serological tubes, 0.5 ml of cells were mixed with 0.5 ml of a 1 to 50 dilution of antiserum. Controls contained saline instead of antiserum. The tubes were incubated for 5 hours at 42°C and overnight at 4°C. Agglutinations were read by patterns formed in the tubes as compared to the buttons in the controls.

All isolates from the blue crab were agglutinated by antiflagellar core antiserum. Flagellar sheath antiserum agglutinated all but 3 of the 200 isolates. Therefore, all 200 isolates possessed the same flagellar core antigen as Inaba and 197 isolates possessed the same sheath antigen. The failure of three isolates (SN) to agglutinate with the sheath antibody could be due to the absence of flagellar sheath or the presence of flagellar sheath composed of protein antigenically distinct from sheath of the vast majority of the isolates.

We investigated the two possibilities on the three isolates not agglutinated by two methods: negative staining and measuring the diameter of the flagellum using an electron microscope and labeling with ferritin-labeled goat anti-rabbit IgG after cells were reacted with rabbit antiserum (Hranitzky et al. 1980). Negative stains of the three showed the presence of a single polar flagellum with a diameter of approximately one-half that of sheathed flagella of isolates which agglutinated with flagellar sheath antiserum. Also, the SN isolates did not show ferritin labeling of flagellum with sheath antibodies, but the flagellum was labeled when flagellar core antibodies were employed. Isolates which showed agglutination with both core and sheath antibodies showed labeling with both kinds of antisera. Therefore, the evidence is that the SN isolates do not possess flagellar sheath.

The SN isolates are motile as indicated by motility medium and by observation of hanging drops. The possession of flagellar sheath must not be required for motility in V. cholerae. The function and importance of the flagellar sheath of V. cholerae is not known. The fact that most motile bacteria do not have flagellar sheath would indicate that sheath has some function other than that associated with motility.

ACKNOWLEDGMENTS

This research was supported by grants from the Louisiana Department of Health and Human Resources and National Oceanic and Atmospheric Administration Office of Sea Grant, Department of Commerce, under Grant NA79AA-D-00128.

REFERENCES

Das, J., and S.N. Chatterjee. 1966. Electron microscopic studies on some ultrastructural aspects of Vibrio cholerae. Indian J. Med. Res. 54:330-338.

Hranitzky. K.W., A. Mulholland, A.D. Larson, E.R. Eubanks, and L.T. Hart. 1980. Characterization of a flagellar sheath protein of Vibrio cholerae. Infect. Immun. 27:597-603.

Subcommittee on Taxonomy of Vibrios. 1972. Report (1966-1970) of the Subcommittee on Taxonomy of Vibrios to the International Committee on Nomemclature of Bacteria. Int. J. Syst. Bacteriol. 22:123.

Yang, Gene C.H., G.D. Schrank, and B.A. Freeman. 1977. Purification of flagellar core Vibrio cholerae. J. Bacteriol. 129:1121-1128.

Pathogenesis

Chapter 7

PATHOGENESIS OF ENTERIC INFECTIONS CAUSED BY VIBRIO

Myron M. Levine, Robert Black, and Mary Lou Clements

Cholera, a diarrheal infection due to noninvasive enterotoxin-producing Vibrio cholerae O1, can occur in explosive outbreaks and can lead to rapid dehydration and death if untreated. Until recently most physicians and microbiologists in the United States viewed cholera as an exotic tropical infection of little practical importance. However, with the recent recognition that there exists an endemic focus of cholera along the coast of the Gulf of Mexico in Texas and Louisiana (Blake et al. 1980; Levine 1980; Weissman et al. 1975), we are compelled to gain familiarity with this disease and its causative agent. Accordingly, the ensuing paragraphs will review current knowledge on the pathogenesis of cholera infection.

The pathogenesis of cholera infection can be regarded as a series of skirmishes between the invading pathogens armed with an array of virulence properties and the human host who possesses an armamentarium of nonspecific as well as specific defense mechanisms.

Inoculum Size, Route, and Role of Gastric Acid

Pathogenic V. cholerae O1 gains access to the human host through ingestion of contaminated food or water. The first (and a very important) nonspecific defense mechanism that the vibrios encounter is gastric acid. Volunteer studies have shown that neither clinical cholera nor asymptomatic infection occurs when fasting, chlorhydric individuals ingest 10^6 or more pathogenic vibrios without food or buffer (Table 1) (Cash et al. 1974; Levine et al. 1981). However, when 10^6 vibrios are consumed with food or NaHCO$_3$ (which serves to buffer gastric acid), clinical cholera occurs in 80-100% of volunteers and the resultant purging may be copious (Table 1) (Cash et al. 1974; Levine et al. 1981).

Volunteer studies have also clearly demonstrated that there exists an inverse relationship between basal levels of gastric acid and severity of cholera diarrhea (Nalin et al. 1978). This relationship is also encountered in field studies. For example, approximately 20-25% of the hospitalized (i.e. severe) cases of cholera during epidemics in Israel (Gitelson 1971) and Italy (Schiraldi et al. 1974) occurred in patients who were hypochlorhydric because of partial gastrectomy or chronic ingestion of antacids. Similarly, the index cases in Guam (Merson et al. 1977) and Port Lavaca, Texas (Weissman et al. 1974) were hypochlorhydric individuals.

Intensive microbiologic studies in households and in the environment in Bangladesh have suggested that the typical inoculum of V. cholerae O1 ingested in nature is 10^2-10^4 organisms (Spira et al. 1980). Dose response data obtained from challenging volunteers with 10^6, 10^5, 10^4, or 10^3 V. cholerae with NaHCO$_3$ demonstrated that inocula of 10^3 and 10^4 indeed readily caused diarrheal illness in two-thirds of individuals but the illness was milder than in volunteers who ingested higher inocula (Table 1) (Levine et al. 1981).

Host-Parasite Interaction in
the Proximal Small Intestine

If V. cholerae survive transit through the adverse gastric environment, they pass through the pylorus and arrive in the proximal small intestine. It is here in the

Table 1. Response of Volunteers to Ingestion of 10^6 Vibrio *Cholerae* El Tor Inaba N16961 With 2.0 grams of NaHCO$_3$, Food or Water

Vehicle	Clinical Attack Rate	Mean Incubation (hours)	Mean Diarrhea Volume[a] (liters)	Mean No. Loose Stools[a]	Vomiting	Culture
NaHCO$_3$	9/10	25.5	3.2 (0.4-13.1)[b]	12.9 (2-39)	2/10	10/10
Food[c]	6/6	24.1	3.5 (0.2-9.1)	13.8 (2-31)	3/6	6/6
Water (300 ml.)	0/7	--	--	--	0/7	0/7

[a] Per ill volunteer.
[b] ( ) = Range.
[c] Standard meal: 4 oz. of fish, 4 oz. rice, 4 oz. custard, 8 oz. skim milk.

duodenum and jejunum that the critical host-parasite interaction occurs as the vibrios interact with intestinal mucosa in a series of events that can culminate in diarrhea.

The proximal small intestine of the healthy individual manifests several defenses against enteric pathogens including: (1) a mucus layer which represents a physical barrier that separates bacteria from mucosal enterocytes; (2) peristalsis which serves to continually clear organisms from the small intestine into the colon; (3) certain normal intestinal flora, particularly lactobacilli, which are indigenous to the proximal small intestine (Drasar and Hill 1974) and are inhibitory to enteric pathogens (Foster 1980; Johnson and Calia 1979).

Overcoming the Mucus Barrier

V. cholerae has multiple virulence properties that allow it to overcome the protective mucus barrier and reach the mucosal enterocytes. Among these virulence properties are chemotaxis, motility, and production of mucinase and other proteolytic enzymes. Nonchemotactic mutants of V. cholerae imbed in the mucus layer like inert particles (Freter et al. 1981a; Freter and O'Brien 1981; Freter et al. 1981b). V. cholerae that show normal chemotaxis and motility rapidly enter and pass through the mucus layer to reach the mucosal surface (Freter et al. 1981a; Freter and O'Brien 1981; Freter et al. 1981b). It has been found that amino acids invoke a chemotactic response in V. cholerae as do certain monosaccharides to a lesser extent (Freter et al. 1981a; Freter and O'Brien 1981). The most potent chemotactic response is elicited by pepsin-digested mucosal scrapings.

Adhesion to Mucosa

Once V. cholerae successfully penetrate the mucus layer and reach the enterocytes of the intestinal mucosa, particularly those in the villus crypts, they must adhere to these cells. Several adhesive mechanisms have been reported. Jones, Abrams, and Freter (1976) showed that broth-grown

V. cholerae adhered to isolated brush border membranes and hemagglutinated human group O but not chicken erythrocytes. Adhesion and hemagglutination required the presence of Ca++ and were inhibited by L-fucose (Jones and Freter 1976). V. cholerae grown on solid agar did not manifest adhesion to brush borders or hemagglutination; nonmotile mutants were also poorly adhesive.

Finkelstein and coworkers (1977; 1982) have described hemagglutinins produced by V. cholerae that react with chicken erythrocytes. They described a cell-associated, mannose-sensitive hemagglutinin that reacts with both human and chicken erythrocytes and is characteristic of vibrios of the El Tor biotype. These investigators confirmed the existence of an L-fucose sensitive hemagglutinin in log phase cultures of classical biotype V. cholerae. A third hemagglutinin that they noted was not cell-associated but was found in supernatants of stationary phase cultures. This soluble hemagglutinin reacts with only certain chicken erythrocytes and poorly with human erythrocytes, and the reaction is unaffected by D-mannose or L-fucose. This substance which has been purified has been called "cholera lectin" by these workers. The purified material consists of subunits of 31,000 molecular weight (MW) which tend to undergo self-aggregation. Antibody prepared against cholera lectin inhibited attachment of V. cholerae.

It is of interest to note that both studies in endemic areas and in volunteers have shown that severe cholera occurs more commonly in persons of blood group O than in others (Levine et al. 1979). It is thus possible that such persons possess "optimal" mucosal receptors for V. cholerae since the blood group glycoproteins are secreted onto the mucosal surface of the intestine. It is also interesting to note that Bengal, the ancestral endemic home of cholera, has the lowest prevalence of blood group O in the world (Bodmer and Cavalli-Sforza 1976).

Cholera Enterotoxin

V. cholerae adheres to mucosal enterocytes and produces an enterotoxin which has a molecular weight of

83,000. It consists of two distinct types of subunits. Subunit A (MW 28,000) is noncovalently attached to five B subunits (each of 11,000 MW). The B subunits bind the toxin to GM_1 ganglioside receptors on the enterocytes which then allows the enzymatically-active (ADP-ribosylating) A subunit to enter the cells and activate intracellular adenylate cyclase resulting in an accumulation of cyclic AMP. The intracellular biochemical events leading to activation of adenylate cyclase have been well-described (Gill 1977).

The intracellular accumulation of cyclic AMP leads to effects on two active ion transport processes: (1) coupled absorption of NaCl is inhibited in villus cells; and (2) active Cl^- secretion is stimulated. The end result of these changes is an outright secretion by villus crypt cells and decreased absorption by villus tip cells (Field 1979); the clinical consequence is the occurrence of watery diarrhea.

In the course of volunteer studies to identify suitable El Tor Ogawa and Inaba challenge strains to use in studies of vaccine efficacy we had an opportunity to gain further insights on the complexity of the pathogenesis of V. cholerae infection in man. Two El Tor Inaba strains, N16961 and P27459, isolated from Bangaldeshi patients with cholera gravis, were fed to volunteers (Levine et al. 1981). Although strain N16961 in vitro produced 30-fold more toxin than strain P27459, the clinical attack rates and total volumes of diarrhea in volunteers given equivalent inocula were indistinguishable (Table 2). These observations demonstrate that the quantity of toxin produced in vitro is not by itself a predictor of virulence of a toxigenic V. cholerae strain.

Two El Tor Ogawa strains--N15870 and N16117--isolated from Bengali patients with cholera gravis were fed to volunteers in doses of 10^5 or 10^6 organisms with $NaHCO_3$ (Table 3). Although both strains were toxigenic in vitro, strain N16117 infected but did not induce clinical diarrhea. Strain N15870 on two different occasions induced a very atypical clinical picture manifested by nausea, vomiting, severe abdominal cramps, and mild or no diarrhea. One wonders what virulence properties were lacking in strain N16117 such that it caused only asymptomatic infection, and

Table 2. Clinical, Bacteriologic and Serologic Response of Healthy Volunteers to Varying Doses of Vibrio cholerae El Tor Inaba Strains that Produce Moderate (N16961) or Low (P27459) Levels of Cholera Toxin In Vitro

Strain and Inoculum	Clinical Attack Rate[a]	Mean Incubation (Hours)	Mean Diarrheal Stool Volume[b] (Liters)	Mean No. Loose Stools[b]	Vomiting	Fever	Positive Stool Culture	Significant Rise in Serum Antibody	
								Antitoxin	Vibriocidal
N16961									
10^6	9/10	25.5	3.2 (0.4-13.1)[c]	12.9 (2-39)	2/10	4/10	10/10	9/10	9/10
10^5	3/5	18	3.1 (0.4-3.7)	15 (9-21)	0/5	0/5	4/5	3/5	5/5
10^4	4/5	36.5	1.1 (0.6-1.5)	6.5 (4-10)	0/5	0/5	4/5	4/5	5/5
10^3	4/6	33.3	0.9 (0.4-1.9)	5.8	0/6	0/6	6/6	6/6	5/6
P27459									
10^6	9/11	37.5	1.9 (0.3-7.6)	11.2 (3-33)	5/11	1/11	10/11	8/11	10/11
10^5	3/5	27.75	4.9 (1.6-9.9)	12.3 (8-18)	0/5	0/5	5/5	5/5	5/5

[a] No. ill/No. volunteers challenged.

[b] Per ill volunteer.

[c] ( ) = Range.

Table 3. Clinical, Bacteriologic and Serologic Response of Healthy Volunteers to Varying Doses of Two Vibrio cholerae El Tor Ogawa Strains

Strain and Inoculum	Clinical Attack Rate[a]	Mean Diarrheal Stool[b] Volume (Liters)	Mean No. Loose[b] Stools	Vomiting	Fever	Moderate or Severe Abdominal Cramps	Positive Stool Culture	Significant Rise in Serum Antibody	
								Antitoxin	Vibriocidal
Ogawa N16117									
10^5	0/4	--	--	--	--	--	2/4	3/4	3/4
10^6	0/5	--	--	--	--	--	1/5	2/5	4/5
Ogawa N15870									
10^5	3/5	0.80 (0.3-1.4)[c]	6 (5-8)	2/15	1/5	2/5	4/5	4/5	4/5
10^5	8/8	1.9 (0.17-5.3)	9 (1-24)	4/8	1/8	4/8	8/8	7/8	8/8

[a] No. ill/No. volunteers challenged.

[b] Per ill volunteer.

[c] ( ) = Range.

what virulence properties were produced by strain N15870 such that it repeatably caused atypical clinical illness. Further observations in this area were made when two nonenterotoxigenic V. cholerae El Tor Ogawa isolates were fed to volunteers with $NaHCO_3$ in doses of 10^6 or 10^8 organisms. These strains failed to cause clinical illness; few recipients had positive coprocultures, and vibriocidal antibody responses were uncommon and meager. Thus, at least these two nonenterotoxigenic environmental V. cholerae strains appeared to lack factors necessary for colonization of the human intestine (Levine et al. 1982).

Immune Responses

More than 90% of individuals infected with V. cholerae manifest rises in serum vibriocidal and antitoxic antibodies (Clements et al. 1982; Levine et al. 1981). Both antibodies are very useful in serodiagnosis of cholera infection, particularly in the United States where symptomatic infections with other enterotoxigenic bacteria are rare. While vibriocidal antibody titers fall rapidly within weeks to approach baseline levels (Clements et al. 1982), IgG antitoxin levels measured by enzyme-linked immunosorbent assay (ELISA) remain elevated for at least two years (Levine et al. 1981). Intestinal SIgA antibody levels also rise in response to infection and are probably the operative mediators of protective immunity. Such immune responses are more difficult to measure, however (Levine et al. 1981).

SUMMARY

The diarrheal disease cholera results from infection of susceptible human hosts with enterotoxigenic Vibrio cholerae, serotype O1. The extent of infection and clinical illness is a consequence of a series of interactions between the virulence properties of the pathogen and defense mechanisms of the human host. Among the bacterial determinants of the outcome of infection are inoculum size, motility, chemotaxis, production of critical enzymes (including mucinase, proteases, and neuraminidase), presence of adhesins, and elaboration of enterotoxin. Arrayed against these properties of V. cholerae are potent nonspecific defenses including gastric acid, gut motility, and intestinal mucus. Immunologically experienced persons manifest both antibacterial and antitoxic antibodies. Known predispositions to severe disease include hypochlorhydria and blood group O.

Inocula as low as 10^3 viable V. cholerae can initiate diarrheal infection in 60% of challenged individuals if the gastric acid barrier can be overcome; illness is mild. Inocula of 10^5 or 10^6 administered with $NaHCO_3$ or food will cause diarrhea in 70-100% of individuals, leading to rice-water purging in some.

The striking serum vibriocidal and antitoxic antibody responses that occur in 90% of infected persons can be used for serodiagnostic and seroepidemiologic purposes. These assays are particularly helpful in the study of cholera along the Gulf Coast of the United States where symptomatic infection with other enterotoxigenic bacteria are rare. Since cholera appears to be endemic in the United States, familiarity with the pathogenesis of the infection and with the etiologic agent is needed.

REFERENCES

Blake, P.A., D.T. Allegra, J.D. Snyder, T.J. Barrett, L. McFarland, C.T. Caraway, J.C. Feeley, J.P. Craig, J.V. Lee, J.D. Puhr, and R.A. Feldman. 1980. Cholera--a possible endemic focus in the United States. N. Engl. J. Med. 302:305-309.

Bodmer, W.F., and L.L. Cavalii-Sforza. 1976. Evolution, human welfare and society. Pages 562-604 in Genetics, evolution and man. W.H. Freeman, New York.

Cash, R.A., S.I. Music, J.P. Libonati, M.J. Snyder, R.P. Wenzel, and R.B. Hornick. 1974. Response of man to infection with Vibrio cholerae. I. Clinical, serologic and bacteriologic responses to a known inoculum. J. Infect. Dis. 129:45-52.

Clements, M.L., M.M. Levine, C.R. Young, R.E. Black, Y-L. Lim, R.M. Robins-Browne, and J.P. Craig. 1982. Magnitude, kinetics and duration of vibriocidal antibody responses in North Americans following ingestion of Vibrio cholerae. J. Infect. Dis. In press.

Drasar, B.S., and M.J. Hill. 1974. Human intestinal flora. Academic Press, New York.

Field, M. 1979. Mechanisms of action of cholera and Escherichia coli enterotoxins. Am. J. Clin. Nutr. 32:189-196.

Finkelstein, R.A., M. Arita, J.D. Clements, and E.T. Nelson. 1978. Isolation and purification of an adhesive factor ("cholera lectin") from Vibrio cholerae. Pages 137-151 in Proc. 12th Joint Conference on Cholera, U.S-Japan Cooperative Medical Science Program, Atlanta, GA. (DHEW Publ. No. 79-1590).

Finkelstein, R.A., and L.F. Hanne. 1982. Hemagglutinins (colonization factors?) produced by Vibrio cholerae in Proc. 17th Joint Conference on Cholera, U.S.-Japan Cooperative Medical Science Program, Baltimore, MD.

Foster, T.L., L. Winans, and T.R. Carski. 1980. Evaluation of lactobacillus preparations on enterotoxigenic E. coli-induced rabbit ileal loop reactions. Am. J. Gastroenterol. 73:238-243.

Freter, R., B. Allweiss, P.C.M. O'Brien, S.A. Halstead, and M.S. Macsai. 1981. Role of chemotaxis in the association of motile bacteria with intestinal mucosa: in Vitro studies. Infect. Immun. 34:241-249.

Freter, R., and P.C.M. O'Brien. 1981. Role of chemotaxis in the association of motile bacteria with intestinal mucosa: chemotactic responses of Vibrio cholerae and description of motile nonchemotactic mutants. Infect. Immun. 34:215-221.

Freter, R., P.C.M. O'Brien, and M.S. Macsai. 1981. Role of chemotaxis in the association of motile bacteria with intestinal mucosa: in vivo studies. Infect. Immun. 34:234-240.

Gill, D.M. 1977. Mechanisms of action of cholera toxin. Advances in cyclic nucleotide research 8:85-118.

Gitelson, S. 1971. Gastrectomy, achlorhydria and cholera. Isr. J. Med. Sci. 7:663-667.

Johnson, D.E., and F.M. Calia. 1979. The effect of Lactinex on rabbit ileal loop reactions induced by enterotoxigenic Escherichia coli. Curr. Microbiol. 2:207-210.

Jones, G.W., G.D. Abrams, and R. Freter. 1976. Adhesive properties of Vibrio cholerae: adhesion to isolated rabbit brush border membranes and hemagglutinating activity. Infect. Immun. 14:232-239.

Jones, G.W., and R. Freter. 1976. Adhesive properties of Vibrio cholerae: nature of the interaction with isolated rabbit brush border membranes and human erythrocytes. Infect. Immun. 14:240-245.

Levine, M.M. 1980. Cholera in Louisiana: Old problem, new light. N. Engl. J. Med. 302:345-347.

Levine, M.M., R.E. Black, M.L. Clements, L. Cisneros, D.R. Nalin, and C.R. Young. 1981. Duration of infection-derived immunity to cholera. J. Infect. Dis. 143:818-820.

Levine, M.M., R.E. Black, M.L. Clements, L. Cisneros, A. Saah, D.R. Nalin, D.M. Gill, J.P. Craig, C.R. Young, and P. Ristaino. 1982. Pathogenicity of nonenterotoxinogenic <u>Vibrio</u> <u>cholerae</u> El Tor isolated from sewage water in Brazil. J. Infect. Dis. In press.

Levine, M.M., R.E. Black, M.L. Clements, D.R. Nalin, L. Cisneros, and R.A. Finkelstein. 1982. Volunteer studies in development of vaccines against cholera and enterotoxigenic <u>Escherichia</u> <u>coli</u>: a review <u>in</u> J. Holmgren and T. Holme (eds.). Acute enteric infections in children: new prospects for treatment and prevention. Elsevier, Amsterdam. In press.

Levine, M.M., D.R. Nalin, M.B. Rennels, R.B. Hornick, S. Sotman, G. Van Blerk, T.P. Hughes, and S. O'Donnell. 1979. Genetic susceptibility to cholera. Ann. Human Biol. 6:369-374.

Levine, M.M., C.R. Young, T.P. Hughes, S. O'Donnell, R.E. Black, M.L. Clements, R. Robins-Browne, and Y-L. Lim. 1981. Duration of serum antitoxin response following <u>Vibrio</u> <u>cholerae</u> infection in North Americans: relevance for sero-epidemiology. Am. J. Epidemiol. 114:348-354.

Merson, M.J., W.T. Martin, J.P. Craig, G.K. Morris, P.A. Blake, G.F. Craun, J.C. Feeley, J.C. Camacho, and E.J. Gangarosa. 1977. Cholera on Guam, 1971. Epidemiologic findings and isolation of non-toxinogenic strains. Am. J. Epidemiol. 105:349-361.

Nalin, D.R., R.J. Levine, M.M. Levine, D. Hoover, E. Bergquist, J. McLaughlin, J. Libonati, J. Alam, and R.B. Hornick. 1978. Cholera, non-vibrio cholera and stomach acid. Lancet II:856-859.

Sack, G.H., Jr., N.F. Pierce, K.H. Hennessey, R.C. Mitra, R.B. Sack, and D.N. Guha Mazumder. 1972. Gastric acidity in cholera and noncholera diarrhoea. Bull. W.H.O. 47:31-36.

Schiraldi, O., V. Benvestito, C. DiBari, R. Moschetta, and G. Pastore. 1974. Gastric abnormalities in cholera:

epidemiological and clinical considerations. Bull. W.H.O. 58:731-740.

Spira, W.M., M.U. Khan, Y.A. Saeed, and M.A. Sattar. 1980. Microbiological surveillance of intra-neighborhood El Tor cholera transmission in rural Bangladesh. Bull. W.H.O. 58:731-740.

Weissman, J.B., W.E. DeWitt, J. Thompson, C.N. Mushnick, B.L. Portnoy, J.C. Feeley, and E.J. Gangarosa. 1975. A case of cholera in Texas. Am. J. Epidemiol. 100:487-498.

Chapter 8

AN ASSESSMENT OF NON-O1 VIBRIO CHOLERAE VIRULENCE IN THE Y-1 MOUSE ADRENAL CELL ASSAY

S.W. Joseph, S.T. Donta, D.R. Maneval, J.B. Kaper, R.R. Colwell and W.M. Spira

Non-O1 Vibrio cholerae, previously termed erroneously non-cholera vibrio (NCV) and nonagglutinating vibrio (NAG), is indistinguishable biochemically from O1 V. cholerae.

While interest in this organism has been of long duration in many countries, including Japan, India, the Philippines, the Sudan, Thailand, Malaysia, Australia, Bangladesh, Sweden, and Russia, there has been an increasing awareness in the United States only within the last few years (Hughes et al. 1978). For example, the numbers of isolates submitted to the Centers for Disease Control for confirmation or identification have been increasing since 1972 and have included not only strains from patient fecal specimens, but from tissues and other body fluids as well.

Non-O1 V. cholerae is associated with food-borne outbreaks (primarily overseas), sporadic gastroenteritis (sometimes associated in the U.S. with foreign travel), septicemia, meningitis, middle ear infection, and soft tissue infection. Reports of gastrointestinal infections far out-number those of extra-intestinal infections. Although this may be a reflection of the organism's inability to colonize, penetrate, or invade body tissue, it could also be a case of underreporting because of lack of awareness by clinicians and microbiologists.

While V. cholerae O1 strain-to-strain variation for the production of cholera toxin has been observed (Kaper et al. 1981), it is well accepted that this is the primary mechanism by which both classical and El Tor V. cholerae cause disease ranging from mild to massive diarrheal discharges; to the extent that absence of supportive therapy during outbreaks can lead to shock and high fatality rates.

The mode of action of cholera toxin is quite clear. The toxin is composed of two subunits, A and B. The A subunit is the biologically active component and is composed of two fragments, A_1 and A_2. The B portion is composed of five fragments and is responsible for toxin binding to intestinal cells. The A subunit elevates the activity of membrane bound adenyl cyclase which converts ATP to cAMP. This, in turn, leads to fluid loss with accompanying unbalanced electrolyte secretion from the mucosal cells of the small intestine. And, of course, this conjures up the vision of the massively dehydrated patient in metabolic acidosis lying on the famous Watten cot producing voluminous diarrheal discharge.

The pathogenicity (and/or toxigenicity) of non-O1 V. cholerae is not nearly so well established. Strains isolated from environmental and human sources have been examined in several biological assays in an attempt to characterize the pathogenicity of this organism and assess its virulence capacity.

Table 1 provides a list of some of the efforts which have been made in the past to measure the virulence of human and environmental strains of non-O1 V. cholerae. Gupta and colleagues (1956) reported that so-called "NCV" strains from humans, but not water, caused fluid accumulation (FA) in the rabbit ileal loop assay (RIL). Dutta et al. (1963) tested those environmental strains in infant rabbits, after previous animal passage, and found them to cause diarrhea. Likewise, McIntyre et al. (1965) and Sakazaki et al. (1967) found similar results with human strains. Bhattacharya et al. (1971) reported positive reactions with human strains in RIL after 10X filtrate concentration, but were unable to demonstrate permeability factor (PF).

Zinnaka and Carpenter in 1972 reported that 100% of patient isolates (10/10) produced positive fluid accumulation in RIL, but with lower FA ratio than did El Tor strains. Only two strains were PF-positive. The "NCV" toxin was similar, if not identical, to cholera toxin and was almost completely neutralized by antisera against purified cholera toxin. Ohashi and coworkers (1972) reported similar findings from cases in India, the Philippines, and the Sudan.

Ciznar et al. (1977) partially purified the non-O1 V. cholerae toxin and isolated a fraction which had permeability factor (PF) and hemorrhagic capabilities and proved lethal for mice, but did not produce fluid accumulation in RIL.

Robbins-Browne et al. (1977) reported on a strain which was able to invade rabbit ileal mucosa, but not the guinea pig cornea. The strain was also positive for enterotoxin and PF.

In 1975 Dunaev and coworkers were unable to show enterotoxic activity in RIL with either human or environmental strains. Conversely, Draskovicova and colleagues (1977) found 12 of 16 strains from human diarrhea and 12 of 20 from water to be positive with the RIL assay.

Other environmental studies by Bisgaard et al. (1975, 1978) on 105 strains isolated from ducks showed both fluid accumulation in RIL and a cytotoxic effect on Y-1 adrenal cells. Several environmental strains tested by Weissman et al. (1975) also caused FA in RIL.

Singh and Sanyal (1978) reported a study of 75 strains of non-O1 V. cholerae, including isolates from the feces of healthy humans, drinking and surface waters, sewage, and domestic animal feces. Examination in the RIL revealed 75% of the human strains, 45% of animal strains, and 64% of the water strains were able to produce fluid accumulation in RIL comparable to that produced by V. cholerae 569B. Culture filtrates of these strains produced similar results.

Spira and coworkers reported (1978) their examination of the pathogenicity of O group-1 V. cholerae from diarrheal and non-diarrheal illness and from environmental sources. In their study of diarrheal patients, 35 isolates of non-O1

Table 1. Results of Assays for Non-O1 Vibrio cholerae Enterotoxicity

Source of Isolates	Rabbit Ileal Loop (RIL)	Infant Rabbit	Permeability Factor (PF)	Y-1 Adrenal Cell	References
		Method of Assay			
Human	+				Gupta et al. (1956)
Environment		+			Dutta (1963)
Human		+(3/3)[a]			McIntyre et al. (1965)
Human		+(10/10)			Sakazaki et al. (1967)
Human	±		-		Bhattacharya et al. (1971)
Human	+(10/10)		+(2/10)		Zinnaka and Carpenter (1972)

Source				Reference
Human	+	+(8/41)		Ohashi, et al. (1972)
Human & Environment	-			Dunaev et al. (1975)
Avian	+		Cyto-toxic	Bisgaard et al. (1975, 1978)
Environment	+			Weissman et al. (1975)
Human	+(12/16)			Draskovicova et al. (1977)
Environment	+(12/20)			
Human	+(75%)			Singh and Sanyal (1978)
Environment	+(64%)			
Animal	+(45%)			
Human	+(23/120)	+(21/120)	+(21/120)	Spira et al. (1978)
Environment	+(75%)		Cyto-toxic (88%)	Kaper et al. (1979)

[a]Values in ( ) indicate number positive/number tested or percent positive.

V. cholerae were recovered. Together with strains of other non-O1 V. cholerae from diverse parts of the globe, they were tested for biological activity. Of 72 diarrheal isolates, 17 (24%) produced a cholera-like toxin which was neutralized by antitoxin prepared against cholera toxin, 6 (8%) were nontoxigenic and 49 (68%) produced enteritis without demonstrable CT-like or ST-like toxins. Of the 30 environmental samples tested, 2 (7%) produced CT-like toxin; 18 (60%) were able to cause enteritis, apparently without production of CT-like or ST-like toxins; and 8 (27%) were nontoxigenic. Of 8 strains from patients with nondiarrheal illness, 2 were found to be cholera toxin-like producers.

The majority of Chesapeake Bay strains (76%) studied by Kaper et al. in 1979 produced fluid accumulation in rabbit ileal loops with positive results similar to those noted by Spira et al. (1978). Significant strain-to-strain variation was noted in fluid accumulation ratios. One strain, V-37, produced fluid accumulation ratios equal to those produced by V. cholerae 569B. Other strains were less reactive and almost uniformly cytotoxic for Y-1 adrenal cells.

Those studies on Y-1 cells, as well as the new data presented here, were based on these criteria: no effect (Figure 1a); a "cytotoxic" effect in which cells are rounded, shrunken, granular, and exhibit vacuolization (Figure 1b); an intermediate reaction which is difficult to define as either cytotoxic or cytotonic (Figure 1c); typical enterotoxic or "cytotonic" rounding identical to that produced by V. cholerae 569B (Figure 1d); "cytolytic" where the cells are pyknotic, free-floating and in many instances, completely lysed with only cellular debris visible.

The results of studies which have been accomplished sequentially since the report of biological activity in the Chesapeake Bay non-O1 V. cholerae strains (Kaper et al.) are reported below. In order we have (1) further titrated these strains in the Y-1 assay; (2) attempted to define by blocking experiments, if there is cholera toxin-like activity; (3) attempted to determine by ELISA if cholera toxin-like material is present in culture filtrates; (4) checked representative strains to determine if the enterotoxic substance

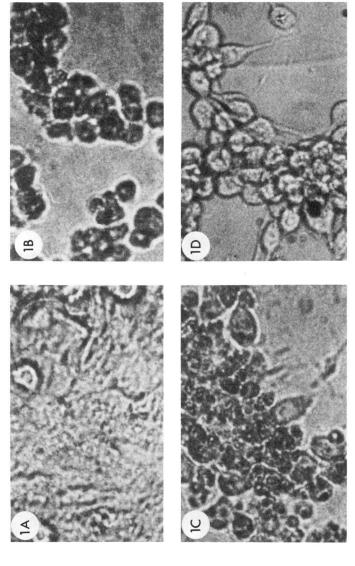

Figure 1. Monolayered Y-1 mouse adrenal cells. (A) Normal appearance of Y-1 monolayer; (B) "cytotoxic" effect in which cells are rounded, shrunken, granular and exhibit vacuolization; (C) an intermediate reaction which contains both types of cellular responses to bacterial toxin described in 1B and 1D; (D) enterotoxic or "cytotonic" effect caused by rounding of cells; typical of reaction caused by V. cholerae 569B or purified choleragen.

is able to stimulate steroidogenesis and increased adenyl cyclase activity in Y-1 adrenal cells.

Y-1 Adrenal Cell Assay

Y-1 tissue culture assays were performed as described previously (Maneval et al. 1980). Briefly, V. cholerae strains were grown at 30°C with shaking (150 rpm) for 18-24 hours in syncase broth (Finkelstein et al. 1966) or syncase plus 1% w/v $(NH_4)_2SO_4$. After centrifugation, 50 μl aliquots of undiluted or serial twofold dilutions of broth supernatant, cholera toxin (CT), or appropriate controls were incubated for 5 minutes at 37°C with subconfluent Y-1 cells in individual wells of microtitration plates. After washing and replacement of medium, Y-1 cell cultures were scored for percentage of cells/wells exhibiting cytotoxic (CX) or typical cholera toxin-like (CT-like) morphologies. Viability of Y-1 cultures with CT-like responses was determined by trypan blue dye exclusion (Tolnai 1975). Neutralization experiments were performed similarly. Before transfer to cell cultures, test materials were preincubated in silanized microtiter plates for 1 hour at 37°C with an equal volume of anti-cholera toxin (Swiss Serum and Vaccine Institute), normal horse serum control, or mixed gangliosides (Sigma) in buffered saline. Concentrations of anti-toxin and gangliosides (0.0156 u/ml and 8 μg/ml, respectively) were chosen to be in excess of the amount required for complete neutralization of any toxin(s) detected previously and were sufficient to neutralize 8 ng/ml of CT. Inactivation of supernatants at 56°C for various times preceded the normal assays in heating experiments.

ELISA Assay

Strains were tested using a modification of the ganglioside-G_{M1} ELISA (enzyme-linked immunosorbent assay) of Sack et al. (1980). For specific antiserum, we used burro anti-CT (prepared by Dr. Z. Dafni) and rabbit anti-CT (prepared by Dr. N. Pierce). Peroxidase-conjugated goat anti-horse IgG or anti-rabbit IgG was obtained from Cappel Laboratories, Inc. (West Chester, PA). Strains to be tested were grown in roller drum culture at 32°C for 24 hours and 50 rpm in casamino acids-yeast extract broth. Supernatant fluids were cleared by centrifugation and frozen at -20°C until tested.

RESULTS AND DISCUSSION

Early studies of effects of environmental <u>V. cholerae</u> supernatants on Y-1 cells indicated that the presence of cytotoxic factors produced by most strains interfered with the detection of CT-like toxins. Cytotoxicity masked any rounding effect in supernatants with purified cholera toxin added and was responsible for loss of viability of the Y-1 cells as shown by their failure to exclude trypan blue. Subsequent use of serial supernatant and CT dilutions in the Y-1 assay (Maneval et al. 1980) not only yielded titers for CX- and CT-like responses and CT equivalents (ng CT-equivalent/ml supernatant) but helped reduce this masking. In some known CX+, CT+ strains, CT morphology could be detected at higher supernatant dilutions where CX was not evident, that is, in strains where CT titers > CX titers. Environmental vibrios in general are enzymatically competent organisms producing a variety of lipases, elastases, nucleases, and proteases. Postulating that extracellular enzymes could be responsible for lysis and death of Y-1 cells, several assay modifications were tested. Limited heat treatment of supernatants usually reduced or eliminated cytotoxicity but also destroyed CT in known CT-producing strains. Protease inhibitors in bacterial media reduced cytotoxicity of some strains but were themselves toxic to Y-1 cells or effective with only a few strains. Inclusion of $(NH_4)_2SO_4$ in media has been reported to suppress bacterial protease formation (Liu and Hsieh 1969), and in our assays reduced cytotoxic titer for most strains tested when incorporated into syncase at a concentration of 1%. Combined use of $(NH_4)_2SO_4$ and serial dilutions enabled us to detect Y-1 CT-like responses.

Table 2. Cytotoxic Titers of Chesapeake Bay $\underline{V}$. $\underline{cholerae}$ Strains

No. Cytotoxic Strains[a]	Cytotoxic Titer (1/dilution)[b]
3	–
3	1
10	2
16	4
10	8
10	16
14	32
9	>32

[a]Syncase broth [without $(NH_4)_2SO_4$] supernatant produced granular, crenated or lysed Y-1 cells which failed to exclude trypan blue.

[b]Supernatant dilution causing cytotoxic effect in 50% of Y-1 cells.

Table 2 provides a summary of the number of strains grown in syncase broth without $(NH_4)_2SO_4$ which were positive at dilutions ranging from undiluted to > 1:32. Of the 75 strains tested using these procedures, 18 had CT-like activities at the final positive dilution as evidenced by morphological appearance, absence of CX, and ability to exclude trypan blue. This was in contrast to the lower dilutions of these same specimens which exhibited only cyto-toxicity.

Of the 18 with CT-like activity, 12 showed absolutely no change in response to ganglioside or anti-toxin neutralization. Six showed some decrease in activity, dropping one or two dilutions, but not demonstrating complete loss of activity as did $\underline{V}$. $\underline{cholerae}$ strain BV-86 and 569-B (Table 3).

A further assessment was made by employing the ELISA test to examine for the presence of cholera toxin using rabbit anti-CT or horse anti-CT. There was remarkably good agreement between the two assays after examination of the filtrates from 10 strains. Only two samples were significantly different from the negative control, V. cholerae 569-B and V-10. The positive finding with V-10 was unexpected since it did not cause a cytotonic-like reaction in Y-1 adrenal cells (Table 4).

The borderline and, occasionally, moderately strong G_{M1}-ELISA responses obtained with certain strains of V. cholerae that have been shown by DNA probe analysis to lack the gene for cholera toxin require further evaluation. We initially assumed that the antisera used were not mono-specific, since they were not prepared against highly purified toxin, and that antibody reactions with other vibrio products may have caused the results observed. We have since retested these strains and others using a fresh lot of rabbit antiserum prepared in our laboratory against highly purified cholera toxin and have found that culture filtrates of certain strains will cross-react with this serum even though they lack the structural gene for CT. They do not react with the rabbit pre-immune serum. This suggests perhaps that these strains may produce a protein that possesses ganglioside-binding sites of sufficient antigenic similarity to an antigenic site of CT (perhaps also the ganglioside binding site?) to cross-react, even though the remainder of primary structure is dissimilar. Such a phe-nomenon would be of interest to document and this possi-bility is currently being examined.

Concurrent with the examination by the ELISA method, the strains listed in Table 5 were examined for the ability to cause increased cAMP accumulation and steroid produc-tion by Y-1 adrenal cells. Ability to inhibit binding of CT to Y-1 cells was tested also.

The Y-1 cells were exposed to undiluted cell free filtrates for 24 hours at 37°C.

The cyclic AMP assay was a simple TCA precipitation and ether extraction followed by collection of appropriate fractions over a Dowex column, drying, reconstitution in acetate buffer, and radioimmunoassay. The steroid assay involved spectrofluorometric assay of methylene-chloride extracted media.

Table 3. Effects of Neutralization on Cytotonic Titers of Chesapeake Bay
V. cholerae Strains Grown in Syncase + 1% $(NH_4)_2SO_4$ Broth

	Titer (1/dilution)[a]			
	Cytotonic[b]			Cytotoxic[c]
	Untreated	Treated		
		Mixed Ganglioside[d]	Swiss-serum Anti-CT[d]	
Strain No.				
V-40	4	1	2	2
V-42	4	2	2	2
V-43	2	1	1	1
V-50	2	1	1	1
V-52	4	1	2	1

V-98	2	—	1	—
BV-86[e]	512	—	—	4
569-B[f]	2048	—	—	—

[a] Supernatant dilution causing morphological changes in 50% of Y-1 cells.

[b] Supernatant which produced CT-like response in Y-1 cells: rounded, refractile morphology.

[c] Supernatant producing granular, crenated or lysed Y-1 cells which failed to exclude trypan blue, with or without treatment.

[d] Supernatant dilutions were preincubated with excess neutralizing agent for one hour at 37°C, before Y-1 assay.

[e] Environmental V. cholerae CT-producing strain from Bangladesh.

[f] Human V. cholerae CT-producing strain.

Table 4. Results of ELISA Assay for Cholera Toxin

Strain No.	Rabbit Anti-CT[a]	Burro Anti-CT[a]
Neg control	0.057	0.055
569-B	0.73[b]	0.98[b]
V-86	0.049	0.060
V-10	0.29[b]	0.38[b]
V-48	0.038	0.013
V-40	0.024	0.072
V-60	0.035	0.043
V-69	0.028	0.039
V-85	0.031	–
V-61	0.066	0.043
V-36	0.099	0.064

[a]O.D. values at 405 nM.
[b]Significantly different from Neg control.

The binding assay was done by incubation of ~10^5 cpm of ^{125}I-labelled cholera toxin (chloramine-T method) with ~10^5 Y-1 cells for 30 minutes, followed by trapping and washing of cells on Millipore EHWP filters and determination of ^{125}I counts present on the filters.

Twelve strains were examined by this technique. Only V-10, V-15, V-31, V-37, and V-69 had been examined in the RIL. FA ratios ranged from 0.21 to 2.11, the highest being caused by V-37. It should be noted that V-69, also examined here, was subsequently identified as an O1 strain of V. cholerae. On three separate occasions, V-69 caused FA ratios of 0.75, 1.0 and 1.0 in the RIL. It is cytotoxic at a dilution of 1:40, but does not cause the appearance of cytotonic activity in Y-1 cells. Kaper et al. (1981) recently reported that this strain does not possess the tox gene for cholera toxin.

As noted in Table 5, none of the test strains were found to stimulate steroidogenesis, whereas V. cholerae

569-B exposure resulted in 24.3 µg/plate and 10 ng/ml of cholera toxin caused 44.99 µg/plate.

The vibrio strains tested for ability to elicit cAMP responses from Y-1 cells were V-10, V-37, V-40, V-48, V-60, V-61, V-69, V-85 and V-86. None of these were able to stimulate more than 208 pMoles of cAMP/10^6 cells/18 hour incubation. In contrast, 0.1 ml of 569-B culture supernatant elicited 820 pMoles of cAMP, 50 ng of cholera toxin elicited 400 pMoles and a partially purified E. coli enterotoxin preparation elicited 990 pMoles.

None of these isolates, including V. cholerae 569-B, could inhibit the binding of ^{125}I-labelled cholera toxin, which probably represents insensitivity of the assay.

SUMMARY AND CONCLUSIONS

Both cytotoxic and cytotonic-like activity have been noted with Y-1 cells. Some of the cytotonic effect can be reduced by neutralization with ganglioside and anti-CT. One strain, unexplainably, was positive for CT in the ELISA assay. None of the strains stimulated steroidogenesis by Y-1 cells, and no significant increase in cAMP was detected.

In conclusion, we have not been able to detect cholera-like "bioactivity" using Y-1 cells. We do, however, have potent cytotoxic effects, which do not appear to manifest through elevated cyclic AMP levels or steroidogenesis. This still does not enable an answer to the question as to how non-O1 V. cholerae in the absence of demonstrable CT-like activity is capable of causing frank enteritis in humans. Obviously, the factors responsible for this ability remain to be identified, purified, and characterized.

Lastly, the very important problem of detection of both CT and non-CT-producing potential pathogens in the environment by simple and rapid methodology is very important to the better understanding of these organisms in their ecological environs and in human pathogenesis. Without such information, we shall find it nearly impossible to

Table 5. Comparison of Results Obtained with the cAMP, Rabbit Ileal Loop, ELISA, and Steroid Assays

Isolate	RIL	ELISA	Y-1 Cytotoxicity Titer	Steroids (μg/plate/18 hr)	cAMP (pMoles)
V-10	0.73	+	1:320	0	0
V-15	0.45	ND	1:640	0	ND
V-31	0.21	ND	1:40	0	ND
V-37	2.11	ND	1:160	0	ND
V-40	ND	–	1:40	0	0
V-48	ND	–	1:40	0	0
V-50	ND	–	1:20	0	ND
V-60	ND	–	1:640	0	0
V-61	ND	–	1:160	0	0

V-69	ND	–	1:40	0	0
V-85	ND	–	1:10	0	0
V-86	ND	–	1:80	0	0
569-B	1.2	–	1:1280[a]	24.3	820
Cholera toxin - 10 ng/ml				44.99	
Cholera toxin - 50 ng/ml					400

[a] V. cholerae 569-B exhibited cytotonic reaction typical of Y-1 response to cholera toxin (CT).

assess the total risk of O1 and non-O1 <u>V</u>. <u>cholerae</u> to human populations in the United States and elsewhere.

ACKNOWLEDGMENT

This work was supported in part by NIH grant AI 14242, a Public Health Service grant through the National Institute of Allergy and Infectious Disease.

REFERENCES

Bhattacharya, S., A.K. Bose, and A.K. Ghosh. 1971. Permeability and enterotoxic factors of nonagglutinable vibrios <u>Vibrio</u> <u>alcaligenes</u> and <u>Vibrio</u> <u>parahaemolyticus</u>. Appl. Microb. 22:1159-1161.

Bisgaard, M., and K.K. Kristensen. 1975. Isolation, characterization and public health aspects of <u>Vibrio</u> <u>cholerae</u> NAG isolated from a Danish duck farm. Avian Path. 4:271-276.

Bisgaard, M., R. Sakazaki, and T. Shimada. 1978. Prevalence of non-cholera vibrios in cavum nasi and pharynx of ducks. Acta path. Microbiol. Scand. Sect. B. 86:261-266.

Ciznar, I., M. Draskovicova, A. Hostacka, and J. Karolcek. 1977. Partial purification and characterization of the NAG vibrio toxin. Zbl. Bakt. Hyg., I. 239:493-503.

Donta, S.T. and J.P. Viner. 1974. Inhibition of the steroidogenic effects of cholera and heat labile <u>Escherichia</u> <u>coli</u> enterotoxins by G_{M1} ganglioside: evidence for a similar receptor site for the two toxins. Infect. Immun. 11:982-985.

Draskovicova, M., J. Karolcek, and D. Winkler. 1977.
Experimental toxigenicity of NAG vibrios. Zbl. Bakt.
Hyg. I. Abt. Orig. A237:65-71.

Dunaev, G.S., L.F. Zykin, and I.N. Bandarev. 1975.
Pathogenicity of non-agglutinating vibrios. Zh. Mikrobiol. Epidemiol. Immunol. 6:81-85.

Dutta, N.K., M.V. Panse, and H.I. Jhala. 1963. Choleragenic property of certain strains of El Tor, non agglu-
tinable and water vibrios confirmed experimentally.
Brit. Med. J. 1:1200-1203.

Finkelstein, R.A., P. Atthasampunna, P. Chatasamaya, and
P. Charunmethee. 1966. Pathogenesis of experimental
cholera: biological activities of purified procholeragen
Am. J. Immunol. 96:440-449.

Gupta, N.P., S.P. Gupta, V.S. Mangalik, B.G. Prasad,
and B.S. Yajnik. 1956. Investigations into the nature
of the vibrio strains isolated from the epidemic of
gastroenteritis in Kumbh Fair at Allahabad in 1954.
Indian J. Med. Sci. 10:781.

Hughes, J.M., D.G. Hollis, E.J. Gangarosa, and R.E.
Weaver. 1978. Non-cholera vibrio infections in the
United States. Clinical, epidemiologic and laboratory
features. Ann. Intern. Med. 88:602-606.

Kaper, J.B., S.L. Moseley, and S. Falkow. 1981. Molecular characterization of environmental and nontoxigenic strains of Vibrio cholerae. Infect. Immun.
32:661-667.

Kaper, J.B., H. Lockman, R.R. Colwell, and S.W. Joseph.
1979. Ecology, serology and enterotoxin production of
Vibrio cholerae in Chesapeake Bay. Appl. Environ.
Microbiol. 37:91-103.

Liu, P.V., and H. Hsieh. 1969. Inhibition of protease
production of various bacteria by ammonium salts: its

effect on toxin production and virulence. J. Bacteriol. 99:406-413.

Maneval, D.R., R.R. Colwell, S.W. Joseph, R. Grays, and S.T. Donta. 1980. A tissue culture method for the detection of bacterial enterotoxins. J. Tissue Culture Meth. 6:85-90.

McIntyre, O.R., J.C. Feely, W.B. Greenough III, A.S. Benensen, S.I. Hassan, and A. Saad. 1965. Diarrhea caused by non-cholera vibrios. Am. J. Trop. Med. Hyg. 14:412-418.

Ohashi, M., T. Shimada, and H. Fukumi. 1972. In vitro production of enterotoxin and hemorrhagic principle by Vibrio cholerae, NAG. Jpn. J. Med. Sci. Biol. 25:179-194.

Robbins-Browne, R.M., C.S. Still, M. Isaacson, H.J. Koornhof, P.C. Applebaum, and J.N. Scragg. 1977. Pathogenic mechanisms of a non-agglutinable Vibrio cholerae strain: demonstration of invasive and enterotoxigenic properties. Infect. Immun. 18:542-545.

Sack, D.A., S. Huda, P.K.B. Neogi, R.R. Daniel, and W.M. Spira. 1980. Microtiter ganglioside enzyme-linked immunosorbent assay for vibrio and Escherichia coli heat-labile enterotoxins and anti-toxin. J. Clin. Microbiol. 11:35-40.

Sakazaki, R., C.Z. Gomez, and M. Sebald. 1967. Taxonomical studies of the so-called NAG vibrios. Jpn. J. Med. Sci. Biol. 20:265-280.

Singh, S.J., and S.C. Sanyal. 1978. Enterotoxicity of the so-called NAG vibrios. Ann. Soc. Belge Med. Trop. 58:133-140.

Spira, W.M., R.R. Daniel, Q.S. Ahmed, A. Huq, A. Yusuf, and D.A. Sack. 1978. Clinical features and pathogenicity of O group I nonagglutinating Vibrio cholerae and other vibrios isolated from cases of diarrhea in Dacca, Bangladesh. Proc. 14th U.S.-Japan Cholera Conference.

Tolnai, S.A. 1975. A method for cell viability count. Procedure 70151. TCA Manual 1:39-40.

Weissman, J.B., W.E. DeWitt, J. Thompson, C.N. Muchnick, B.L. Portnoy, J.C. Feeley, and E.J. Gangarosa. 1975. A case of cholera in Texas. 1973. Am. J. Epidemiol. 100:487-498.

Zinnaka, Y., and C.C.J. Carpenter, Jr. 1972. An enterotoxin produced by non-cholera vibrios. Hopkins Med. J. 131:403-411.

Chapter 9

RESPONSES IN SUCKLING MICE INDUCED BY
VIBRIO VIRULENCE FACTOR(S)

Mitsuaki Nishibuchi and Ramon J. Seidler

In the genus Vibrio, V. cholerae serovar O1 has been
thoroughly studied and its precise pathogenic mechanisms
are generally understood (Finkelstein 1976). There are,
however, other potentially human pathogenic vibrios in the
environment with unknown virulence mechanisms (Blake et
al. 1980). V. fluvialis and V. cholerae O1 are considered
important because both organisms are known to be widely
distributed in the aquatic environment and the number of
gastroenteritis cases caused by these vibrios has been
increasing. Some strains of non-O1 V. cholerae produce
cholera-like toxin (Zinnaka and Carpenter 1972) and possess
genes similar to Escherichia coli heat-labile enterotoxin genes
(Kaper et al. 1981). There are other unknown virulence
factors involved in non-O1 V. cholerae as demonstrated by
guinea pig or rabbit skin tests (Ohashi et al. 1972; Spira
et al. 1979), rabbit ileal loop tests (Singh and Sanyal 1978;
Spira et al. 1979), intraintestinal inoculation of cultures in
infant rabbits (Spira et al. 1979; Twedt et al. 1981; Madden
et al. 1981), intraperitoneal injection of cultures into adult
mice (Spira et al. 1979), and inoculation of culture filtrates
into suckling mice (Ohashi et al. 1972; Spira et al. 1979).
Group F vibrios, or Vibrio fluvialis, produce virulence
factor(s) that give positive rabbit ileal loop tests (Sanyal et
al. 1980). Oral administration of bacterial cultures into

145

suckling mice, however, has the advantage of simulating the actual course of gastroenteritis and is a relatively economical and convenient assay to perform. This method has been used to study the pathogenesis of V. cholerae O1 by others (Ujiiye and Kobari 1970; Chaicumpa and Rowley 1972; Guentzel and Berry 1974; Baselski et al. 1977). In the present study this approach is used to compare and define virulence factors produced by clinical and environmental isolates of O1 and non-O1 V. cholerae and V. fluvialis.

METHODS AND RESULTS

Responses in the suckling mouse were measured by three parameters: fluid accumulation ratio (FA ratio) in the intestine, mortality, and stained feces as an indicator of diarrhea. The test organism was grown in tryptic soy broth (Difco) supplemented with 0.5% sodium chloride (TSB'), and shaken (200 rpm) at 37°C for 18 hours. Three-day-old mice were removed from their mothers and submitted to experimental protocols within 2 hours. A group of five animals was used for each test. One-tenth milliliter of the bacterial culture in 0.01% Evans blue dye was orally administered into the milk-filled stomach of each animal by way of flexible polyethylene tubing (PE60, Clay Adams). Supernates of some cultures obtained by centrifugation and filtration through a membrane filter (0.2 μm pore size, Gelman) were also orally inoculated. The inoculated animals of each test group were incubated on white filter paper at 25°C for 4 to 18 hours. FA ratios were determined by the ratio of the weight of pooled stomachs plus intestines to the rest of the body weight. Mortality was recorded as negative (-) for 0-1 dead animal, positive (+) for 2-3 dead animals, and strongly positive (++) for 4-5 dead animals. Spots of stained feces collected on the filter paper were counted and recorded as negative (-), positive (+), and strongly positive (++) for 0-1, 2-3, and 4 or more stained feces, respectively. Two different strains of mice, Swiss Webster and CF1, were obtained from Laboratory Animal Resources of Oregon State University. There was no significant difference in their responses as measured by mortality and stained feces. FA ratios in the CF1 strain, however, were consistently lower than those of the Swiss Webster strain but only 0.005 on the average.

The assay system provided consistent and repeatable results with negative and positive controls (Table 1). The negative controls employed were culture medium (TSB') and two bacterial isolates from drinking water, namely, Citrobacter freundii strain 3321 and Escherichia coli strain 701. FA ratios for the negative controls ranged from 0.0620 to 0.0755. No mortality and no stained feces were recorded for the negative controls. Positive controls included enterotoxigenic E. coli strain H10407, a well-known heat-stable and heat-labile enterotoxin producer, purified cholera toxin (Sigma), and V. cholerae O1 strains 569B (clinical isolate) and SG-N-7277 (water isolate)--both of which produce cholera toxin. As documented by Dean et al. (1972) the culture supernate of E. coli H10407 containing heat-stable enterotoxin induced a high FA ratio of 0.117 as early as 4 hours postinoculation. Whole cell cultures of toxigenic strains of V. cholerae O1 caused significant increases in the FA ratios as previously reported (Baselski et al. 1977), but culture supernates did not. Cholera toxin elicited a higher FA ratio at 12 hours than at 4 hours in agreement with Baselski et al. (1977). From these results, FA ratios of 0.08 or more were considered significantly positive in the assay system. Mortality and stained feces assays for the positive controls were positive or strongly positive. However, cholera toxin did not kill animals even though massive amounts of stained feces were observed.

FA Ratios

Orally administered cultures of V. cholerae O1 that produce toxin induced significantly high FA ratios at 8 hours or later (Baselski et al. 1977). In our assay system, however, nontoxigenic, V. cholerae non-O1 strains as well as toxigenic strains of V. cholerae O1, regardless of their origin of isolation, caused positive FA ratios as early as 4 hours postinoculation. At 12 hours FA ratios were not as high as at 4 hours except for a toxigenic strain, SG-N-7277

Table 1. Results of Suckling Mouse Bioassays Obtained for Control Cultures

Organism[b]	Whole Culture (C) or Culture Supernate (S)[c]	FA Ratio[d] at 4 hours	12 hours	Mortality[e]	Stained Feces[f]
TSB'[g]		0.0686 ± 0.0061	0.0640 ± 0.0070	–	–
Citrobacter freundii 3321	C	0.0694	0.0634	–	–
	S	0.0694	0.0620	–	–
Escherichia coli 701	C	0.0625	0.0668	–	–
	S	0.0633	0.0631		
E. coli H10407	C	0.1177	0.1276	++	++
	S	0.1104	0.0861		
01 Vibrio cholerae 569B	C	0.0870	0.0822	+	+
	S	0.0708	0.0632		
01 V. cholerae SG-N-7277	C	0.0845	0.0991	++	++
	S	0.0700	0.0635		
Cholera toxin[h]		0.0920	0.1120	–	++

[a]Each of five three-day-old mice received 0.1 ml of the test material per os.
[b]Test organism was grown in TSB' for 18 hours at 37°C with shaking at 200 rpm.
[c]Culture supernate was obtained by centrifugation of the bacterial culture followed by filtration through membrane filter (0.2 μm).
[d](Weight of pooled stomachs plus intestines) ÷ (Remaining body weight).
[e]0-1 dead animal, –; 2-3 dead animals, +; 4-5 dead animals, ++. Results were recorded 18 hours post-inoculation.
[f]0-1 stained feces, –; 2-3 stained·feces, +; 4-5 stained feces, ++. Results were recorded 18 hours postinoculation.
[g]Tryptic soy broth (Difco) supplemented with 0.5% sodium chloride.
[h]Purified cholera toxin (Sigma) diluted in TSB' (100 μg protein/ml).

(Table 2). Strain DJVP6957 of V. fluvialis exhibited the same tendency. None of the culture supernates induced positive FA ratios (data not shown). Rapid fluid accumulation in 4 hours was also recorded when whole cell cultures of four other strains (one clinical and three environmental) of V. fluvialis were tested (data not shown). These data suggest that a virulence factor other than cholera toxin is being produced early in the infection. This assumption was made more clear by experiments quantitating the kinetics of fluid accumulation.

The time course of FA ratios induced by cholera toxin were compared with those induced by toxin-producing strains of V. cholerae O1, 569B and SG-N-7277 (Figure 1). The elevated level of fluid accumulation ratios seen at 12 hours with the toxin-producing strains coincides with the time of maximum fluid accumulation ratios induced by cholera toxin alone. Selected strains of non-O1 V. cholerae were also submitted to the time-course experiments (Figure 2). A toxigenic non-O1 strain N-2002H exhibited a shallow but significant plateau of fluid accumulation at 12 hours analogous in level to that of strain 569B. However, the 4-hour peaks in FA ratios are especially apparent with both non-O1 strains. These results indicate that peaks at 12 hours are due to cholera toxin produced in vivo. Therefore, the peaks at 4 hours are caused by a different factor(s). The distinctiveness of the peaks at 4 versus 12 hours are influenced by the relative amounts of cholera toxin and other FA factor(s) produced by each test strain. The early peak at 4 hours may be masked by a large amount of cholera toxin production as seen in Figure 1 with strain SG-N-7277.

The distinct nature of the early FA factor(s) was immunologically confirmed by in vivo neutralization tests using anticholeragenoid (Table 3). The FA ratios at 12 hours induced by cholera toxin or by toxigenic strains of V. cholerae O1 (569B, SG-N-7277) dropped significantly due to the reaction with anticholeragenoid. Interestingly, the FA ratios at 12 hours due to the toxigenic non-O1 strain N-2002H was not affected by the addition of anticholeragenoid. This may be related to the fact that the toxin genes of this strain are somewhat different from those of O1

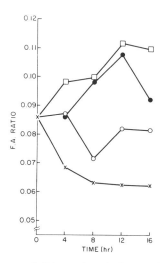

Figure 1. Time course of FA ratios induced by <u>Vibrio</u> <u>cholerae</u> O1. Test organism was grown in TSB' (see text) for 18 hours at 37°C with agitation at 200 rpm. Each animal was given 0.1 ml of the test material per os. Five animals were sacrificed for each FA ratio determination. □-□ Strain SG-N-7277 (toxigenic), ○-○ Strain 569B (toxigenic), ●-●Cholera toxin (100 µg/1 ml of TSB'), X-X Control (TSB').

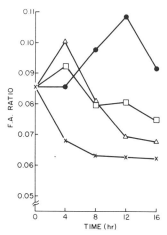

Figure 2. Time course of FA ratios induced by non-O1 <u>Vibrio</u> <u>cholerae</u>. Test organism was grown in TSB' (see text) for 18 hours at 37°C with agitation at 200 rpm. Each animal was given 0.1 ml of the test material per os. Five animals were sacrificed for each FA ratio determination. □-□ Strain N-2002H (toxigenic), △-△ Strain N-2030H (nontoxigenic), ●-● Cholera toxin (100 µg/1 ml of TSB'), X-X Control (TSB').

150

Table 2. FA Ratios[a] Determined for Whole Cultures of O1 and Non-O1 Vibrio cholerae and V. fluvialis 4 hours and 12 hours Postinoculation

Test Organism				FA Ratio at	
Species	Strain No.	Cholera Toxin Production	Origin	4 hours	12 hours
O1 Vibrio cholerae	569B	+	Clinical	0.0870	0.0822
	SG-N-7277	+	Environmental	0.0845	0.0991
Non-O1 V. cholerae	N-2030H	-	Clinical	0.0872	0.0664
	WA-0-001	-	Environmental	0.0914	0.0858
	WA-0-028	-	Environmental	0.0993	0.0887
V. fluvialis	DJVP6957	-	Clinical	0.0909	0.0729

[a]See Table 1.

Table 3. Effects of Anticholeragenoid on FA Ratios Induced by Vibrio cholerae in the Suckling Mouse

Test Organism[b]	FA Ratio[a] at					
	4 hours			12 hours		
	Culture	Culture + Anti-[c] choleragenoid	Difference[d]	Culture	Culture + Anti-[c] choleragenoid	Difference[d]
Cholera toxin[e]	0.0920±0.0122	0.0654±0.0055	+ (p<0.006)	0.1120±0.0133	0.0676±0.0051	+ (p<0.005)
Control (TSB')	0.0678±0.0041	0.0668±0.0045	–	0.0625±0.0024	0.0640±0.0016	–
01 V. cholerae 569B (Toxigenic)	0.0870±0.0081	0.0820±0.0160	–	0.0822±0.0106	0.0713±0.0088	+ (0.050<p < 0.100)
01 V. cholerae SG-N-7277	0.0862±0.0048	0.0912±0.0105	–	0.0922±0.0052	0.0808±0.0094	+ (0.010<p < 0.025)
Non-01 V. cholerae N-2002H (Toxigenic)	0.0917±0.0111	0.0958±0.0051	–	0.0819±0.0087	0.0800±0.0051	–
Non-01 V. cholerae N-2030H (Nontoxigenic)	0.0872±0.0178	0.0897±0.0129	–	0.0664±0.0082	0.0677±0.0091	–

[a] FA ratio of each of five animals was determined. Each animal was given 0.1 ml of the test material.
[b] Test organism was grown in TSB' (see text) for 18 hours at 37°C with agitation at 200 rpm.
[c] Culture:anticholeragenois = 9:1 (v/v).
[d] Compared by t-test using a pooled sample estimator of population variance.
[e] Diluted in TSB' (100 µg protein/ml).

V. cholerae strains (personal communication, Dr. James B. Kaper of Center for Vaccine Development, University of Maryland School of Medicine). In any event, it is evident from these results that high FA ratios observed at 4 hours are not associated with cholera toxin produced in vivo since they are not affected by anticholeragenoid.

Mortality and Stained Feces

There were two different types of diarrhea scored as stained feces. Watery diarrhea was induced by enterotoxigenic E. coli strain H10407 and purified cholera toxin. Mucoid, pasty feces was excreted from the mice administered nontoxigenic strains of non-O1 V. cholerae and strains of V. fluvialis. The diarrhea caused by toxigenic strains of V. cholerae consisted of both types of feces, indicating watery diarrhea is due to cholera toxin and mucoid feces is induced by some other factor possessed by all strains of O1 and non-O1 V. cholerae and V. fluvialis. Results of mortality and stained feces assays obtained for O1 and non-O1 V. cholerae and V. fluvialis isolated from clinical and environmental origin are summarized in Table 4. Also included in Table 4 are the results of assays involving Y-1 mouse adrenal cells performed by a modification of Maneval et al. (1980). The results indicate, regardless of serovar (O1 and non-O1) and origin of isolation, that all strains of V. cholerae were positive or strongly positive in both mortality and stained feces assays in the suckling mouse, and produced a very strong cytotoxic response in the Y-1 assay. The cytotoxic factor was present in culture supernates and was inactivated by heating at 56°C for 10 minutes. Regardless of their source of isolation, all V. fluvialis strains, except one which lost motility, induced death and were positive or strongly positive in the stained feces assay; 5 out of these 8 strains also produced an extracellular, heat-labile, cytotoxic factor detected in the Y-1 assay. The degree of cytotoxicity to Y-1 cells was weaker with V. fluvialis than with V. cholerae. When other species belonging to the genera Vibrio and Aeromonas were assayed for mortality and stained feces in suckling mice,

Table 4. Mortality and Stained Feces in Suckling Mice and Cytotoxic Effect to Y-1 Mouse Adrenal Cells Caused by Vibrio cholerae and V. fluvialis

Organism	Origin	No. Strains Tested	Suckling Mouse Assay[a]		Cytotoxic Effect to Y-1 Cells[b] Due to		
			Mortality	Stained Feces	Whole Culture	Culture Supernatant	Heated Supernatant[c]
O1 Vibrio cholerae	Clinical	1	+	+	4+[d]	4+	-
	Environmental	3	++	++	4+	4+	-
Non-O1 V. cholerae	Clinical	5	+(1)[e],++(4)	+(3),++(2)	4+	4+	-
	Environmental	7	++	+(1),++(6)	4+	4+	-
V. fluvialis	Clinical	4	+(1),++(3)	+(2),++(2)	-(2),1+(1), 3+(1)	-(2),1+(1), 3+(1)	-
	Environmental	5	-(1),++(4)	-(1),++(4)	-(1),1+(1), 2+(2),3+(1)	-(1),1+(1), 2+(3)	-

[a] see Table 1. Whole culture was administered to the test animals.
[b] Test was performed by the method of Maneval et al. (1980) with minor modifications.
[c] Culture supernatant was heated at 56°C for 10 minutes.
[d] Scored as 1+ to 4+, corresponding to 25%, 25-50%, 50-75%, or 75-100% cells exhibiting cytotoxic morphology.
[e] Number of test strains.

10 out of 15 strains caused mortality but only 3 of them induced a positive stained feces response. These included a V. vulnificus strain ATCC 27562 (= CDCB9629) of clinical origin, unidentified Vibrio strains HOG3 isolated from oysters incriminated in a gastroenteritis case, and WA-0-27 isolated from water.

In order to investigate the relationship between mortality and the stained feces response, representative strains of V. cholerae and V. fluvialis were examined for their LD_{50} and the effective oral dose producing stained feces (SF_{50}). LD_{50} was determined by the method of moving averages (Meynell and Meynell 1965). SF_{50} was defined as the number of colony-forming units (cfu) that caused 50% stained feces (2 or 3 out of 5 mice) response. Negative (0-1), positive (2-3), and strongly positive (4-5) feces response was graded as 0%, 50%, and 100% response, respectively, in calculating the SF_{50}. It can be seen in Table 5 that LD_{50} values were generally one-log higher than SF_{50} values with one exception; V. cholerae strain 569B which had an extremely high LD_{50} value as reported by other workers (Guentzel and Berry 1974). These data suggest that mortality results from the gastrointestinal infection and production of stained feces is generally a good indicator of virulence. A stained feces response without mortality could result from a bacterial strain having few virulence-associated factors. The results (Table 5) also show that LD_{50} values and SF_{50} values are higher for V. fluvialis than for V. cholerae with the exception of strain 569B. There is a good quantitative correlation among the parameters used to measure virulence responses in the suckling mouse and the Y-1 cytotoxic response. This indicates these responses (early FA ratios, mortality, diarrhea, Y-1 cytotoxicity) may be due to the same factor(s).

Internal symptoms of the mice given purified cholera toxin or enterotoxigenic E. coli strain H10407 were limited to the accumulation of fluid in the upper bowel. The animals administered most O1 and non-O1 V. cholerae and V. fluvialis showed a distended stomach and duodenum in addition to fluid accumulation in the upper bowel. It is not yet clear whether the distended stomach/duodenum is

Table 5. LD_{50} and SF_{50} in Suckling Mice for Representative Strains of Vibrio cholerae and V. fluvialis

Test Organism[a]

Species	Strain	LD_{50}	SF_{50}[b]
O1 Vibrio cholerae	569B	>1.06 x 10^9 cfu	3.35 x 10^6 cfu
Non-O1 V. cholerae	N-53	1.11 x 10^7	1.11 x 10^6
	N-3	7.02 x 10^7	1.41 x 10^7
	WA-0-028	3.94 x 10^8	4.96 x 10^7
V. fluvialis	DJVP6957	6.01 x 10^8	3.79 x 10^7
	H-5	1.61 x 10^8	4.05 x 10^7
	LSU10-41C	1.88 x 10^9	1.49 x 10^8

[a]Test organism was grown in TSB' (see text) at 37°C for 18 hours with agitation at 200 rpm. The culture was diluted tenfold in 0.01 M phosphate-buffered saline, pH 7.2. Five three-day-old mice were orally administered 0.1 ml of each dilution. Inoculated animals were incubated at 35°C for 18 hours.

[b]Effective dose for stained feces; see text for definition.

caused by the same factors responsible for intestinal fluid accumulation, mortality, and stained feces.

Occasionally moribund animals manifested hemorrhagic intestines. Ohashi and his associates (1972), in this skin test in guinea pigs, found a virulence factor termed the "hemorrhagic principle" which was produced by both O1 and non-O1 V. cholerae strains. The culture filtrate containing this factor, when injected in the skin of guinea pigs, caused hemorrhagic lesions. Later Spira et al. (1979) made a similar observation in a skin test using rabbits. Production of a hemorrhagic factor was tested in the present study by injection of culture supernates into the skin of guinea pigs. Only 9 out of 16 strains of O1 and non-O1 V. cholerae tested were found to produce the hemorrhagic response. This factor was resistant to heating at 56°C for 30 minutes as previously reported (Ohashi et al. 1972). The hemorrhagic principle was not produced by all strains of O1 and non-O1 V. cholerae tested, and it did not lose its biological activity by heating at 56°C for 30 minutes. It was concluded that these factors are distinct from the virulence factor(s) causing early fluid accumulation and cytotoxicity in the Y-1 assay.

CONCLUSIONS

Oral administration of bacterial cultures to three-day-old suckling mice demonstrated that, regardless of the origin of isolation and toxigenic property, O1 and non-O1 V. cholerae and V. fluvialis produced virulence factor(s) which are responsible for intestinal fluid accumulation, stained feces, and mortality in suckling mice. The organisms also produced cytotoxic factors as evidenced by the Y-1 adrenal cell assay. There were correlations in the various assays in the degree of virulence response to these organisms, indicating that the responses may be due to a common factor. Although the heat-sensitive cytotoxic factor demonstrated by the Y-1 assay was present in culture supernates, the culture supernates administered to suckling mice per os did not induce any detectable symptoms of disease. This may be due to the differences in the sensitivity of each assay system.

The virulence factor(s) were shown to be different from the already known cholera toxin and hemorrhagic principles by the kinetics of FA ratios, in vivo neutralization test, symptomatology (type of stained feces, distended stomach and duodenum), and the skin test in guinea pigs.

Other Vibrio species of clinical and environmental origin were found to cause mortality and stained feces in the suckling mouse assay. This suggests there may exist a wide variety of potentially enteropathogenic vibrios in the environment.

ACKNOWLEDGMENTS

This work was supported by the Oregon State University Sea Grant College Program, National Oceanic and Atmospheric Administration Office of Sea Grant, U.S. Department of Commerce, under Grant NA79AA-D-00106, project R/FSD8. The assistance provided by Dr. Sam Joseph and Dave Rollins in conducting the Y-1 mouse adrenal cell assays is gratefully appreciated. Oregon State University Agricultural Experiment Station Technical Paper No. 6387.

REFERENCES

Baselski, V., R. Briggs, and C. Parker. 1977. Intestinal fluid accumulation induced by oral challenge with Vibrio cholerae or cholera toxin in infant mice. Infect. Immun. 15:704-712.

Blake, P.A., R.E. Weaver, and D.G. Hollis. 1980. Diseases of humans (other than cholera) caused by vibrios. Ann. Rev. Microbiol. 34:341-367.

Chaicumpa, W., and D. Rowley. 1972. Experimental cholera in infant mice: protective effects of antibody. J. Infect. Dis. 125:480-485.

Dean, A.G., Y. Ching, R.G. Williams, and L.B. Harden. 1972. Test for Escherichia coli enterotoxin using infant mice: application in a study of diarrhea in children in Honolulu. J. Infect. Dis. 125:407-411.

Finkelstein, R.A. 1976. Progress in the study of cholera and related enterotoxins. Pages 54-84 in A.W. Bernheimer (Ed.), Mechanisms in bacterial toxinology. John Wiley, New York.

Guentzel, N.M., and L.J. Berry. 1974. Protection of suckling mice from experimental cholera by maternal immunization: comparison of the efficacy of whole-cell, ribosomal-derived, and enterotoxin immunogens. Infect. Immun. 10:167-172.

Kaper, J.B., S.L. Moseley, and S. Falkow. 1981. Molecular characterization of environmental and nontoxigenic strains of Vibrio cholerae. Infect. Immun. 32:661-667.

Madden, J.M., W.P. Nematollahi, W.E. Hill, B.A. McCardell, and R.M. Twedt. 1981. Virulence of three clinical isolates of Vibrio cholerae non-O1 serogroup in experimental infections in rabbits. Infect. Immun. 33:616-619.

Maneval, D.R., Jr., R.R. Colwell, S.W. Joseph, R. Grays, and S.T. Donta. 1980. A tissue culture method for the detection of bacterial enterotoxins. J. Tiss. Cult. Meth. 6:85-90.

Meynell, G., and E. Meynell. 1965. Theory and practice in experimental bacteriology. Cambridge University Press, Cambridge, Great Britain.

Ohashi, M., T. Shimada, and H. Fukumi. 1972. In vitro production of enterotoxin and hemorrhagic principle by Vibrio cholerae NAG. Jpn. J. Med. Sci. Biol. 25:179-194.

Sanyal, S.C., R.K. Agarwal, E. Annapurna, and J.V. Lee. 1980. Enterotoxicity of Group F vibrios. Jpn. J. Med. Sci. Biol. 33:217-222.

Singh, S.J., and S.C. Sanyal. 1978. Enterotoxicity of the so-called NAG vibrios. Ann. Soc. Belge. Med. Trop. 58:133-140.

Spira, W.M., R.R. Daniel, Q.S. Ahmed, A. Huq, A. Yusuf, and D.A. Sack. 1979. Clinical features and pathogenicity of group 1 non-agglutinating Vibrio cholerae and other vibrios isolated from cases of diarrhea in Dacca, Bangladesh. Pages 137-153 in Proc. 14th Joint Conference, U.S.-Japan Cooperative Medical Science Program, Karatsu, Japan, 1978. Toho University.

Twedt, R.M., J.M. Madden, J.M. Hebert, S.G. McCay, C.N. Roderick, G.T. Spite, and T.J. Wazenski. 1981. Characterization of Vibrio cholerae isolated from oysters. Appl. Environ. Microbiol. 41:1475-1478.

Ujiiye, A., and K. Kobari. 1970. Protective effect on infections with Vibrio cholerae in suckling mice caused by the passive immunization with milk of immune mothers. J. Infect. Dis. 121:S50-55.

Zinnaka, Y., and C.C.J. Carpenter, Jr. 1972. An enterotoxin produced by noncholera vibrios. Johns Hopkins Med. J. 131:403-411.

Chapter 10

MONOCLONAL ANTIBODIES TO CHOLERA TOXIN

E.F. Remmers, R.R. Colwell and R.A. Goldsby

Precise detection of low concentrations of cholera toxin is important for identifying toxin-producing strains of Vibrio cholerae and for molecular and biochemical characterization of toxin production and mode of action. Biological assays, e.g., rabbit skin and ligated ileal loop (Craig 1965; De 1959), suckling infant mouse (Baselski et al. 1977), and CHO and Y-1 adrenal cell assays (Guerrant et al. 1974; Donta et al. 1974), have been used to detect cholera toxin, but are expensive, tedious to carry out, and may be subject to interference by cytotoxins and related substances. Immunological assays for cholera toxin, such as the radioimmunoassay (RIA) (Ceska 1978; Hejtmancik et al. 1977) and reversed passive hemagglutination reaction (Holmes et al. 1978), provide some advantage over biological assays, but the specificity of these assays is dependent upon the specificity of the antiserum used.

Preparation of conventional antisera to cholera toxin requires an elaborate methodology and can result in the production of reagents that vary greatly from preparation to preparation, depending upon the immunization and purification steps involved. Even greater difficulties are encountered in the production of conventional antisera that are specific for the individual A and B subunits of cholera toxin (Hejtmancik et al. 1977). Whether the difficulties encountered in the production of subunit-specific antisera are due to contamination of the subunit preparations or to the presence of shared determinants on A and B subunits was not determined.

Monoclonal antibody technology pioneered by Kohler and Milstein (1975, 1976) provides a means of overcoming the limitations inherent in conventional antisera production. Because a monoclonal antibody is a single molecular species, it can specifically detect a particular epitope of a set of antigenic determinants displayed by a complex antigen, such as cholera toxin. Thus, monoclonal antibody preparations do not require the protocols of adsorption and purification necessary to render conventionally prepared polyclonal antisera epitope-specific. With monoclonal antibodies, toxin subunit specificity is not a problem if the antibodies are specific for unshared A or B subunit determinants.

Monoclonal antibodies are produced by hybrid cells (hybridomas) derived from the fusion of mouse myeloma cells and lymphocytes from the spleens of mice that have been previously immunized with a particular antigen. The resulting hybridomas display the cellular immortality of the tumor cell parent and the immunoglobulin production of the mouse B lymphocyte lineage cell parent.

In this paper we report the derivation, stabilization, and characterization of 15 hybridoma cell lines which produce antibody specific for the determinants of cholera toxin.

Production of Monoclonal Antibody-Secreting Hybridomas

In order to obtain predominantly IgM-producing hybridomas, approximately 8-week-old female BALB/cJ mice were intraperitoneally primed with 50 µg alum-precipitated purified cholera toxin (Sigma Chemical Co., St. Louis, MO) in complete Freund's adjuvant. Four days after priming, spleen cells from these mice were fused to the nonsecreting mouse myeloma cell line SP 2/0 with polyethylene glycol by the procedure of Goldsby et al. (1977). The cells were plated in 96-well microtiter plates and hybrid cells selected using Littlefield's (1967) hypoxanthine-aminopterin-thymidine medium in which only hybrid cells will grow.

In order to obtain predominantly IgG-producing hybridomas, approximately 8-week-old female BALB/cJ mice were multiply immunized with cholera toxin, according to the method of Svennerholm et al. (1978). The hyperimmunized mice were allowed to rest two months, after which they were boosted with alum-precipitated cholera toxin four days before their spleen cells were fused to SP 2/0 cells and plated, as above.

Approximately two weeks after fusion, microtiter wells containing single or double macroscopic clones were tested for specific antibody production using an indirect-solid-phase RIA. Flexible, polyvinyl chloride, 96-well microtiter plates were coated with the antigen (20 µl of 10 µg cholera toxin or toxin subunit/ml PBS) and incubated for one hour at room temperature. The plates were washed three times with PBS-bovine serum albumin (PBS-BSA; PBS containing 0.1% BSA and 0.01% NaN_3) to remove unbound antigen and to block unoccupied sites on the polyvinyl chloride well. Approximately 50 µl of culture supernatant or serum dilution was added to duplicate wells, incubated one hour and washed three times with PBS-BSA. Bound antibody was detected with ^{125}I-labeled sheep antibody to murine immunoglobulins, (IgA, IgG_1, IgG_{2a}, IgG_{2b}, and IgM), which had been purified by adsorption to a mouse immunoglobulin affinity column. Twenty µl (approximately 10,000 cpm) of the labeled reagent was added to each well and incubated one hour at room temperature. Unbound label was removed by washing three times with PBS-BSA. The wells were cut apart with a hot wire device (D. Lee Co., Sunnyvale, CA) and counted on a gamma counter (Beckman Gamma 4000, Irvine, CA). Samples with a signal-to-noise ratio greater than or equal to 2 were considered positive. The initial clonal response of hybrids from these two fusions are shown in Figures 1 and 2.

Culture wells containing positive clones were recloned by limiting dilution at least three times to ensure mono-clonality. Fifteen positive hybridoma cell lines were stabilized. All of the stabilized hybridoma lines were pre-served by freezing cell cultures and the solid tumors

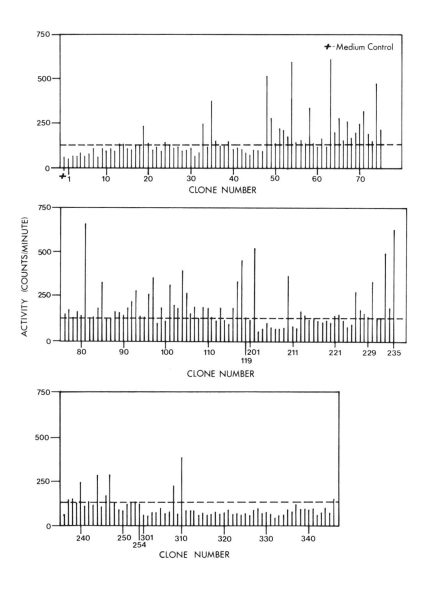

Figure 1. Initial clonal response of hybrids derived from primed mouse spleens. Bar height indicates activity of bound ^{125}I-labeled sheep antimouse immunoglobulin. The horizontal broken line indicates a signal-to-noise ratio of 2. The medium control (✦) is shown. Clone numbers 1-119, 201-254, 301-345 represent clones tested on the first, second and third days, respectively.

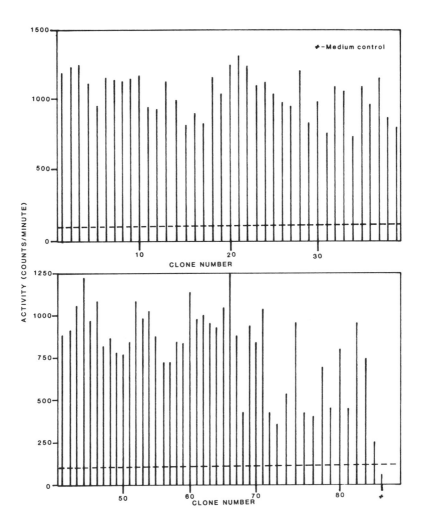

Figure 2. Initial clonal response of hybrids derived from multiply-boosted mouse spleens. See Figure 1 legend.

produced by subcutaneous injection of hybridoma cells into BALB/cJ mice. All have been successfully thawed and demonstrated to continue antibody secretion.

Characterization of Monoclonal
Antibodies to Cholera Toxin

The 15 monoclonal antibodies derived were characterized by testing specificity to cholera toxin, by determination of heavy and light chain classes, and by determination of subunit specificity.

All 15 monoclonal antibodies were tested for specificity to cholera toxin by determining reactivity against the unrelated antigen, bovine serum albumin (BSA), which was a component of the RIA washing protocol. The results of the indirect-solid-phase RIA, using BSA-coated plates, showed that all 15 monoclonal antibodies were specific for cholera toxin.

The heavy and light immunoglobulin chain classes of each of the antibodies were determined using heavy chain and light chain specific antisera (Litton Bionetics, Kensington, MD) and polyacrylamide gel electrophoresis. The heavy and light chain specific antisera were used to coat plates in the indirect-solid-phase RIA described above. All the antibodies contained the predominant murine light chain, kappa. Of the antibodies tested, 4 contained the μ heavy chain and 11 contained the γ_1 heavy chain. Results are given in Table 1.

Subunit specificity of the monoclonal antibodies was determined using purified A and B subunit, kindly provided by Dr. R. Finkelstein (University of Missouri, Columbia). The subunits were coated on plates used in the indirect-solid-phase RIA described above. The reactivities of each antibody against the purified A and B subunits of cholera toxin are shown in Figure 3. Of the antibodies tested, 3 were specific for the A subunit of cholera toxin, 10 were specific for the B subunit and 2 appeared to react with both subunits. A summary of the results (Table 1) lists the subunit specificity and the isotype of each of the monoclonal antibodies. A-specific, B-specific, and

Table 1. Summary of Monoclonal Antibody Subunit Specificity and Heavy Chain Class[a]

Monoclonal Antibody Number	Toxin Subunit Specificity[b]	Heavy Chain Class
LHR-117-63	B	M
LHR-117-233	B	M
LHR-117-235	A & B	M
LHR-227-2	B	G_1
LHR-227-6	B	G_1
LHR-227-8	B	G_1
LHR-227-13	B	G_1
LHR-227-32	A	M
LHR-227-45	B	G_1
LHR-227-53	B	G_1
LHR-227-58	A	G_1
LHR-227-59	B	G_1
LHR-227-62	A	G_1
LHR-227-65	B	G_1
LHR-227-77	A & B	G_1

[a]Reprinted, by permission, from Remmers, E.F., R.R. Colwell, and R.A. Goldsby. 1982. Infect. Immun. 37:70-76.
[b]Subunits A and B of cholera toxin (see text).

A+B-specific antibodies of each isotype--IgM and IgG_1--were stabilized and characterized.

CONCLUSIONS

A total of 15 monoclonal antibodies specific for cholera toxin were derived and stabilized. Both IgG_1 and IgM isotypes were obtained. The IgG antibodies are particularly well suited to affinity column techniques since the antigen-antibody complex can be disassociated by gentle means. Thus, the toxin and its individual subunits should be readily purified by affinity column techniques. The IgM antibodies, on the other hand, are useful as binding reagents in ELISA (enzyme-linked immunosorbent assay) or RIA because of their decavalent nature and subsequent high avidity for antigen. The results of the two hybridizations described here demonstrate that it is possible to tailor monoclonal antibodies of a desired class by the immunization scheme used. Thus, the LHR-117 series of antibodies, derived from primed mice, are all of the IgM class and the LHR-227 series of antibodies, derived from multiply boosted mice, are predominantly of the IgG class. Within each isotype class, both A subunit and B subunit specific anti-bodies were derived. These reagents should prove useful in the detection of cholera toxin and its subunits.

Since monoclonal antibodies detect specific antigenic determinants, the battery of monoclonal antibodies produced using the toxin of the classical strain of Vibrio cholerae, 569 B, can be employed to determine the antigenic related-ness of toxins, elaborated by other strains, to that of 569 B. Also, functionally or biochemically related toxin mole-cules from other sources can be examined for antigenic relatedness to the classical cholera toxin.

SUMMARY

Monoclonal antibody-producing cell lines were derived from the fusion of mouse myeloma cells and spleen cells from mice immunized with cholera toxin. A total of 15 cell lines which produced antibody specific for cholera toxin were stabilized in culture and immortalized by freezing cultured cells and tumor cells which had been grown subcutaneously in mice. All cell lines continued antibody secretion upon thawing. The antibodies produced by the hybridoma cell lines were characterized by determination of the class of light and heavy chain components and by determination of specificity for cholera toxin subunit A or B. All the anti-bodies contained the kappa light chain; 4 contained the μ

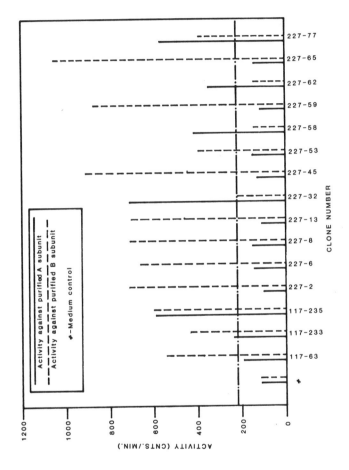

Figure 3. Subunit specificity of monoclonal antibodies prepared against cholera toxin. The solid bars indicate activity against purified A subunit. The broken bars indicate activity against purified B subunit. The horizontal bar represents a signal-to-noise ratio of 2. The medium control (✦) is shown. Reprinted, by permission, from Remmers, E.F., R.R. Colwell, and R.A. Goldsby. 1982. Infect. Immun. 37:70-76.

heavy chain, and the remaining 11 the γ_1 heavy chain. Ten of the monoclonal antibodies were specific for the B subunit of cholera toxin and three were specific for the A subunit. The remaining two appear to react with both subunits.

ACKNOWLEDGMENTS

This work was supported by the University of Maryland Graduate School and the National Science Foundation in a graduate fellowship awarded to Elaine F. Remmers. Additional support for this investigation was supplied by Public Health Service Grant R22-AI-14242, awarded under the U.S.-Japan Cooperative Medical Science Program by the National Institute of Allergy and Infectious Diseases. This work is from a dissertation to be submitted to the Graduate School, University of Maryland, by E.F. Remmers in partial fulfillment of the requirements for the Ph.D. degree in Microbiology.

REFERENCES

Baselski, V., R. Briggs, and C. Parker. 1977. Intestinal fluid accumulation induced by oral challenge with Vibrio cholerae or cholera toxin in infant mice. Infect. Immun. 15:704-712.

Ceska, M., F. Effenberger, and F. Grossmuller. 1978. Highly sensitive solid-phase radioimmunoassay suitable for determination of low amounts of cholera toxin antibodies. J. Clin. Microbiol. 7:209-213.

Craig, J.P. 1965. A permeability factor (toxin) found in cholera stools and cultures filtrates and its neutralization by convalescent cholera sera. Nature 207: 614-616.

De, S.N. 1959. Enterotoxicity of bacteria-free culture-filtrate of Vibrio cholerae. Nature 183:1533-1534.

Donta, S.T., H.W. Moon, and S.C. Whipp. 1974. Detection of heat-labile Escherichia coli enterotoxin with use of adrenal cells in tissue culture. Science 183:334-336.

Goldsby, R.A., B.A. Osborne, E. Simpson, and L.A. Herzenberg. 1977. Hybrid cell lines with T-cell characteristics. Nature 267:707-708.

Guerrant, R.L., L.L. Brunton, T.C. Schnaitman, L.I. Rebhun, and A.G. Gilman. 1974. Cyclic adenosine monophosphate and alteration of Chinese hamster ovary cell morphology: a rapid, sensitive in vitro assay for the enterotoxins of Vibrio cholerae and Escherichia coli. Infect. Immun. 10:320-327.

Hejtmancik, K.E., J.W. Peterson, D.E. Markel, and A. Kurosky. 1977. Radioimmunoassay for the antigenic determinants of cholera toxin and its components. Infect. Immun. 17:621-628.

Holmes, R.K., W.B. Baine, and M.L. Vasil. 1978. Quantitative measurements of cholera enterotoxin in cultures of toxigenic wild-type and nontoxigenic mutant strains of Vibrio cholerae by using a sensitive and specific reversed passive hemagglutination assay for cholera enterotoxin. Infect. Immun. 19:101-106.

Kohler, G. and C. Milstein. 1975. Continuous cultures of fused cells secreting antibody of predefined specificity. Nature 256:495-497.

Kohler, G. and C. Milstein. 1976. Derivation of specific antibody producing tissue culture and tumor lines by cell fusion. Eur. J. Immunol. 6:511-519.

Littlefield, J.W. 1964. Selection of hybrids from matings of fibroblasts in vitro and their presumed recombinants. Science 145:709-710.

Svennerholm, A.-M., S. Lange, and J. Holmgren. 1978. Correlation between intestinal synthesis of specific immunoglobulin A and protection against experimental cholera in mice. Infect. Immun. 21:1-6.

Chapter 11

PRELIMINARY OBSERVATIONS ON VIBRIO FLUVIALIS INDURATION FACTOR(S)

Susan L. Payne, Ronald J. Siebeling,
and Alworth D. Larson

In 1980, we began to assay the hemolymph and feces of live blue crabs for the presence of Vibrio cholerae. More than 50 V. cholerae non-O1 serovars as well as other species of Vibrio were isolated. Numerous isolates were identified as Vibrio fluvialis or group F vibrios (Lee et al. 1981). The identifications were confirmed by D. Tison at Oregon State University (personal communication). We set up an enzyme-linked immunosorbent assay (ELISA) to assay for cholera toxin production by the V. cholerae non-O1 isolates re-covered from crabs. Toxin production by V. cholerae reference strains was tested by the rabbit skin test assay (Craig 1965). During one assay, the concentrated filtrate of a V. fluvialis isolate, DJVP 6957, was injected along with V. cholerae filtrates. The isolate originated from a case of human gastroenteritis in Indonesia and was sent to us by R. Seidler, Oregon State University. The DJVP 6957 culture filtrate produced a large, red indurated reaction similar to, but not identical to, those produced by purified cholera toxin (Sigma Chemical Co., St. Louis, MO). V. fluvialis has been isolated from patients with diarrhea and produces an "enterotoxin" which provokes positive reactions in the Y-1 adrenal cell assay and in rabbit ileal loop assays (Seidler et al. 1980). We have found that these organisms also produce "toxins" detectable by the rabbit skin test, and we are now using this assay to test isolates from both environmental and clinical sources.

V. fluvialis isolates which were tested for toxin activity were grown in Casamino Acids-glucose media with yeast extract (Sack et al. 1980). The cultures were grown on a rotary shaker at 37°C for 18 to 24 hours. Cells were pelleted and the supernatant fluids were filtered through 0.45-μm filters. Filtrates were lyophilized and dissolved in dH_2O at one-tenth the original volume and dialyzed against phosphate-buffered saline (PBS), pH 7.4. Eight-to-ten-week-old rabbits were shaved and depilated 12 to 24 hours prior to skin testing. One-tenth ml volumes of each concentrated filtrate to be tested were injected intradermally in a random fashion. The area of each induration was measured at 18 to 24 hours postinjection. Table 1 shows the mean and range of 3 to 12 injections for each organism tested. Most filtrates were tested in two or more rabbits. The skin reactions were measured in two directions and the skin results are reported as mm^2 induration. Environmental and clinical V. fluvialis isolates produced similar reactions as did both aerogenic and anaerogenic biotypes. Strain 10-19b is a non-O1 V. cholerae crab isolate. This organism was negative for cholera toxin in the ELISA assay yet provoked a skin reaction. It appears that many environmental vibrios may produce toxic factors.

When skin-tested rabbits were injected intravenously with 2% Trypan blue dye, the indurated reactions turned blue (results not shown)--indicating that culture filtrates produced increased capillary permeability. However, we found that, in our hands, the blueing response was inconsistent. When dye was injected 18 hours after skin testing, small indurated skin test sites were more likely to blue than large reactions. As a result, we chose to measure induration directly rather than blueing as a measure of toxin production.

Preliminary attempts were made to isolate the induration factors (IFs) present in culture supernatant fluids of DJVP 6957. Culture filtrates were prepared as described above and then concentrated by lyophilization (whole, concentrated fraction) or by passage over a diaflo XM-50

Table 1. Induration Factor Activity of Concentrated Vibrio fluvialis Filtrates

Strain	Source	mm^2 Induration Mean	Range
6957[a]	Human gastroenteritis	210	200–225
2386[a,b]	River water	555	375–690
2391[a,b]	River water	300	225–375
9-4[b]	Crab feces, May 1980	47	16–100
9-26a	Crab feces, May 1980	33	9–36
9-48c	Crab feces, May 1980	80	36–100
10-2e	Crab feces, June 1980	82	25–121
10-50d	Crab feces, June 1980	280	25–1200
12-1h[b]	Crab feces, August 1980	214	144–400
12-3k	Crab feces, August 1980	144	81–225
12-5e[b]	Crab feces, August 1980	498	400–595
12-6j	Crab feces, August 1980	120	36–225
12-9f	Crab feces, August 1980	81	36–144
10-19b	V. cholerae non-O1, crab feces	400	180–750

[a]Received through R. Seidler, Oregon State University.
[b]Aerogenic biotype.

membrane (Amicon Corp., Lexington, MA). The membrane-retained fraction was washed extensively with PBS. Table 2 shows the effect of heat on both the whole concentrated and the membrane-retained fractions. Argarwal and Sanyal (1981) reported that V. fluvialis filtrates retained

Table 2. Effect of Heat on Induration Factor Activity in Rabbit Skin Tests

Temp °C	Minutes	mm^2 Induration	
		Whole Filtrate 10X	XM-50 Retained 10X
56	0	280	400
	15	–	200
	30	–	135
	60	76	200
65	0	210	210
	15	121	0
	30	90	0
	60	85	0
80	0	210	210
	10	0	0
	30	0	0

enterotoxin activity after being heated for 30 minutes at 65°C, whereas 85°C destroyed toxin activity. They suggested that the heat stability of their enterotoxin preparations may be due to some undefined protecting factor(s) present in the culture supernatant fluids. The results in Table 2 show a difference in the heat sensitivity of the membrane-retained fractions versus whole concentrated filtrates. The membrane-retained fraction remained active after heating for 1 hour at 56°C but was inactivated by heating at 65°C for 15 minutes. Whole concentrated filtrates retained partial activity after heating at 65°C for 1 hour. Both preparations lost all detectable IF activity when heated for 10 minutes at 80°C. Some yet to be defined substance in whole filtrates may protect IF activity since the more purified membrane-retained preparation was more heat sensitive. Another possibility for the observed difference in heat sensitivity between whole and XM-50 retained fractions may be due to the presence of more than one IF in culture filtrates. We have recently separated three IF activities from crude concentrated filtrate by gel filtration (see Author's Note). It is possible a heat-stable IF was separated from a heat-labile IF during the concentration and washing steps.

Table 3 shows the results of a few early attempts to characterize IF activity. Whole concentrated filtrates were dialyzed and treated with Pronase at pH 8.0, DNase at pH 5.5, or RNase at pH 8.0 for 60 minutes at 37°C. The final concentration of each enzyme used was 1 µg of enzyme per 100 µg of total protein. None of these enzymes reduced IF activity when compared to control IF incubated under the same conditions at the appropriate pH. Controls of each enzyme plus media were negative by the skin test assay. Table 3 also shows the results of EDTA treatment of IF activity. Filtrates were dialyzed extensively at 4°C, and Na$_2$EDTA was added to give 0.2 M. The EDTA was dissolved by stirring at room temperature and the filtrate was concentrated by passage through an XM-50 membrane. The membrane-retained material was washed two times with 100 ml of deionized water. EDTA treatment appeared to have no effect on IF activity.

CONCLUSIONS

We have reported preliminary results of studies of an induration or permeability factor(s) present in V. fluvialis filtrates. It has not been established if IF activity is identical to the enterotoxin activity reported for some V. fluvialis isolates although this is clearly a possibility. We hope to purify and characterize the IF(s) produced by V. fluvialis DJVP 6957 and compare these to the IF(s) produced by environmental isolates. The role of an enterotoxin or other toxic factors has not been established in the pathogenicity of V. fluvialis. It may be of interest to attempt to study the role of the induration factors as an environmental survival factor since all isolates recovered

Table 3. Effects of Various Treatments on V. fluvialis Induration Factor Activity

	Treatment	Mean mm^2 Induration
1.	Whole Filtrate (10X)	310
	Plus Pronase	225
	Plus RNase	225
	pH 8.0 control	130
	Plus DNase	175
	pH 5.5 control	110
2.	Media	
	Plus Pronase	0
	Plus RNase	0
	Plus DNase	0
3.	Dialyzed Filtrate (10X)	280
	Plus EDTA (7X)	208

from the environment to date appear to produce these factors.

Author's Note

Since the initial presentation of this data we have separated from culture filtrates three induration factors by gel filtration. Crude concentrated filtrates were applied to a 46 x 1.5 cm column of Sephadex G-100 (Pharmacia Fine Chemicals, Piscataway, NJ) and were eluted with .02 M phosphate buffer, pH 7.4. One-ml fractions were collected and assayed for absorbence at 280 nm and for IF activity in the rabbit dermis. The column was calibrated with molecular weight standards for estimation of the MW of IF activity peaks. Three peaks of activity were observed, one eluting in the void volume, a second eluted at 45-50,000 MW, and the third in the range of 15-20,000 MW. These peaks did not correspond to discrete A_{280} peaks. The presence of more than one induration factor makes the characterization of IF activity in whole filtrates of questionable value.

ACKNOWLEDGMENTS

This research was supported by grants from the Louisiana Department of Health and Human Resources and the National Oceanic and Atmospheric Administration Office of Sea Grant, U.S. Department of Commerce, under Grant NA79AA-D-00128.

REFERENCES

Argarwal, R.K., and S.C. Sanyal. 1981. Experimental studies on enteropathogenicity and pathogenesis of group "F" vibrio infections. Zentralbl. Backteriol. Parasitenkd. Infektionski. Hyg. 249:392-399.

Craig, J.P. 1965. A permeability factor (toxin) found in cholera stools and culture filtrates and its neutralization by convalescent cholera sera. Nature 207:614-616.

Lee, J.V., P. Shread, and A.L. Furniss. 1981. Taxonomy and description of Vibrio fluvialis sp. nov. (Synonym group F vibrios, group EF-6). J. Appl. Bacteriol. 50:73-94.

Sack, D.A., S. Huda, P.K.B. Neogi, R.R. Daniel, and W. Spira. 1980. Microtiter ganglioside enzyme-linked immunosorbent assay for vibrio and Escherichia coli heat-labile enterotoxin and antitoxin. J. Clin. Microbiol. 11:35-50.

Seidler, R.J., D.A. Allen, R.R. Colwell, S.W. Joseph, and O.P. Daily. 1980. Biochemical characteristics and virulence of environmental group F bacteria isolated in the United States. Appl. Environ. Microbiol. 40:715-720.

Molecular Genetic
Aspects of Vibrios

Chapter 12

PLASMIDS IN MARINE VIBRIO SPP.: INCIDENCE AND DETERMINATION OF POTENTIAL FUNCTIONS USING NUMERICAL TAXONOMIC METHODS

Howard S. Hada and Ronald K. Sizemore

There have been relatively few comprehensive studies examining the ecology of extrachromosomal DNA elements, or plasmids, in marine bacteria. Surveys determining the distribution of plasmids in the environment have dealt largely with nonmarine bacteria (Kelch and Lee 1978; Smith 1970; Sturtevant et al. 1971). The few reports concerning marine bacteria have described primarily R plasmids, which mediate resistances to antibiotics (Sizemore and Colwell 1977; Timoney et al. 1978). Many of the bacterial plasmids discovered in the marine ecosystem are cryptic in nature and have unknown functions (Guerry and Colwell 1977). In view of the lack of information concerning plasmids in marine bacteria and the potential ecological significance, this study was conducted to screen a large number of Vibrio spp. for the incidence of plasmids and to attempt to determine plasmid functions using a numerical taxonomic approach (Sneath and Sokal 1973).

METHODS AND RESULTS

Marine vibrios were isolated from two areas of the Gulf of Mexico, a site located about 50 km south-southeast of

183

Galveston Island, Texas, and a rock jetty extending about 0.25 km from the island into the Gulf. Four collections (spring, summer, fall, and winter) were taken at the offshore location and a single summer collection was taken at the near-shore site. Isolation and identification of vibrios has been previously described (Hada and Sizemore 1981).

Plasmid screening included a technique for the isolation of large molecular weight plasmids (Hansen and Olsen 1978) and a modification of the "cleared lysate" method (Clewell and Helinksi 1969). Detection of plasmids was accomplished by agarose gel electrophoresis (Hada and Sizemore 1981; Meyers et al. 1976). Plasmid sizes (average molecular masses) were estimated by comparing migration distances with plasmid standards included in each agarose gel experiment. Figure 1 illustrates a standard curve derived from the relative mobilities of plasmids with previously characterized molecular weights. Four reference strains of Escherichia coli containing plasmids Col El (4.2 megadaltons [Mdal]), R6-K (24.7 Mdal), RP 4 (34 Mdal), and R6-5 (61 Mdal) were provided by D. Zink, Texas A&M University, College Station, Texas. G. Thorn of Tufts University in Boston, Massachusetts provided a strain of E. coli containing plasmid 3ΔSm (6 Mdal).

Determination of potential plasmid functions by numerical taxonomy required tests which allowed separation of the vibrios into phenetic groups. Preparation and composition of media employed--SWYE, MSWYE, YE broth and agar, and three-salts solution--has been described elsewhere (Colwell and Wiebe 1970). Vibrios were tested for ability to grow at temperatures of 10°C, 15°C, 37°C, and 42°C by inoculating SWYE broth and incubating for 72 hours. Isolates were also tested for ability to grow at 0, 4, 6, 8, and 10% salinity by inoculating YE broth containing appropriate concentrations of NaCl. Cultures were incubated at 25°C for 72 hours. To test for bacterial bioluminescence, isolates were inoculated onto SWYE agar plates and incubated at 25°C for 36 hours. Luminescence was determined by examining colonies in the dark.

Marine isolates were tested for the ability to utilize 64 single carbon sources for growth. Single carbon source

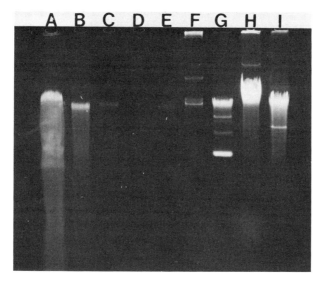

Figure 1. Ethidium bromide stained agarose gel photographed under an ultraviolet transilluminator. Lanes A, B, C, D, E, G, and I contained cleared lysates from marine Vibrio spp. Lanes F and H contained lysates from strains of E. coli with plasmids R6-K and R6-5 respectively.

utilizations serve as taxonomic distinctions and as tests for possible plasmid-mediated functions. Glassware was cleaned in a chromic acid bath to prevent organic contamination. Each medium consisted of three-salts solution and 2% agar supplemented with 0.001 M potassium nitrate, 0.001 M potassium phosphate, and 100 mg/ml of each filter-sterilized substrate, pH 8.0. Inoculated cultures were incubated at 25°C for 120 hours.

Hydrocarbon utilization was tested by transferring each isolate into a chromic acid-cleaned test tube containing three-salts solution with 0.001 M potassium nitrate, 0.001 M potassium phosphate, and 0.1 ml whole crude oil obtained from Buccaneer Gas and Oil field (Jackson 1979). Cultures were incubated at 25°C for 692 hours.

Tests to determine other potential plasmid functions included antibiotic and heavy metal resistance and plasmid-mediated antibiotic production. Resistances to 11 antibiotics

were determined by inoculating SWYE agar plates, dis-
pensing antibiotic discs (BBL Microbiology Systems, Cockeysville, MD), and allowing to incubate at 25°C for 36
hours. Sensitivity patterns were interpreted using information from a chart supplied by the manufacturer. A list of
antibiotics tested and a zone interpretation chart are
included in Table 1.

Resistance to either lead nitrate, mercuric chloride, or
zinc chloride was tested by inoculating cultures onto a
medium consisting of MSWYE agar containing an appropriate
concentration of each filter-sterilized heavy metal. Appropriate concentrations of each metal were determined by
testing for levels which inhibited growth of nonplasmid-
containing marine isolates and selected standard strains
(Beneckea harveyi KN 96 [K. Nealson, Scripps Institute of
Oceanography, San Diego, CA] and Vibrio parahaemolyticus
Sak 4 [R.R. Colwell, University of Maryland, College Park,
MD]). Cultures inoculated onto heavy metal-containing
plates were incubated at 25°C for 120 hours.

Vibrios were tested for the ability to produce antibacterial agents (i.e. bacteriocin and microcin [McCall and
Sizemore 1979; Baquero et al. 1978]) using strips of cellulose dialysis membrane, preconditioned according to manufacturer's instructions, embedded in SWYE agar. Each
isolate was spotted on four areas of a plate; two were above
the membrane. Plates were incubated at 25°C until dense
growth was observed. Agar was inverted and indicator
organisms (KN 96 and Sak 4) were streaked onto halves so
that each was both above embedded membrane and areas
lacking the material. Plates were incubated an additional 24
to 36 hours. Isolates producing bacteriocin, a nondializable
substance, caused clearing of an indicator lawn over an
area lacking, but not under, the membrane. Production of
microcin, a dializable antibacterial substance, caused
clearing in all areas of a plate.

Computer analysis to group vibrios was based on
phenetic data comprising more than 100 bits of information
including taxonomic tests, potential plasmid-mediated
functions, and plasmid incidence and characteristics (i.e.
molecular weight and multiplicity). The computer method
employed was a cluster analysis based on a two-dimensional

matrix or table of strains by features (Walczak and Krichevsky 1980). Data were clustered using simple matching coefficient, and the clustering method was unweighted average linkage (Sneath and Sokal 1973). Correlations between high plasmid incidence and phenetic traits were made by visually searching for distinguishing characteristics in clustered strains.

A total of 543 isolates were judged to be Vibrio spp. according to the identification procedures employed. Of that total, 512 strains yielded lysates which could be analyzed for the presence of plasmids. Figure 2 shows an ethidium bromide-stained agarose gel photographed over an ultraviolet transilluminator. Lanes A, B, C, D, E, G, and I contained cleared lysates from marine vibrios. Lanes F and H contained lysates from two E. coli strains containing either plasmids R6-K or R6-5. Among the isolates examined, 143 (28%) demonstrated distinct plasmid bands. Percentages of plasmid-containing strains among groups of offshore vibrios isolated on a seasonal basis were not significantly different ($P > 0.05$). A 12% rate of plasmid carriage among near-shore isolates, however, appeared to be significantly different ($P = 0.025-0.01$).

More than half of all plasmids detected were estimated to have molecular masses in a range of 0 to 12 Mdal. Most of the plasmids in that size class were either 0 to 2 or 9 to 11 Mdal. There was a fairly even distribution of numbers of plasmids in size classes to 80 Mdal. While there were a few plasmids estimated to have masses greater than 80 Mdal, none larger than 100 Mdal were observed.

Plasmid multiplicity (i.e. different plasmids carried by a single strain) was observed in almost half of the plasmid-containing strains. Multiple plasmid bands ranging from 2 to 7 were observed in individual isolates.

Large percentages (> 30%) of the vibrios tested demonstrated resistance to six antibiotics. The frequency of plasmid-containing strains among each group of resistant strains was determined (Table 1). Eight of eleven of the resistant groups were determined to have frequencies of plasmid-containing strains greater than 30%.

A low percentage (< 10%) of the strains were resistant to the three heavy metals tested. Within the group of

Table 1. Antibiotic Sensitivity Patterns of Vibrio spp. and the Incidence of Plasmids in the Resistant Strains

Antibiotic	% Resistant[a]	% Intermediate	% Sensitive	% Plasmid Incidence Among Resistant Strains
Ampicillin	32.9	1.4	65.2	32.9
Bacitracin	87.9	1.3	10.8	18.0
Chloramphenicol	4.7	2.9	92.4	40.0
Kanamycin	51.4	37.3	11.3	34.4
Nalidixic Acid	19.1	43.7	37.2	46.0
Neomycin	19.2	40.0	40.8	35.1
Novobiocin	37.9	30.1	32.0	40.2
Polymyxin-B	19.0	7.9	73.1	16.1

Streptomycin	62.7	20.1	17.2	27.6
Tetracycline	44.9	21.3	33.8	40.5
Triple Sulfa	20.1	8.7	71.2	36.0

[a]Resistance and sensitivity patterns were interpreted using information from BBL Zone Size Interpretation Chart. Inhibition zones were established with nonmarine bacteria by BBL.

resistant strains however, more than 40% contained detectable plasmids.

Few (< 3%) of the vibrios demonstrated the ability to produce antibacterial agents. Plasmids were observed in 21% of the vibriocin-producing and in 13% of the microcin-producing strains.

Computer analysis of phenetic data using simple matching average linkage resulted in 27 strain clusters based on relatedness at an 80% level. The 2 largest clusters contained 135 and 130 strains respectively and 10 clusters were doublets. Plasmid frequency was unevenly distributed among the clusters with 9 having a plasmid frequency of 0%.

Table 2 lists 3 clusters which demonstrated plasmid frequencies greater than the overall plasmid incidence of 28%. Cluster C demonstrated a 93% incidence of plasmids contained in strains within the group. Phenetic characteristics associated with the group are resistance to lead nitrate (17%) and luminescence (52%). Strains in cluster D had a 41% plasmid incidence. Growth at 15°C was a positive feature (83%) in this group. Strains in cluster I had a 72% plasmid incidence. Chloramphenicol resistance (28%) and polymyxin B resistance (50%) were distinguishing characteristics of strains in this group.

DISCUSSION

This survey of plasmid incidence has shown that these elements occur frequently in marine Vibrio spp. This result is somewhat unexpected since the marine ecosystem has been characterized as a nutrient deficient environment (Carlucci 1974). It seems reasonable that energy limitations might reduce the rate of carriage of nonessential factors such as plasmids. The frequency observed compares to rates discovered in other groups of both terrestrial (Smith 1971) and marine bacteria (Guerry and Colwell 1977; Dastidar et al. 1977). However, it was also observed that plasmids in marine vibrios tend to have small molecular weights. Whether or not this characteristic of vibrio plasmids can be attributed to nutrient levels remains to be

Table 2. Groups of Vibrio spp. which Cluster at the 80% Level and have Plasmid Frequencies Greater than 28%

Cluster Designation	No. of Strains in the Cluster	Distinguishing Taxonomic Characteristics	Plasmid Frequency
C	45	Lead nitrate resistance, Luminescence	93%
D	27	Growth at 15°C	41%
I	18	Chloramphenicol resistance, Polymyxin-B resistance	72%

seen. The small molecular weight of many vibrio plasmids indicated that transmissible plasmids in this group of organisms may be uncommon since exchange of these elements has been related to their size (Novick 1969). The study has also shown that plasmids do not occur homogeneously among vibrios, but appear to be group related. Genetic flexibility in groups of marine vibrios may be enhanced with the carriage of small plasmids which often occur in multiple forms.

Determination of potential plasmid functions included testing for well-documented plasmid-mediated traits. Plasmid frequencies were determined for each group of strains demonstrating specific functions. If the percentage of plasmids was higher in the group than the average plasmid incidence (28%), then the group was assumed to have some strains exhibiting plasmid-mediated functions. Most notable were groups of strains demonstrating resistance to a number of antibiotics and to all of the heavy metals tested. Such comparisons do not, however, rule out the possibility of plasmid-mediated functions in groups with low incidences of plasmid-containing strains.

Numerical taxonomy was used in this study as an approach to determine potential plasmid functions. Numerical taxonomy is used to form natural phenotypic clusters from a variety of unweighted characters. This approach is useful to separate chromosomal traits from plasmid traits in that the cluster is biased toward overall similarity or chromosomal traits. If plasmid occurrence is recorded for each strain and included with the data, the clusters should form without much input from the plasmid characters (i.e. occurrence of plasmid and an unknown plasmid trait). Therefore, the technique removes the taxonomic or chromosomal traits by clustering and permits correlations between non-chromosomal traits (i.e. plasmid traits). Plasmid occurrence correlated with unique traits exhibited by members of a cluster should be detected more easily.

Computer analysis of phenetic data helped confirm correlations between antibiotic and heavy metal resistances and plasmid occurrence in groups of clustered vibrios. Since numerical taxonomy theoretically separates chromosomal from plasmid functions, these correlations give strong indications that the traits are plasmid mediated. This approach can greatly reduce the multitude of potential tests for plasmid curing experiments, which are more substantial proof of function. The incidence and computer data give an insight as to the ecology of plasmids in marine Vibrio spp.

REFERENCES

Baquero, F., D. Bouanchaud, M.C. Martinez-Perez, and C. Fernandez. 1978. Microcin plasmids: a group of extra-chromosomal elements coding for low-molecular-weight antibiotics in Escherichia coli. J. Bacteriol. 135: 342-352.

Carlucci, A.F. 1974. Nutrients and microbial response to nutrients in seawater. Pages 245-248 in R.R. Colwell and R.Y. Morita (Eds.), Effect of the ocean environment on microbial activities, University Park Press, Baltimore.

Clewell, D.B., and D.R. Helinksi. 1969. Supercoiled circular DNA-protein complex in Escherichia coli: purification and induced conversion to an open circular DNA form. Proc. Natl. Acad. Sci. U.S.A. 62:1159-1166.

Colwell, R.R., and W.J. Wiebe. 1970. "Core" characteristics for use in classifying aerobic, heterotrophic bacteria by numerical taxonomy. Bull. Ga. Acad. Sci. 28:165-185.

Dastidar, S.G., R. Poddar, R. Kumar, and A.N. Chakrabarty. 1977. Incidence and elimination of R plasmids in Vibrio cholerae. Antimicrob. Agents and Chemother. 11:1079-1080.

Guerry, P., and R.R. Colwell. 1977. Isolation of cryptic plasmid deoxyribonucleic acid from Kanagawa-positive strains of Vibrio parahaemolyticus. Infect. Immun. 16:328-334.

Hada, H.S., and R.K. Sizemore. 1981. Incidence of plasmids in marine Vibrio spp. isolated from an oil field in the northwestern Gulf of Mexico. Appl. Environ. Microbiol. 41:199-202.

Hansen, J.B., and R.H. Olsen. 1978. Isolation of large bacterial plasmids pMG1 and pMG5. J. Bacteriol. 135:227-238.

Jackson, W.B. (Ed.). 1979. Environmental assessment of an active oil field in the northwestern Gulf of Mexico, 1977-1978. Volume III: Chemical and physical investigations. NOAA Annual Report to EPA, NTIS, Springfield, VA.

Kelch, W.J., and J.S. Lee. 1978. Antibiotic resistance patterns of gram-negative bacteria isolated from environmental sources. Appl. Environ. Microbiol. 36:450-456.

McCall, J.O., and R.K. Sizemore. 1979. Description of a bacteriocinogenic plasmid in Beneckea harveyi. Appl. Environ. Microbiol. 38:974-979.

Meyers, J.A., D. Sanchez, L.P. Elwell, and S. Falkow. 1976. Simple agarose gel electrophoretic method for the identification and characterization of plasmid deoxyribonucleic acid. J. Bacteriol. 127:1529-1537.

Novick, R.P. 1969. Extrachromosomal inheritance in bacteria. Bact. Rev. 33:210-235.

Sizemore, R.K., and R.R. Colwell. 1977. Plasmids carried by antibiotic resistant marine bacteria. Antimicrob. Agents and Chemother. 12:373-382.

Smith, H.W. 1970. Incidence in river water of Escherichia coli containing R factors. Nature 228:1286-1288.

Sneath, P.H.A., and R.R. Sokal. 1973. Numerical taxonomy: the principles of numerical taxonomy. W.H. Freeman and Co., San Francisco.

Sturtevant, A.B., G.H. Cassell, and T.W. Feary. 1971. Incidence of infectious drug resistance among fecal coliforms isolated from raw sewage. Appl. Environ. Microbiol. 21:487-491.

Timoney, J.F., J. Port, J. Giles, and J. Spanier. 1978. Heavy-metal and antibiotic resistance in the bacterial flora of sediments of New York Bight. Appl. Environ. Microbiol. 36:465-472.

Walczak, C.A., and M.I. Krichevsky. 1980. Computer methods for describing groups from binary phenetic data: preliminary summary and editing of data. Int. J. Sys. Bacteriol. 30:615-621.

Chapter 13

THE MOLECULAR GENETICS OF
CHOLERA TOXIN

John J. Mekalanos

Over the last decade a variety of mutations have been described which affect the production of cholera toxin by Vibrio cholerae. Mutations which cause either an increase or a decrease in toxin production have been isolated in the classical strain 569B, and some of these regulatory mutations have been mapped on the V. cholerae chromosome. However, mutations in the structural genes for the toxin have never been described for this strain. An explanation for this inability to obtain toxin structural gene mutations in 569B has come from DNA hybridization experiments in which the cholera toxin genes are detected with radioactive probes derived from the heat-labile enterotoxin (LT) genes of Escherichia coli. These studies indicate that strain 569B contains a duplication of the cholera toxin A and B subunit genes. Similar studies indicate that genetic duplication of the cholera toxin operon is a common phenomenon in both classical and El Tor strains of V. cholerae. Although many strains contain toxin operon duplications which appear to have similar chromosomal locations, other strains contain one or more operon copies which occupy unique chromosomal sites. The variation in chromosomal location and copy number of the toxin operon suggests that the toxin genes may be associated with a genetic element capable of amplification and transposition.

This paper reviews published observations relating to the genetics of toxin production in V. cholerae and attempts to integrate these findings with our most recent results concerning the molecular structure and organization of the cholera toxin genes.

Regulatory Mutations Affecting
Toxin Production in V. cholerae

The highly toxinogenic strain, 569B, has been the most widely used strain of V. cholerae for studies addressing the protein chemistry and genetics of cholera toxin (Collier and Mekalanos 1980). Baine et al. (1978) reported the mapping of several mutations which resulted in a three log drop in toxin production by this strain. The site at which these mutations mapped was designated the tox locus and showed genetic linkage to the his region of the V. cholerae chromosome. We have also mapped a number of similar mutations causing coordinate depression of A and B subunit production in 569B. These all appear to map in between his and cys markers and are presumably allelic mutations in the tox locus. The phenotype of mutations in the tox locus can be explained by a number of models, three of which are presented on the right half of Figure 1. Recent evidence in my laboratory favors the first model in which the tox locus codes for a positive control element required for toxin expression in strain 569B. We have shown that the tox locus does not define any toxin structural genes by performing Southern blot hybridization analysis on certain tox genetic recombinants (see below). Moreover, we have shown that this regulatory site exists in at least one El Tor strain which does not possess toxin structural genes in the cys his region.

Another interesting regulatory site has been mapped which mediates the elevation of toxin production in hypertoxinogenic mutants of V. cholerae (Mekalanos and Murphy 1980). This site, called htx, has the characteristics of a negative control site since mutations in this locus cause an increase in toxin production. Furthermore, potentially allelic mutations in the ltx locus map very close to the htx

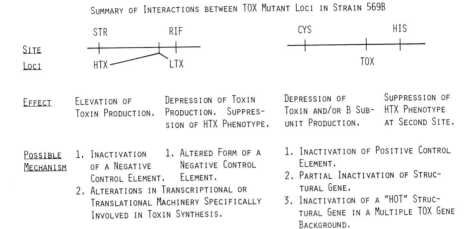

Figure 1. Toxin regulatory mutations. The htx, ltx, and tox loci are genetic sites which map as shown and which mediate the effects on toxin production noted. Some possible molecular mechanisms responsible for these effects are given.

locus but mediate the opposite effect--depression of toxin production. The relative frequency of htx and ltx mutations are consistent with a model in which the htx locus codes for a toxin operon repressor (Figure 1). However, the location of this site in the str-rif region also suggests that these mutations may define some alteration in the translational or transcriptional machinery which is specific to toxin expression.

The notable absence of mutations in 569B that abolish toxin synthesis or result in production of a structurally altered toxin molecule has until recently been a mystery and suggested the toxin might play some indispensable role in the physiology of V. cholerae.

Cross Hybridization of the LT Genes and V. cholerae DNA

The heat-labile enterotoxin of E. coli (LT) has recently been shown to be markedly similar to cholera toxin in its protein chemistry (Clements and Finkelstein 1979). More-over, the cloned A and B subunit genes of LT have been shown to hybridize to V. cholerae DNA restriction frag-ments under conditions of reduced stringency (Moseley and Falkow 1980). That these LT-homologous, V. cholerae restriction fragments code for cholera toxin was demon-strated by two recent results. We have shown that several phage-induced, nontoxinogenic mutants of the El Tor strain RV79 have lost all or part of the LT-homologous sequences (Mekalanos et al. 1982). Apparently, these nontoxinogenic mutants have deletion mutations in the cholera toxin genes induced by the mutagenic phage. A more straight forward proof that these LT-homologous sequences code for cholera toxin was demonstrated by our experiments involving the molecular cloning of these sequences. We have shown that a 5 kilobase fragment containing LT-homologous sequences derived from strain 569B does indeed code for production of cholera toxin in E. coli K12 (Pearson and Mekalanos 1982). This result leaves no doubt that the LT-homologous sequen-ces in V. cholerae are the genes coding for cholera toxin. Physical analysis of the cloned fragment has shown that the cholera toxin operon, like the LT operon (Dallas et al. 1979), is polycistronic with the A gene proximal to the B gene.

Multiple Toxin Gene Copies
in V. cholerae 569B

Moseley and Falkow (1980) have reported that Southern blot analysis utilizing LT-A and LT-B probes indicated that V. cholerae might contain multiple toxin gene copies. We have recently completed a detailed analysis of 569B and have concluded that this strain contains a duplication of the toxin A and B subunit genes (Pearson and Mekalanos 1982). This conclusion is based primarily on the observation that most restriction enzymes give two bands which hybridize to both the LT-A and B probes when analyzing 569B DNA by the Southern method (Figure 2). One of the two 569B toxin operons has been cloned and characterized (Pearson and Mekalanos 1982).

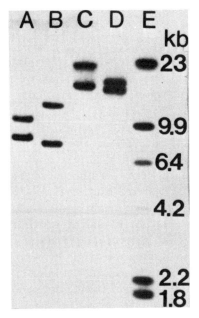

Figure 2. Southern blot hybridization. 569B DNA was digested with the indicated restriction enyzmes, and analyzed by the Southern method using the radioactively labeled LT-A probe (5). Lane A, Xba I; B, Bgl II; C, Sal I; D, Hind III; E, ^{32}P-labeled λ Hind III standards.

The existence of a toxin operon duplication in 569B offers a plausible explanation for why it has been difficult to isolate nontoxinogenic mutants of this strain. If both gene copies are biosynthetically active, then only regulatory mutations which simultaneously affect both gene copies would give rise to altered toxinogenic phenotypes in 569B. Accordingly, mutations in the tox, htx, and ltx loci most likely define regulatory alterations which coordinately affect both copies of the toxin operon in strain 569B. Consistent with this observation, we have found that a regulatory region proximal to the toxin's A cistron is conserved in both copies of the toxin operon present in strain 569B and is probably the location of the toxin promoter and operator sites.

Incidence of Toxin Gene
Duplication in V. cholerae

Analysis of a variety of other strains of V. cholerae isolated in many different geographical locations throughout the last 30 years has revealed that toxin operon duplications are very common among V. cholerae strains of the classical biotype (Figure 3). Moreover, the chromosomal location of the toxin gene copies is highly conserved in these strains. About 75% of the V. cholerae El Tor strains we tested possessed only a single copy of the toxin operon. However, several El Tor strains have been identified which also contain toxin operon duplications (Figure 3). Some of these latter strains have toxin genes which occupy positions similar to those seen in classical strains (Figure 3). This result suggests that a preference exists for the location of the cholera toxin genes on the V. cholerae chromosome. This preference is not absolute inasmuch as several other strains have one or more toxin operon copies at unique sites on the V. cholerae chromosome. Indeed, we have observed triplication (Figure 3, lane 9) and even further amplification of the toxin operon in other strains of V. cholerae. We think that the marked variation in copy number and chromosomal location of the cholera toxin genes may indicate that the toxin operon resides on a genetic element associated with some form of illegitimate recombination. If such an element was also capable of genetic transposition (e.g., a cholera toxin transposon) it would also provide a possible mechanism by which the toxin gene has become widely distributed in nature.

It has been shown that strains of V. cholerae exist in the environment which lack the structural genes for the toxin (Kaper et al. 1981). Sporadic outbreaks of toxinogenic cholera near these environmental sources suggest that acquisition of the toxin genes by previously nontoxinogenic V. cholerae might be associated with these isolated cases. The delivery of a toxin transposon into a nontoxinogenic strain by a transducing phage or conjugative plasmid might be one possible means of attaining this conversion.

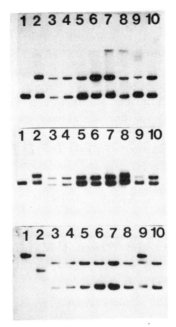

Figure 3. Southern blot hybridization. DNA from 10 different strains of V. cholerae was digested with Pst I (upper set), Xba I (middle set), or Ava I (lower set). Southern blot analysis with LT-A probe was performed on these digestions after electrophoresis in a 0.7% agarose gel (5). Strains 1-3 are of the El Tor biotype and strains 4-10 are of the classical biotype.

CONCLUSION

The cholera toxin operon has been shown to exist in duplicated form in most classical strains of V. cholerae. El Tor strains may contain single or multiple copies of the toxin operon which occupy either similar or unique sites on the V. cholerae chromosome. A strong conservation of the location at which the duplications exist in classical strain suggests that the genetic element responsible for the gene duplication might have site-specific insertion properties. Specific localization of the toxin genes might also be important to its expression if these locations define cis acting regulatory sites at which toxin positive or negative control elements bind. The possible existence of the toxin genes on a transposable genetic element also provides a mechanism by which these genes might be disseminated in nature to nontoxinogenic strains of V. cholerae and other procaryotic species.

The same evolutionary pressures responsible for selection and maintenance of toxin operon duplications in epidemic strains of V. cholerae may also act to strongly select rare genetic recombinants of environmental strains of V. cholerae which have acquired the cholera toxin genes.

ACKNOWLEDGMENTS

This work was supported by U.S. Public Health Service Grant AI-18045 from the National Institute of Allergy and Infectious Disease and also by the Medical Foundation, Inc. of Boston, Massachusetts.

REFERENCES

Baine, W.B., M.L. Vasil, and R.K. Holmes. 1978. Genetic mapping of mutations in independently isolated nontoxinogenic mutants of Vibrio cholerae. Infect. Immun. 21:194-200.

Clements, J.D., and R.A. Finkelstein. 1979. Isolation and characterization of homogeneous heat-labile enterotoxins with high specific activity from Escherichia coli cultures. Infect. Immun. 24:760-769.

Collier, R.J., and J.J. Mekalanos. 1980. ADP-ribosylating exotoxins. Pages 261-291 in Multifunctional proteins. H. Bisswanger and E. Schmincke-Ott (Eds.), John Wiley and Sons, New York.

Dallas, W.S., D.M. Gill, and S. Falkow. 1979. Cistrons encoding Escherichia coli heat labile toxin. J. Bacteriol. 139:850-858.

Kaper, J.B., S.L. Moseley, and S. Falkow. 1981. Molecular characterization of environmental and nontoxinogenic strains of Vibrio cholerae. Infect. Immun. 32:661-667.

Mekalanos, J.J., and J.R. Murphy. 1980. Regulation of cholera toxin production in Vibrio cholerae: genetic analysis of phenotypic instability in hypertoxinogenic mutants. J. Bact. 141:570-576.

Mekalanos, J.J., S.L. Moseley, J.R. Murphy, and S. Falkow. 1982. Isolation of enterotoxin structural gene deletion mutations in Vibrio cholerae induced by two mutagenic vibriophages. Proc. Natl. Acad. Sci. U.S.A. 79:151-155.

Moseley, S.L. and S. Falkow. 1980. Nucleotide sequence homology between the heat-labile enterotoxin gene of Escherichia coli and Vibrio cholerae deoxyribonucleic acid. J. Bact. 144:444-446.

Pearson, G.D.N., and J.J. Mekalanos. 1982. Molecular cloning of Vibrio cholerae enterotoxin genes in Escherichia coli K-12. Proc. Natl. Acad. Sci. U.S.A. 79:2976-2980.

Chapter 14

EXTRACHROMOSOMAL DNA IN
VIBRIO CHOLERAE

D.L. Glassman, L.B. Edelstein,
and L.A. McNicol

Our laboratory is studying the extent and nature of genetic exchange in naturally occurring populations of microorganisms. We have particularly wanted to examine the ways in which information can be mobilized across species or generic boundaries in the environment. Vibrio cholerae has been one of the model systems we are looking at because of what we know about the genetics of the toxin genes: The major virulence factor of V. cholerae is a multi-subunit enterotoxin protein (tox), encoded by chromosomal genes. Tox sequences occur in multiple copies in some V. cholerae strains, but are totally missing in others (Kaper et al. 1981). The cholera tox protein shares extensive sequence homology and immunologic cross-reaction with a heat-labile enterotoxin (elt) produced by certain strains of Escherichia coli. As expected, the elt and tox DNA sequences show a high degree of cross-hybridization, but the elt genes are carried on an extrachromosomal genetic element (So et al. 1978). These facts suggest that at some time V. cholerae and E. coli exchanged the genetic information for elaboration of toxic protein. And we'd like to find out how.

Transposable Elements in
Vibrio cholerae

A major mechanism for the mobilization of DNA is the presence of transposable genetic sequences (Kleckner 1977). We surveyed a number of Vibrio type strains, as well as clinical and environmental V. cholerae, for the presence of known IS or tn elements. DNA from bacteriophage lambda containing inserts of IS1 or tn5 in the b2 region was radio-labelled by nick translation (Maniatis et al. 1975) and used as a probe against colony (Grunstein and Hogness 1975) or Southern (Southern 1975) blots of Vibrio DNA. Table 1 summarizes this data. The tn5 element is found in both the Enterobacteriaceae and Pseudomonadaceae organisms tested. And IS1 is present in the enteric strains studied. However, V. cholerae and strains from six other Vibrionaceae genera did not contain either of these common transposable elements.

Extrachromosomal Elements in
Indigenous Estuarine Microorganisms

The Vibrionaceae are a significant component of the aquatic estuarine microflora. In order to have a background against which to assess the extent of plasmid carriage by V. cholerae, we have characterized the plasmid DNA species found in microorganisms indigenous to the Chesapeake Bay estuarine system. Random isolates totaling 248 collected from three different locations over a three-year period were screened for the presence of extrachromosomal DNA using a horizontal in-the-well lysis agarose gel electrophoretic technique (Newland et al. 1980). Forty-four percent of these organisms carried at least one plasmid species. The identity of strains which demonstrated plasmid carriage was investigated by a limited taxonomic study of 14 standard tests. The isolates could be clustered into 12 groups (Table 2). The largest group was identified as the family Vibrionaceae. Other major clusters included Flavobacterium, Enterobacteriaceae, and Bacillus organisms. The relationship between taxonomic group and

Table 1. Incidence of IS1 and tn5 Translocatable Elements

Organism	Strain	IS1	tn5
Escherichia coli	CR63	+	+
	H10407	+	+
	PRC107	NT	+
	PRC116	NT	+
	RP4	+	+
	W3110	+	+
Salmonella typhimurium	LT2	+	+
Shigella dysenteriae	SH16	+	+
Aerobacter aerogenes		+	+
Pseudomonas marina		−	+
Pseudomonas aeruginosa	ATCC10145	−	+
	ATCC27853	−	+
Aeromonas hydrophila	A17	−	−
	ATCC7966	−	−
	M2C7	−	−
	8AE	−	−
Aeromonas sobria	A16	−	−
Vibrio cholerae	ATCC14033	−	−
	ATCC14035	−	−
	CA401	−	−
	569B	−	−
	LSU3−35a	−	−
	2927A	−	−
	1878G	−	−
	SGN7077	−	−
	1881	−	−
	1880	−	−
	1878A	−	−
	152B−4	−	−
	1521	−	−
	1191−1A2	−	−
Vibrio fisheri	ATCC7744	−	−
Vibrio fluvialis	C5125	−	−
Vibrio parahaemolyticus	ATCC17749	−	−
	ATCC17802	−	−
	SAK8	−	−
	VpCR	−	−

the presence of large (greater than 10^6 daltons) plasmids and multiple plasmid species is also documented in Table 2. An unusually high proportion of the vibrios were among the strains carrying multiple extrachromosomal DNA bands.

Low molecular weight plasmids (3-5 x 10^6) formed the most prevalent class found among estuarine bacteria (85% of the total extrachromosomal DNA species). The relationships between these plasmids were assessed by DNA-DNA hybridization, using plasmids purified by CsCl-ethidium bromide density gradient centrifugation (Davis et al. 1980) as probes. Table 3 summarizes the results of these experiments. The Vibrionaceae plasmid species probe cross-reacted with plasmids found in other vibrios, but also showed homology with plasmids from enteric and unidentified oxidase-positive, catalase reference plasmids of known incompatibility groups, nor did it contain IS1 or tn5 sequences. The function of the vibrio plasmids was not identified. They do not code for elaboration of bacteriocins or for resistance to ampicillin, chloramphenicol, erythromycin, kanamycin, nalidixic acid, streptomycin, tetracycline, $HgCl_2$, $CdCl_2$, $NiCl_2$, or $PbCl_2$.

Plasmid Carriage in Vibrio cholerae

We have used the same techniques to examine plasmid carriage in 108 strains of V. cholerae. These organisms were from both clinical (32%) and environmental (68%) sources and came from such diverse regions as Bangladesh, India, Great Britain, the Chesapeake Bay, Florida, Louisiana, and Oregon. As Table 4 demonstrates, 15% of these isolates carried extrachromosomal DNA. The molecular weights of these plasmids ranged from 25 to 3 x 10^6, but the majority were small. All were cryptic in function.

There was a striking correlation between serovar (as tested by the LSU and Sakazaki typing systems) and plasmid carriage among the V. cholerae isolates we have studied. Table 5 documents the low occurrence of extra-chromosomal DNA among strains of the O1 serovar, which is traditionally associated with virulence (Finkelstein 1973). The non-O1 plasmid-bearing strains fell into 18 different

Table 2. Taxonomic Grouping of Plasmid-Bearing Estuarine Bacteria

Taxonomic Group	Number of Strains	Number of Strains Carrying Large Plasmids	Number of Strains Carrying Multiple Plasmids
1. Bacillus spp.	13	2	2
2. Micrococcaceae	3	1	1
3. Acinetobacter spp.	3	2	2
4. Alcaligenes spp.	8	0	1
5. Pseudomonas spp.	5	1	1
6. Vibrionaceae	20	4	10
7. Enterobacteriaceae	12	3	3
8. Flavobacterium-Cytophage-Flexibacter (Chromogens)	16	2	2
9. Fermentative, oxidase (+), catalase (+), nitrate (-), Gram (-) rods	12	0	0
10. Fermentative, oxidase (+), catalase (-), Gram (-) rods	6	2	2
11. Fermentative, oxidase (-), catalase (+), nitrate (-), Gram (-) rods	6	1	2
12. Atypical	4	1	0
TOTAL	108		

Table 3. Hybridization of Estuarine Plasmid DNA Probes to DNA from Colony and Southern Blots of Estuarine Bacteria

Taxonomic Group[a]	Strain[b]	Group 9 (Ox+ Cat+) pDG128	Plasmid Probe Vibrionaceae pDG1-pDG2	Flavobacterium pDG64
1. Bacillus spp.	T3	+	−	−
	T5	−	−	NT[c]
	B8	+	−	−
	S22	−	−	−
	S42	−	−	NT
	BP146	+	−	NT
2. Micrococcaceae	BP184	−	NT	NT
	JF32	−	−	NT
3. Acinetobacter spp.	JF19	−	−	NT
4. Alcaligenes spp.	BP58	−	−	+
	BP62	−	−	+
	BP120	−	−	−
	JF14	NT	−	+
5. Pseudomonas spp.	JF28	−	−	−
6. Vibrionaceae	T2	−	+	−
	T87	−	+	+
	T89	−	+	−
	T102	−	+	−
	BP199	−	−	NT

		Col 1	Col 2	Col 3
7. Enterobacteriaceae	T64	−	−	NT
	T104	−	+	NT
	S39	−	−	−
	JF7	−	−	NT
8. _Flavobacterium_	T100	−	−	NT
	B17	−	NT	NT
	S4	−	−	+
	JF4	−	−	−
	JF6	−	−	−
9. Ox$^+$ Cat$^+$	T13	+	−	−
	T72	−	−	+
	JF8	+	−	+/−^{d}
	JF17	−	−	+
10. Ox$^+$ Cat$^-$	T88	+	NT	NT
	T93	−	+	−
	T98	−	NT	NT
	T101	NT	+	NT
11. Ox$^-$ Cat$^+$	BP181	+	−	−
	BP192	+	−	NT
12. Atypical	S53	−	−	NT

^{a}From Table 2.
^{b}BP, Bloody Point sediment; JF, Jones Falls top water; and at Eastern Bay: T, top water; B, bottom water; and S, sediment.
^{c}NT, not tested.
^{d}+/−, equivocal results, weak hybridization.

211

Table 4. Correlation between Serovar and Plasmid Carriage in Vibrio cholerae

Source	Serovar		
	O1	non-O1	
Clinical	1/30 (3%)	2/5 (40%)	
Environmental	0/11 (0%)	14/62 (23%)	
Totals	1/41 (2%)	16/67 (24%)	16/108 (15%)

serovar groups. All five isolates of the W serovar which we have examined carried a small 3 megadalton plasmid. Although this is a small number of strains, we are currently attempting plasmid curing and DNA hybridization experiments to determine whether a unique plasmid species is associated with the group W antigen.

CONCLUSIONS

Our most significant finding has been the virtual absence of plasmid DNA in V. cholerae organisms of the O1 serovar. Of the 41 such strains isolated in the past ten years from clinical and environmental sources in various parts of the world, 1 contained extrachromosomal DNA. Using the same experimental procedures we can clearly demonstrate the frequent existence of plasmids in non-O1 serovars of V. cholerae, other Vibrio species, other genera within the Vibrionaceae family, and other gram-negative organisms.

This observation is consistent with a large body of work on antibiotic resistance in V. cholerae. Although plasmid-mediated drug resistance is extraordinarily common among other gram-negative enteric pathogen (Falkow 1974), it is rare among V. cholerae Ol organisms (Prescott et al. 1968; Kuwahara et al. 1967; Sack 1979). R-factors can be transferred to V. cholerae Ol strains by conjugation, but they are extremely unstable and show abnormal expression of plasmid encoded genes (Abe et al. 1966; Yokota et al. 1972; Hedges et al. 1977; Hedges and Jacob 1975).

The molecular basis for the absence of small cryptic plasmids or the instability of large R factors in Ol V. cholerae is not known. We examined membrane proteins of 24 Ol and non-Ol V. cholerae strains but could find no evidence of an "exclusion" or "immunity" protein in Ol serovars (Kelley, Colwell and McNicol, submitted). It has been observed that plasmids can reduce the growth rate of V. cholerae host cells (Yokota et al. 1975) and can sup-press the synthesis or release of cholera toxin in Ol V. cholerae (Sinha and Srivastava 1978). Therefore, it may be that Ol V. cholerae transcriptional or translational systems are particularly susceptible to interference by plasmid encoded genes.

REFERENCES

Abe, H., S. Goto, and S. Kuwahara. 1966. Transmission of multiple drug-resistance from Shigella to Aeromonas and non-agglutinable Vibrio through conjugation. Jap. J. Bacteriol. 21:266-273.

Davis, R.W., D. Botstein, and J.R. Roth. 1980. A manual for genetic engineering: advanced bacterial genetics. Cold Spring Harbor Laboratory. Cold Spring Harbor, New York.

Falkow, S. 1974. R Factors. Pion. London.

Finkelstein, R.A. 1973. Cholera. CRC Crit. Rev. Microbiol. 2:553-623.

Grunstein, M., and D.S. Hogness. 1975. Colony hybridiza-tion: a method for the isolation of cloned DNA's that contain a specific gene. Proc. Nat. Acad. Sci. U.S.A. 72:3961-3965.

Hedges, R.W., and A.E. Jacob. 1975. A 98 megadalton R factor of compatibility group C in a Vibrio cholerae El Tor isolate from southern U.S.S.R. J. Gen. Microbiol. 89:383-386.

Hedges, R.W., J.L. Vialard, N.J. Pearson, and F. O'Grady. 1977. R plasmids from Asian strains of Vibrio cholerae. Antimicrob. Agts. Chemother. 11:585-588.

Kaper, J.B., S.L. Moseley, and S. Falkow. 1981. Molecular characterization of environmental and nontoxigenic strains of Vibrio cholerae. Infect. Immun. 32:661-667.

Kleckner, N. 1977. Translocatable elements in procaryotes. Cell 11:11-23.

Kuwahara, S., S. Goto, M. Kimura, and H. Abe. 1967. Drug-sensitivity of El Tor Vibrio strains isolated in the Philippines in 1964 and 1965. Bull. W.H.O. 37:763-771.

Maniatis, T., A. Jeffery, and D.G. Kleid. 1975. Nucleotide sequence of the rightward operator of phage λ Proc. Nat. Acad. Sci. U.S.A. 72:1184-1188.

Newland, J.W., L.A. McNicol, M.J. Voll, and R.R. Colwell. 1980. Rapid screening for plasmids in environmental isolates of Vibrio cholerae by an in-the-well lysis technique using horizontal gel electrophoresis. Plasmid 3:238-239.

Prescott, L.M., A. Datta, and G.C. Datta. 1968. R-factors in Calcutta strains of Vibrio cholerae and members of the Enterobacteriaceae. Bull. W.H.O. 39:971-973.

Sack, R.B. 1979. Prophylactic antibiotics? The individual versus the community. New Engl. J. Med. 300:1107–1108.

Sinha, V.B., and B.S. Srivastava. 1978. Plasmid-induced loss of virulence in <u>Vibrio cholerae</u>. Nature 276: 708–709.

So, M., W.S. Dallas, and S. Falkow. 1978. Characterization of an <u>Escherichia coli</u> plasmid encoding for synthesis of heat-labile toxin: molecular cloning of a toxin determinant. Infect. Immun. 21:405–411.

Southern, E.M. 1975. Detection of specific sequences among DNA fragments separated by gel electrophoresis. J. Molec. Biol. 98:503–517.

Yokota, T., T. Kasuga, M. Kaneko, and S. Kuwahara. 1972. Genetic behavior of R factors in <u>Vibrio cholerae</u>. J. Bacteriol. 109:440–442.

Yokota, T., R. Kuwahara, and S. Kuwahara. 1975. Genetic and biological characterization of an R plasmid obtained from <u>Vibrio cholerae</u>. Pages 144–153 in Proc. 11th U.S.-Japan Joint Conf. Cholera.

Chapter 15

MOLECULAR TAXONOMY OF LACTOSE-FERMENTING VIBRIOS

David L. Tison, John Greenwood,
Mitsuaki Nishibuchi, and Ramon J. Seidler

The significance of a halophilic, lactose-fermenting Vibrio as an agent of septicemia and wound infection in humans is becoming increasingly apparent (Blake 1979; Kelly and Avery 1980; Kelly and McCormick 1981). This organism has been referred to as the lactose-positive (L+) Vibrio (Hollis et al. 1976), Beneckea vulnifica (Reichelt et al. 1976), and Vibrio vulnificus (Baumann et al. 1980; Farmer 1979, 1980). This organism is not the only vibrio capable of fermenting lactose, however. Vibrio cholerae and Vibrio nigripulchritudo (a former Beneckea species) can also ferment lactose; however, these Vibrio species can be distinguished phenotypically from V. vulnificus. Vibrio cholerae requires only trace amounts of Na$^+$ for growth and lactose fermentation is delayed if it occurs at all; V. nigripulchritudo produces a blue-black pigment. Vibrio vulnificus is non-pigmented and can be readily distinguished from V. cholerae on the basis of NaCl requirements and sucrose fermentation. The lactose phenotype is also present in an number of taxonomically undefined vibrios readily isolated from estuarine habitats (Oliver et al. 1981; Tison et al. 1981). Therefore, it is desirable to define V. vulnificus taxonomically in order to recognize this agent in both clinical and environmental sources.

217

In 1976 Hollis and coworkers showed that a group of halophilic organisms isolated from serious human infections, which they called the L+ Vibrio, could be distinguished phenotypically from V. parahaemolyticus and V. alginolyticus. Later in 1976 Reichelt, Baumann, and Baumann showed that the L+ Vibrio was distinct from other Vibrio species based on DNA-DNA hybridization studies and proposed the name Beneckea vulnifica. They also reported that B. vulnifica had a DNA base composition of about 47 mol% quanine + cytosine (mol% G+C). In 1977 Clark and Steigerwalt presented results of DNA-DNA hybridization experiments which confirmed the conclusion that the L+ Vibrio was distinct from other Vibrio species. However, these authors reported a DNA base composition of 50-53 mol% G+C for the lactose-positive Vibrio. In 1979, Farmer proposed that Beneckea vulnifica be classified in the genus Vibrio as V. vulnificus. However, Beneckea vulnifica appeared on the Approved Lists of Bacterial Names in 1980 while Vibrio vulnificus did not. Later in 1980 Baumann et al. proposed that the genus Beneckea be abolished and its species transferred to the genera Vibrio and Photobacterium. In the October 1980 issue of the International Journal of Systematic Bacteriology, Vibrio vulnificus was published as a revived name giving it valid standing in bacterial nomenclature (Farmer 1980).

As knowledge of the clinical significance of V. vulnificus as an agent of septicemia and wound infections has increased, interest in the ecology of this organism has been stimulated. Kelly and Avery (198) reported the isolation of V. vulnificus (referred to as L+ Vibrio in their paper) from seawater near Galveston, Texas. A study of the distribution of V. vulnificus in waters along the East Coast of the United States is currently underway (Oliver et al. 1981). The occurrence of V. vulnificus and other pathogenic vibrios is also being studied in Oregon, Maryland, Louisiana, and Florida estuaries by Sea Grant-sponsored research groups.

As a result of the apparent widespread distribution of V. vulnificus in estuarine environments, we became interested in determining the relatedness of clinical and environmental strains of V. vulnificus and identifying other lactose-fermenting vibrios from estuarine habitats, many of which were phenotypically different from V. vulnificus.

MATERIALS AND METHODS

Bacterial Strains Tested. From the Oregon State University (OSU) Vibrio culture collection, 137 strains were tested for lactose fermentation in Hugh-Leifson O/F medium (Difco) containing 0.5% NaCl. Selected strains of V. fluvialis, V. anguillarum and a taxonomically undefined arginine dihydrolase-positive (ADH), lactose-fermenting vibrio are listed in Table 1. Selected V. vulnificus and reference strains of other taxa in the family Vibrionaceae are shown in Table 5.

Biochemical Characteristics. Methods used to test biochemical characteristics are explained in Table 2. Test cultures were grown on trypticase soy agar (Difco) for approximately 24 hours prior to inoculation into test media. All test media contained 0.5% NaCl except 1% peptone water for the NaCl tolerance test.

Mouse LD_{50}. Test organisms were grown in tryptic soy broth without dextrose (Difco) supplemented with 0.5% sodium chloride (TSB') for 10 hours at 25°C. Tenfold dilutions made in 0.01 M phosphate-buffered saline (pH 7.2) were injected intraperitoneally into Swiss-Webster mice weighing 17-20 g. After 72 hours, mortality was recorded and LD_{50} values were determined by the method of moving averages (Maynell and Maynell 1965).

Pathogenicity for Eel. Eel pathogenicity tests were performed as described by Muroga et al. (1976).

DNA Studies. Cells were grown in TSB' for 24 hours at 37°C on a reciprocal shaker. Cells were harvested by centrifugation, washed with 0.01 M phosphate-buffered saline, and stored frozen until DNA extraction was done. DNA was extracted and purified with phenol using conventional techniques previously published (Johnson

Table 1. Characteristics of Selected ADH-Positive Vibrios

Strain	Source	Mol% G+C	0/129 Sensitivity (MIC)	NaCl Tolerance (Maximum)	Arabinose	Lactose
Vibrio fluvialis						
DJVP 7092	Feces-Indonesia	50	150 µg/ml	10%	+	+
F43[a]	Water-Louisiana	51	150 µg/ml	7%	+	-
F16	Sediment-Louisiana	51	150 µg/ml	7%	+	-
LADHHR 75	Water-Louisiana	50	150 µg/ml	7%	+	-
WA-0-010	Water-Oregon	51	50 µg/ml	10%	+	-
VFL strains						
HOG-3[a]	Oyster-Louisiana	46	10 µg/ml	7%	+	-
OY-0-005	Oyster-Oregon	46	10 µg/ml	7%	+	-
CL-0-001	Clam-Washington	45	10 µg/ml	7%	+	-
WA-0-017	Water-Oregon	44	10 µg/ml	7%	+	-
V. anguillarum						
LS 174	Salmon-Oregon	44	10 µg/ml	7%	-	-
ALP strains						
OY-0-002[a]	Oyster-Oregon	43	10 µg/ml	5%	-	+
OY-0-004	Oyster-Washington	44	10 µg/ml	5%	-	+
OY-0-006	Oyster-Oregon	44	10 µg/ml	5%	-	+

[a]Reference strains.

Table 2. Biochemical Characteristics for Four Groups of Lactose-Fermenting Vibrios

Test or Substrate	V. vulnificus	V. cholerae	Unidentifiable ADH + vibrios	Unidentifiable ADH - vibrios
Oxidase (Kovacs)	+[a]	+	+	+
Gelatin Hydrolysis				
0% NaCl	-[b]	+	-	-
3% NaCl	+	+	+	+
O/129 sensitive (10 µg/ml)	+	+	+	+
Moellers' Decarboxylase Medium				
Arginine dihydrolase (ADH)	-	-	+	-
Ornithine decarboxylase (ODC)	+	+	-	d[c]
Lysine decarboxylase (LDC)	+	+	-	d
Indole Production	+	+	-	d
Voges-Proskauer	-	+	-	-
Fermentation of				
Sucrose	-	+	+	-
D-Glucose	+	+	+	+
Lactose	d	(+)[d]	+	(+)
D-Mannitol	d	+	d	d
L-Arabinose	-	-	-	-
Amygdalin	+	-	-	-

[a] + = > 90% of strains positive.
[b] - = > 90% of strains negative.
[c] d = 11-89% of strains positive.
[d] (+) = reaction delayed $\geq$ 3 days.

1981). Labeled reference DNA was prepared by growing cells in 200 ml of TSB' and 5 mCi of ^{3}H-thymidine (New England Nuclear). Cultures were incubated 18 hours at 37°C on a shaker. Cells were harvested and the DNA purified as described above. Purified ^{3}H-labeled reference DNA had a specific activity of 4 to 5 x 10^4CPM/μg DNA.

The DNA base composition (mol% G+C) was determined by the thermal melting technique, employing the relationship between mid-point temperature (Tm) and mol% G+C described by Mandel et al. (1970). DNA-DNA competition hybridization experiments were done using the membrane filter technique (Johnson 1981). Renaturation buffer consisted of 2X SSC (SSC is 0.15 M NaCl and 0.015 M trisodium citrate, pH 7) plus 40% dimethyl sulfoxide (DMSO). Renaturation was carried out at a temperature of 15° or 25°C below the DNA thermal denaturation temperature as measured in the renaturation buffer.

RESULTS AND DISCUSSION

Lactose-fermenting vibrios from the OSU Vibrio culture collection could be placed into four groups based on phenotypic characteristics. V. vulnificus strains fermented lactose in 48 hours or less while lactose fermentation by V. cholerae strains were generally delayed (5-10 days) as stated previously. Two groups of taxonomically undefined Vibrio also fermented lactose. One group was arginine dihydrolase-positive (ADH) and fermented lactose rapidly (< 48 hours) while the other group fermented lactose in 2-5 days, was ADH-negative and exhibited some divergence in a number of other traits. Because of the limited number of strains and the phenotypic heterogeneity of the last group these strains were not examined further.

In order to determine the taxonomic and genetic relationship between the ADH-positive, lactose-positive vibrios and other phenotypically similar (ADH-positive) vibrios these strains were compared to V. fluvialis, V. anguillarum, and a group of vibrios which were tentatively identified as 0/129 sensitive (10 μg/ml) V. fluvialis.

Based on characteristics listed in Table 1, the ADH positive vibrios fall into four general groups: (1) V. fluvialis strains which are more resistant to the vibriocidal compound 0/129 and have a DNA base composition of 50-51 mol% G+C; (2) V. fluvialis-like (VFL) strains which are arabinose-positive, sensitive to low concentrations (10 µg/ml) of 0/129, and have a DNA base composition of 44-46 mol% G+C; (3) V. anguillarum strains which are arabinose negative, 0/129 sensitive (10 µg/ml), and have a DNA base composition of 44-46 mol% G+C: and (4) ADH-positive, lactose-positive (ALP) strains which are arabinose-negative, less tolerant of high NaCl concentrations (5% maximum), and have a DNA base composition of 43-44 mol% G+C.

The results of DNA-DNA competition experiments conducted at stringent temperature (Tm-15°C) using V. fluvialis, a VFL strain, and an ALP strain as references are shown in Tables 3, 4, and 5, respectively. The data in Table 3 show that all of the V. fluvialis strains are related at the species level [> 75% relative reassociation at stringent temperature is indicative of species level of relatedness (Brenner 1969)]. They are also genetically distinct from the VFL and ALP strains, and V. vulnificus. Table 4 presents data which indicates the VFL strains are in fact atypical V. anguillarum Type I. These strains were originally identified as V. fluvialis which were sensitive to 0/129 (10 µg/ml), however, the genetic data indicate that these strains which are arabinose-positive and indole-negative are atypical V. anguillarum. The results in Table 5 show that the ALP strains are related at the species level and are genetically distinct from V. fluvialis (see Table 3), V. anguillarum, and V. vulnificus--indicating that these strains may represent a previously undescribed species in the genus Vibrio.

In order to determine the relationship between clinical and environmental isolates of V. vulnificus these strains are compared for phenotype, for pathogenicity to mice, for DNA base composition, and for DNA-DNA homology. Strains tested and their sources are listed in Table 6. Clinical and environmental V. vulnificus strains were phenotypically indistinguishable (Table 7), and the DNA base composition of about 47-48 mol% G+C is comparable to that reported in

Table 3. Reassociation of V. fluvialis Environmental Isolate F43 DNA with Other Vibrio spp.

Competitor DNA	% RR[a]
Vibrio fluvialis	
F43	100
DJVP 7092	90
F16	91
LADHHR 75	93
WA-0-010	94
VFL strain	
HOG 3	23
ALP strains	
OY-0-005	19
OY-0-002	15
OY-0-004	16
OY-0-006	23
V. vulnificus	
ATCC 27562	13

[a]% RR = Percent relative reassociation.

the original description of the species (Reichelt et al. 1976).

The results of DNA-DNA competition experiments between clinical and environmental V. vulnificus strains and other Vibrionaceae are shown in Table 8. These data show that clinical and environmental strains of V. vulnificus are genetically related with > 85% relative reassociation at stringent temperature indicative of the species level of relatedness. These results support the conclusion of others (Clark and Steigerwalt 1977; Reichelt et al. 1976) that V. vulnificus is genetically distinct from other valid Vibrio species. Based on these results, it can be concluded the V. vulnificus strains which are present in a wide range of geographically distinct estuarine habitats are phenotypically

Table 4. Reassociation of VFL strain HOG 3 DNA with Other Vibrio spp.

Competitor DNA	% RR[a]
VFL strains	
HOG 3	100
OY-0-005	98
WA-0-012	98
CL-0-001	90
V. anguillarum Type I	
LS-174	92
V. anguillarum Type II	
MSC-275	71
V. fluvialis	
F43	27
V. fluvialis	
WA-0-010	23
V. vulnificus	
11-3M-30	22

[a]% RR = Percent relative reassociation.

and genetically indistinguishable from clinical V. vulnificus isolates and may be of public health significance, either as agents of septicemia due to the consumption of contaminated shellfish or in wound infections following exposure to seawater.

It should be noted however that one strain not classified as V. vulnificus did show significant reassociation (97% at stringent temperature) with the environmental V. vulnificus reference strain (Table 8). This strain was isolated from diseased eels cultured in Japan (Muroga et al. 1976) and classified as V. anguillarum type B according to the description of Nybelin (1935). Since this biotype did not have valid taxonomic standing, Muroga et al. (1976) suggested that these strains be classified as V. anguillicida

Table 5. Reassociation of ALP strain OY-0-022 DNA with Other Vibrio spp.

Competitor DNA	% RR[a]
ALP strains	
OY-0-002	100
OY-0-004	100
OY-0-006	86
VLF strains	
OY-0-005	23
CL-0-001	1
WA-0-017	16
Vibrio anguillarum LS174	24
V. vulnificus ATCC 27562	20

[a] % RR = Percent relative reassociation.

as described by Bruun and Heiberg (1932). The name V. anguillicida was not validly proposed under the current rules of bacterial nomenclature, however. DNA-DNA homology studies indicated that these strains were not genetically related to other Vibrio species tested, although V. vulnificus was not included in those experiments (Nishibuchi et al. 1979). In order to confirm the initial observation that the eel isolate was genetically related to V. vulnificus, additional DNA-DNA competition experiments were done. The results of these experiments shown in Table 9 indicate that the three eel isolates are genetically related to the reference V. vulnificus strains at the species level (there was > 90% relative reassociation between these strains at stringent temperature). The phenotypic characteristics of V. vulnificus and the eel isolates are shown in Table 10. As a whole these strains are quite similar phenotypically with the major difference being that V. vulnificus strains were indole-positive while the eel isolates were negative. The eel isolates were also variable in the fermentation of lactose and arabinose and negative for mannitol fermentation

Table 6. Sources of Strains Used in the Comparison of Clinical and Environmental V. vulnificus Strains

Organism	Strain	Source
Vibrio (Beneckea) vulnificus	ATCC 27562 (CDC B9629)	Blood-Florida
V. vulnificus	CDC B51	Blood-Hawaii
V. vulnificus	11-3M-30	Crab feces-Louisiana
V. vulnificus	A38	Crab feces-Oregon
V. vulnificus	CDC A8694 (ATCC 29307)	Blood-Florida
V. vulnificus	79-11-114	Seawater-Texas
V. vulnificus	80-02-125	Blood-Texas
V. cholerae[a]	WA-0-18	Seawater-Oregon
V. parahaemolyticus[a]	CDC A8659	Gastroenteritis-Maryland
V. alginolyticus[a]	ATCC 17749	Seawater-Japan
V. anguillarum[a]	LS-174	Salmon-Oregon
V. anguillicida	ET-7617	Eel-Japan
V. fluvialis[a]	2386	River water-UK
Aeromonas hydrophila[a]	NMRI 7	Wound infection-Maryland

[a]strains included in DNA-DNA homology experiments only.

Table 7. Phenotypic Characteristics of Selected Clinical and Environmental Isolates of V. vulnificus

Test or Substrate	Clinical Isolates (n=4)	Environmental Isolates (n=3)
Oxidase (Kovacs)	+[a]	+
Indole production	+	+
Voges-Proskauer	-[b]	-
Simmons' Citrate	+	+
ADH	-	-
LDC + ODC	+	+
Growth in 1% Peptone Plus		
0% + 7% NaCl	-	-
3% + 5% NaCl	+	+
D-Glucose	+	+
Sucrose	-	-
Lactose	+	+
Salicin	+	+
Amygdalin	+	+
D-Mannitol	d[c]	d
D-Mannose	+	+
L-Arabinose	-	-
mol% G+C	46.8-47.8	47.3-47.5
Mouse LD_{50}	10^5-10^7	10^7-10^8

[a] + = > 90% of strains positive.
[b] - = > 90% of strains negative.
[c] d = 11-89% of strains positive.

while the V. vulnificus strains were positive for lactose, negative for arabinose, and variable for mannitol fermentation. Both of these groups were pathogenic to mice although the V. vulnificus strains of both clinical and environmental origin were not pathogenic to eels.

The results of the DNA-DNA competition experiments indicate that V. vulnificus and the eel isolates were the

Table 8. Reassociation of DNA from Clinical (B51) and Environmental (11-3M-30) Isolates of V. vulnificus with Other Members of the Family Vibrionaceae

| Source of the Unlabeled | Relative % Reassociation | | | |
| | V. vulnificus BST[a] | | V. vulnificus 11-3M-30[a] | |
Competitor DNA	Tm-25°	Tm-15°	Tm-25°	Tm-15°
V. vulnificus B51	100	100	85	88
V. vulnificus 11-3M-30	82	95	100	100
V. vulnificus ATCC 27562	86	87	88	95
V. vulnificus A38	109	87	98	92
V. vulnificus A8694	103	92	92	87
V. vulnificus 79-11-114	82	90	95	90
V. vulnificus 80-02-125	102	95	72	85
V. cholerae WA-0-18	_b	-	-	3
V. parahaemolyticus A8659	-	-	-	19
V. aglinolyticus ATCC 17749	-	-	-	4
V. anguillarum LS-174	-	-	-	4
V. anguillicida ET-7617	-	-	-	97
V. fluvialis 2386	-	-	-	28
Aeromonas hydrophila NMRI 7	-	-	-	0

[a]Source of labeled reference DNA.
[b]- = Not determined.

229

Table 9. Reassociation of Vibrio vulnificus DNA with the Vibrio Eel Isolate DNA at Stringent Temperature (T_M-15°C)

| Competitor DNA | V. vulnificus B51 | Relative % Reassociation | |
		V. vulnificus CDC B9629 (ATCC 27562)	V. vulnificus 11-3M-30
Eel Isolates			
ES-7601	106	94	100
ET-7617	103	93	97
KV-1	104	91	99

Table 10. Phenotypic Characteristics of _Vibrio_ _vulnificus_ and the _Vibrio_ Eel Isolates

Test or Substrate	_Vibrio_ _vulnificus_	_Vibrio_ Eel Isolates
Oxidase (Kovacs)	+[a]	+
Growth in 1% peptone w/		
0% + 7% NaCl	−[b]	−
0.5%, 3% + 5% NaCl	+	+
Indole production	+	−
VP	−	−
ADH	−	−
ODC	d[c]	−
LDC	+	+
Simmons' Citrate	+	+
D-Glucose, Acid	+	+
D-Glucose, Gas	−	−
Fermentation of		
Lactose	+	d
Sucrose	−	−
L-Arabinose	−	d
Amygdalin	+	+
Salacin	+	+
D-Mannitol	d	−
D-Mannose	+	+
Maltose	+	+
Sensitivity to 0/129 (10 µg/ml)	+	+
Pathogenic to Eels	−	+
Mouse LD_{50}	10^5-10^8	10^5-10^6

[a] + = > 90% of strains positive.
[b] − = > 90% of strains negative.
[c] d = 11-89% of strains positive.

same species while the phenotypic differences, particularly the pathogenicity to eels, indicate that these groups represent different biotypes or subspecies of V. vulnificus. Therefore, we propose that those strains phenotypically resembling the eel isolates be classified as V. vulnificus biotype anguillicidus. Characteristics which distinguish the biotypes of V. vulnificus from other phenotypically similar pathogenic Vibrio species are shown in Table 11.

CONCLUSIONS

The results of these studies reveal the power of the genetic approach to bacterial taxonomy. The ability to ferment lactose was found in not only strains of the "lactose-positive vibrio," V. vulnificus, but also in a number of phenotypically distinct vibrio strains including a group of genetically related strains (ALP strains) which apparently represent a new species of Vibrio. A group of vibrios isolated from a number of sources in Gulf and Pacific Northwest estuaries originally characterized 0/129 sensitive Vibrio fluvialis (VFL strains) were identified as atypical V. anguillarum by DNA-DNA homology. Genotypic characterization of a group of vibrio strains isolated from diseased eels revealed that, although these strains are phenotypically different from V. vulnificus in a number of traits, genetically they are V. vulnificus which differ in host range from the human pathogens of the species.

These results emphasize the heterogeneity of strains within species of the genus Vibrio and the need for thorough characterization of strains from seafood and clinical sources before decisions are made regarding the public health and etiological significance of Vibrio species from these sources. Vibrio strains isolated from oysters incriminated in cases of gastroenteritis which were characterized as 0/129 sensitive V. fluvialis are actually atypical strains of the fish pathogen V. anguillarum. The mistaken identification of vibrio strains from shellfish as species pathogenic to humans could lead to unwarranted conclusions by public health officials as to the quality of commercially marketed products. On the other hand, the failure to

Table 11. Differentiation of Phenotypically Similar Pathogenic Vibrio species

Test or substrate	V. vulnificus	V. vulnificus biotype anguillicidus	V. parahaemolyticus	V. cholerae	V. alginolyticus
ADH	$-^a$	-	-	-	-
LDC	$+^b$	+	+	+	-
ODC	d^c	-	+	+	d
ONPG	+	+	-	+	-
Indole production	+	-	+	+	+
Voges-Proskauer	-	-	-	d	+
Fermentation of					
lactose	+	$(+)^d$	-	(+)	-
salacin	+	+	-	-	-
sucrose	-	-	-	+	+
Growth in 1% peptone w/					
0% NaCl	-	-	-	+	-
0.5% to 5% NaCl	+	+	+	+	+
7% to 10% NaCl	-	-	+	-	+
> 10% NaCl	-	-	-	-	+

^{a}- = > 90% of strains negative.
^{b}+ = > 90% of strains positive.
^{c}d = 11-89% of strains positive.
^{d}(+) = positive reaction delayed $\geq$ 3 days.

recognize pathogenic Vibrio species from environmental and clinical sources would adversely effect the diagnosis of infections and epidemiological studies. This is of particular importance in the recognition of V. vulnificus because of the severity of the infection by this organism. Clinicians must be able to differentiate V. vulnificus not only from other Vibrio species must also consider the possibility that the eel pathogen biotype, Vibrio vulnificus biotype anguillicidus, may be the etiologic agent of infections in humans and recognize that, although these strains differ from the original species description in several characteristics, they are V. vulnificus. The pathogenic characteristics exhibited by these strains in eels and the LD_{50} of these strains to mice, which is comparable to that of clinical isolates of V. vulnificus, indicate that significant virulence is expressed by these strains. However, we know of no strains with the phenotypic characteristics of the eel pathogen biotype of V. vulnificus which have been isolated from human infections.

Vibrio species should be considered as the etiologic agent of not only gasteroenteritis but also septicemia and wound infections, particularly in cases where exposure to the marine environment has occurred. This requires an increased awareness by clinicians, physicians, and public health officials of the ecology, pathology, and taxonomy of the genus Vibrio.

ACKNOWLEDGMENTS

We thank Dr. K. Muroga for performing the eel pathogenicity tests and J. Baross, D. Hollis, M. Kelly, S. Payne, and N. Roberts for supplying bacterial strains.

This work is a result of research sponsored by the Oregon State University Sea Grant College Program supported by National Oceanic and Atmospheric Administration Office of Sea Grant, U.S. Department of Commerce, under grant NA79AA-D-00106, project number R/RSD 8. Oregon State University Agricultural Experiment Station Technical Paper No. 6365.

REFERENCES

Baumann, R., L. Baumann, S.S. Bang, and M.J. Woolkalis. 1980. Reevaluation of the taxonomy of Vibrio, Beneckea and Photobacterium. Curr. Microbiol. 4:127-132.

Blake, P.A., M.H. Merson, R.E. Weaver, D.G. Hollis, and P.C. Heublein. 1979. Disease caused by a marine vibrio: clinical characteristics and epidemiology. N. Engl. J. Med. 300:1-5.

Brenner, D.J., G.R. Fanning, K.E. Johnson, R.V. Citarella, and S. Falkow. 1969. Polynucleotide sequence relationships among members of Enterobacteriaceae. J. Bacteriol. 98:637-650.

Bruun, A., and B. Heiberg. 1932. The "red disease" of the eel in Danish waters. Meddelelser fra Kommissionen for Danmarks Fikeriog Havundersøgelser, Serie:Fisheri, Bind IX, Nr. 6, København, 1-19.

Clark, W.A., and A.G. Steigerwalt. 1977. Deoxyribonucleic acid reassociation experiments with a halophilic, lactose-fermenting vibrio isolated from blood culture. Int. J. System. Bact. 27:194-199.

Farmer, J.J. III. 1979. Vibrio ("Beneckea") vulnificus, the bacterium associated with sepsis, septicemia, and the sea. Lancet 2:902.

Farmer, J.J. III. 1980. Revival of the name Vibrio vulnificus. Int. J. System. Bact. 30:656.

Hollis, D.G., R.E. Weaver, C.N. Baker, and C. Thornberry. 1976. Halophilic Vibrio species isolated from blood culture. J. Clin. Microbiol. 3:425-431.

Johnson, J.L. 1981. Genetic characterization in P. Gerhardt et al. (Eds.) Manual of methods for general bacteriology. American Society for Microbiology, Washington, D.C.

Kelly, M.T., and D.M. Avery. 1980. Lactose-positive *Vibrio* in seawater: a cause of pneumonia and septicemia in a drowning victim. J. Clin. Microbiol. 11:278-280.

Kelly, M.T., and W.F. McCormick. 1981. Acute bacterial mylositis caused by *Vibrio vulnificus*. J. Am. Med. Assn. 246:72-73.

Mandel, M., L. Igambi, J. Bergendahl, M.L. Dodson, Jr., and E. Scheltgen. 1970. Correlation of melting temperature and cesium chloride buoyant density of bacteria deoxyribonucleic acid. J. Bacteriol. 101:333-338.

Meynell, G., and E. Meynell. 1965. Theory and practice in experimental bacteriology. University Press, Cambridge, England.

Muroga, K., Y. Jo, and M. Nishibuchi. 1976. Pathogenic *Vibrio* isolated from cultured eels. I. Characteristics and taxonomic status. Fish Pathol. 11:141-145.

Nishibuchi, M., K. Muroga, R.J. Seidler, and J.L. Fryer. 1979. Pathogenic *Vibrio* isolated from cultured eels. IV. Deoxyribonucleic acid studies. Bull. Jpn. Soc. Sci. Fish. 45:1469-1473.

Nybelin, O. 1935. Untersuchungen uber den bei Fischen Krankheitserregenden Spaltpilz *Vibrio anguillarum*. Medd. Statens Unders Forsoganst Sotvattenfisket, Nr. 8, 5-62.

Oliver, J.D., D.R. Cleland, and R.A. Warner. 1981. Lactose-fermenting vibrios in the marine environment. Abst. Ann. Mtg. Am. Soc. Microbiol. N16.

Reichelt, J.L., P. Baumann, and L. Baumann. 1976. Study of genetic relationships among marine species of the genus *Beneckea* and *Photobacterium* by means of *in* vitro DNA/DNA hybridization. Arch. Microbiol. 110:101-120.

Tison, D.L., M. Nishibuchi, and R.J. Seidler. 1981. Isolation and characterization of potentially pathogenic vibrios from Oregon estuaries. Abst. Ann. Mtg. Am. Soc. Microbiol. Q97.

Chapter 16

MOLECULAR TOXIGENIC CHARACTERIZATION OF ENVIRONMENTAL V. CHOLERAE

James B. Kaper

In recent years, many isolates of nonenterotoxigenic Vibrio cholerae O1 have been isolated from environmental sources in areas such as the U.S. Gulf Coast, the Chesapeake Bay, Brazil, Guam, and Great Britain. The significance of these isolates in terms of an environmental reservoir of cholera is uncertain. It has been postulated that they could be mutants of toxigenic strains which have the potential to revert to toxigenicity and therefore serve as a source of infection. Conversely, they could be merely natural inhabitants of aquatic environments which are aberrant not in their toxigenicity, but rather in their serological characteristics.

Because conventional biological assays for toxigenicity such as animal virulence assays and tissue culture systems gave inconclusive results with these strains (Joseph, this volume), a molecular approach using the techniques of recombinant DNA was employed.

This approach utilized the similarity of Escherichia coli heat-labile toxin (LT) to cholera toxin (CT). Both toxins share structural, enzymatic activity, and antigenic similarity. LT has been cloned and characterized by Dallas and coworkers (Dallas and Falkow 1980; Spicer et al. 1981); and the amino acid sequence for the protein was found to be very similar to CT. Because of the high amino acid sequence homology present between these two proteins, the genetic information encoding LT and CT were presumed to be highly homologous also. Related DNA sequences can be studied by the use of DNA/DNA hybridization techniques whereby the two different DNAs are denatured by heat or high pH so that the two strands of the double-stranded DNA molecule are separated. The denatured strands from each sample are mixed and conditions adjusted so that the strands can reanneal, that is, seek out similar DNA sequences from the other sample and join together to become an intact, double-stranded molecule. By radioactively labeling a specific DNA sequence, a highly specific probe for that sequence is obtained.

Such a probe for LT was obtained by purifying DNA from the cloned LT genes, which are carried on the recombinant plasmid pEWD299. Plasmid DNA was cut with restriction endonucleases to yield gene fragments specific for the LT A or LT B subunits. The purified fragments were then labeled in vitro with ^{32}P. Total DNA from V. cholerae strains was prepared, cut with restriction endonucleases and the resulting fragments separated by agarose gel electrophoresis. The cut DNA was then denatured and transferred to nitrocellulose filter paper by the method of Southern (1975). The paper containing the V. cholerae DNA was then incubated overnight in a solution containing the labeled LT DNA probe. The labeled DNA will hybridize to homologous sequences on the filter paper and, after the paper is washed and dried, can then be visualized by autoradiography. Thus, any DNA sample containing sequences similar to LT will be seen as a darkening of the X-ray film after the autoradiograph is developed (see Figure 1). All toxigenic strains of V. cholerae hybridized with the LT probe owing to the homology between the CT and LT genes. All nonenterotoxigenic strains isolated from throughout the world showed no such homology. Thus, the reason for their nonenterotoxigenicity is due to the lack of structural genes encoding toxin. They are not simple mutants that were once enterotoxigenic but rather, they lack the entire gene for toxin production and therefore cannot revert to enterotoxigenicity. Thus, the nonenterotoxigenic strains of V. cholerae found in areas such as

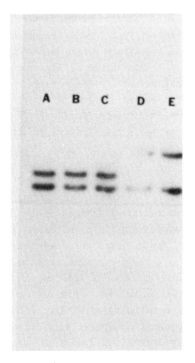

Figure 1. Autoradiograph showing hybridization of the LT probe to Hind III restriction fragments of V. cholerae strains. Chromosomal DNA was extracted from each strain, digested with Hind III restriction endonuclease, separated on an agarose gel and transferred to nitrocellulose paper. The LT probe was labeled with ^{32}P, and where it has hybridized to DNA from V. cholerae is indicated by darkening of the X-ray film. a) E506; b) 4808; c) SGN7277; d) 2002H; e) 2011H.

England, Brazil, or Maryland cannot serve as a reservoir of cholera since they lack the genes for cholera toxin. In addition, they lack other necessary virulence factors such as colonization factors and have been shown to be avirulent in human volunteers (Levine et al. 1982).

When DNA extracted from a toxigenic strain of V. cholerae was examined further by use of restriction endonucleases, certain differences were noted. All strains of the El Tor biotype examined in an earlier study possessed only one <u>Hind</u> III restriction fragment homologous to LT with the exception of strain 4808, isolated from the 1978 outbreak in Louisiana (Kaper et al. 1981).

This strain yielded two small fragments when cut with the enzyme <u>Hind</u> III, rather than the single fragment seen with other El Tors. The sum of the molecular weights of the two smaller fragments of 4808 was approximately equal to that of the single large fragment of other El Tor strains. When cut with other enzymes such as <u>Eco</u> RI, strain 4808 yielded only one fragment as did other El Tors. Thus, the Louisiana strain possessed a unique <u>Hind</u> III restriction site within the toxin gene in addition to the unique phage type reported for the Louisiana strains (Blake et al. 1980).

This analysis was performed on other enterotoxigenic <u>V. cholerae</u> O1 strains isolated from the U.S. Gulf Coast and the same pattern was seen. In addition to strain 4808 from the 1978 outbreak, E506 from an isolated case in Texas in 1973 and SGN7277, a 1980 sewer isolate from Louisiana, were both found to possess a unique <u>Hind</u> III restriction endonucleases site within the toxin gene which caused two small fragments to hybridize with the LT probe rather than a single large fragment (Figure 1). More recent isolates such as the strains from two cases in Texas in Spring 1981 (Shandera et al. in press) and the most recent outbreak in Fall 1981 all exhibit the identical pattern (Kaper, unpublished observations). No other strains so far examined from sources elsewhere in the world have possessed this pattern. This indicates that the toxin gene base sequence has undergone evolutionary divergence and that slightly different base sequences are to be found among different strains. How recently this divergence occurred is not known but it indicates that there is an "American" strain of <u>V. cholerae</u> O1 unique to the Gulf Coast. A second reservoir of cholera toxin genes in the Gulf Coast is found in strains of <u>V. cholerae</u> of serotypes other than O1. Strains 2002H and 2011H are non-O1 strains isolated from cases in Louisiana which produce CT and possess CT genes (Figure 1). They also possess a <u>Hind</u> III site in the middle of the gene but are not identical to the O1 strains with other restriction enzymes (Kaper et al. 1982).

The similarity of the Gulf Coast strains is so striking that the use of a radioactive probe is not even necessary. Figure 2 shows total chromosomal DNA of various V. cholerae strains digested with Hind III and separated by agarose gel electrophoresis. The restriction pattern for strains SGN7700, an enterotoxigenic V. cholerae O1 isolated from sewage in 1981; 4808; and E506 are identical, reflecting highly similar, if not identical, DNA sequences in their chromosomes. A number of differences can be seen in other strains. None of the various strains of V. cholerae isolated throughout the world that we have examined possessed the exact restriction pattern seen in the enterotoxigenic U.S. strains (Figure 2). Of particular interest is strain SGN7730, a nonenterotoxigenic O1 Ogawa strain which did not hybridize with the LT probe. Strain SGN7730 was isolated at the same site as SGN7700, but one week later. It clearly possesses a number of genetic dissimilarities from the earlier isolate, as evidenced by the restriction pattern. The nonenterotoxigenic strain SGN7730 is also quite different in phage type from the enterotoxigenic strains (J. Lee, personal communication). Similarly, strain 2002H, a non-O1 strain of V. cholerae, shows a distinctly different restriction pattern from the O1 strain (Figure 2).

Differences among strains in restriction endonuclease patterns, particularly those fragments hybridizing with the LT probe, can be exploited as a very sensitive "molecular fingerprinting" tool for V. cholerae. At the present time, phage typing is the chief epidemiological typing system employed for V. cholerae, and the preliminary evidence suggests considerable common ground between these methods. The 1973, 1978, 1980, and 1981 isolates are of the same phage type, which is extremely uncommon in other strains isolated throughout the world. By examining different phage types of V. cholerae with different restriction enzymes and noting different numbers and sizes of homologous fragments, a comprehensive typing scheme could be devised. Such a study relating phage type to restriction fragment differences is currently underway (Kaper and Lee, in progress). In at least one instance, however, the restriction fragment analysis has proven more reliable than phage typing. Recent isolates of V. cholerae O1 from

A B C D E F G H I J

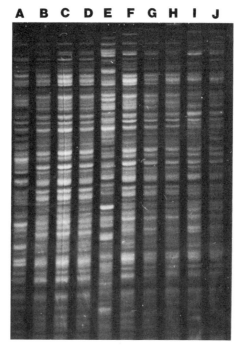

Figure 2. Restriction endonuclease pattern of V. cholerae chromosomal DNA digested with Hind III and separated by agarose gel electrophoresis. a) SGN7730; b) SGN7700; c) 4808; d) E506; e) 2002H; f) 62746; g) Stokes 1; h) E9120; i) E9950; j) 569B.

Florida were of the same phage type as the 1973, 1978, 1980 and 1981 isolates (J. Lee, personal communication), but did not produce cholera toxin and were negative with the LT gene probe (Kaper, unpublished observations).

These techniques of DNA hybridization can be simplified by the use of colony blots (Grunstein and Hogness 1975) whereby bacterial colonies grown on filter paper can be tested for homology with the LT probe (Figure 3). This technique allows the testing of hundreds of isolates in a single day. Thus, molecular epidemiological studies can be carried out on a large scale with great accuracy. Such a project is currently underway in a collaboration between the Center for Vaccine Development and scientists in Louisiana

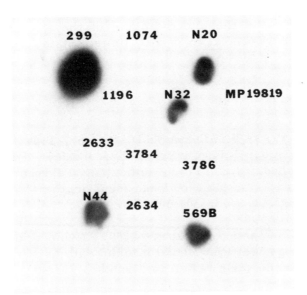

Figure 3. Colony hybridization of V. cholerae O1 strains on nitrocellulose filters after hybridization with ^{32}P-labeled LT probe. Only those colonies possessing DNA sequences homologous to LT bind the probe, subsequently darkening the film. Strains 299, N26, N32, N44 and 569B are positive while 1074, 1196, MP19819, 2633, 3784, 3786 and 2634 are negative.

whereby thousands of environmental isolates of V. cholerae are grown and treated on filters in Louisiana and then sent to Baltimore for DNA hybridization. By testing isolates for the presence of toxin genes on a scale difficult to match by conventional techniques, environmental reservoirs of toxigenic V. cholerae could be detected.

The use of such molecular techniques for the study of the epidemiology of diseases due to V. cholerae was recently advanced by the cloning of the genes encoding cholera toxin (Kaper and Levine 1981). These cloned genes are now available as a direct probe for CT genes rather than the indirect use of LT genes. The results obtained with the CT gene probe have been identical to those obtained with the LT probe, thus validating earlier studies (Kaper et al. 1981). The CT gene probe, along with the many powerful techniques of recombinant DNA, should greatly advance the understanding of the epidemiology and ecology of V. cholerae in the United States and other countries.

REFERENCES

Blake, P.A., D.T. Allegra, J.D. Snyder, T.J. Barrett, L. McFarland, C.T. Caraway, J.C. Feeley, J.P. Craig, J.V. Lee, N.D. Puhr, and R.A. Feldman. 1980. Cholera--a possible endemic focus in the United States. N. Engl. J. Med. 302:305-309.

Dallas, W.S., and S. Falkow. 1980. Amino acid sequence homology between cholera toxin and Escherichia coli heat-labile toxin. Nature (London) 288:499-501.

Grunstein, M., and D.S. Hogness. 1975. Colony hybridization: a method for the isolation of cloned DNAs that contain a specific gene. Proc. Nat. Acad. Sci. USA 72:3961-3965.

Kaper, J.B., H.B. Bradford, N.C. Roberts, and S. Falkow. 1982. Molecular epidemiology of Vibrio cholerae resident in the U.S. Gulf Coast. J. Clin. Microbiol. 16:129-134.

Kaper, J.B., and M.M. Levine. 1981. Cloned cholera enterotoxin genes in study and prevention of cholera. Lancet ii:1162-1163.

Kaper, J.B., S.L. Moseley and S. Falkow. 1981. Molecular characterization of environmental and nontoxigenic strains of Vibrio cholerae. Infect. Immun. 32:661-667.

Levine, M.M., R.E. Black, M.L. Clements, L. Cisneros, A. Saah, D.R. Nalin, D.M. Gill, J.P. Craig, C.R. Young, and P. Ristaino. 1982. Pathogenicity of non-enterotoxigenogenic Vibrio cholerae El Tor isolated from sewage water in Brazil. J. Infect. Dis. 145:296-299.

Shandera, W.X., B. Hafkin, D.L. Martin, J.P. Taylor, D.L. Maserang, J.G. Wells, M. Kelly, K. Ghandi, J.B. Kaper, J.V. Lee, and P.A. Blake. 1982. Persistence of cholera in the United States: implications for control measures. Lancet. In press.

Southern, E.M. 1975. Detection of specific sequences among DNA fragments separated by gel electrophoresis. J. Mol. Biol. 98:503-517.

Spicer, E.K., W.M. Kavanaugh, W.S. Dallas, S. Falkow, W.H. Konigsberg, and D.E. Schafer. 1981. Sequence homologies between A subunits of Escherichia coli and Vibrio cholerae enterotoxins. Proc. Natl. Acad. Sci. USA 78:50-54.

Methods for Isolation, Characterization and Identification

Chapter 17

TACTICS FOR DETECTING PATHOGENIC VIBRIOS IN THE ENVIRONMENT

William M. Spira

The detection of pathogenic vibrios in the environment involves a four-part strategy: (1) collect the proper environmental samples; (2) recover vibrios from these samples; (3) identify the vibrios recovered; and (4) confirm that they are pathogenic. The methods used to do this will vary with the specific Vibrio species under investigation, the nature of the environment being scrutinized, and the purpose for which the search is being carried out.

The members of the genus Vibrio present a spectrum of virulence that is impressive. Three species clusters within the genus are of actual or potential public health significance. The first is the nonhalophilic, arginine dihydrolase-negative group of V. cholerae, both O group-1 and non-O1, and V. mimicus (Fanning et al. 1981), a very closely allied species until recently included with V. cholerae. The second group, the halophilic, arginine-negative vibrios, contains V. parahaemolyticus, V. vulnificus, and V. alginolyticus. The third group consists of arginine-positive vibrios and related genera. It contains V. fluvialis, a recently described species earlier identified as EF-6 or group F organisms (Lee et al. 1981), whose potential as an etiologic agent is still unclear. The same conclusion applies to the two related organisms, Plesiomonas shigelloides and Aeromonas hydrophila. There is no published evidence that other members of the third group, including V. anguillarum and V. metschnikovii, are human pathogens.

These vibrios are aquatic microorganisms, generally inhabiting estuarine and brackish water environments. Even for the toxigenic El Tor biotype of V. cholerae, traditionally thought to be highly adapted to the human intestine, there is now evidence for a free-living existence under, at least, certain limited circumstances (Rogers et al. 1980). In any case, there is no doubt of the overwhelming aquatic component to the epidemiology of vibrio infections. The common risk factor in all is the ingestion of, or exposure to, contaminated water, fish, or shellfish.

Collection and Handling of Samples

The successful recovery of pathogenic vibrios from the environment depends substantially on how closely the types and time of sample collection parallel the natural cycle of the target organism. For example, V. parahaemolyticus in temperate waters can be isolated from sediments during winter months though at the same time they are frequently undetectable in the water column. As warmer weather approaches, V. parahaemolyticus are found associated with zooplankton; they then proliferate in the water column during the warm summer months. A surveillance based solely on water sampling might seriously misconstrue the actual situation.

Though the ecology of other Vibrio spp. has not been established to the extent of that of V. parahaemolyticus, the data that are available on the association of vibrios with various environmental and biological surfaces suggest the prudence of expanding the scope of routine sampling beyond the collection of water to include plankton, plants, and animals in the area under surveillance.

This point is illustrated by our data from Bangladesh concerning the relative efficiency of two types of sampling in revealing the presence of V. cholerae biotype El Tor in ponds or rivers used a day or two previously by persons suffering from cholera (Spira et al. 1981). The two samples collected from each water source within 5 feet of one another were: a 1-liter water sample and a single water hyacinth, a plant that is ubiquitous in the waters of this region. Plants were homogenized, then enriched and plated in an identical fashion to the water sample. For the pairs in which only one sample was positive, plants yielded V. cholerae over three times more frequently than did the water sample. Water sampling alone would have missed identifying over half of the contaminated water sources.

Since we know little of the ecology of most pathogenic vibrios in aquatic environments, the conservative approach to surveillance would include sampling from as wide a variety of microenvironments as possible. The list would include water (with and without filtration), sediment, zoo- and phytoplankton, surface plants, shellfish, annelids, and intestinal contents of fish, reptiles, and aquatic birds. As our knowledge of the ecology of specific Vibrio species becomes more precise, we will be able to focus our surveillance on the samples with the highest likelihood of harboring pathogens. At present, however, we need to maintain a broad scope.

How samples are handled after collection also influences the recovery of pathogenic vibrios. If samples must be held for some time before being processed, this aspect should be considered carefully. The methods to be employed should first be tested with representative samples seeded with the organism of interest to ensure that its viability is not severely reduced during holding.

A dramatic example of the effect of holding conditions has recently been published by Dr. James Oliver (1981), who examined lethal cold stress of V. vulnificus in oysters. The combination of exposure to oysters and 4°C was extremely detrimental to V. vulnificus, but either condition alone had little or no effect. Whole oysters contaminated with V. vulnificus and held for 24 hours on ice (0.5°C) showed a three-log decrease in viable cells. An even more dramatic drop occurred when V. vulnificus was held in homogenized oyster samples: greater than a five-log drop in 12 hours. It appears that some lethal factor is released from oysters upon homogenization. This may be selective for V. vulnificus, however, since the viability of V.

parahaemolyticus held under similar conditions appeared to be little affected.

Though this is an extreme case, it indicates the importance of careful consideration and pretesting of holding conditions. The ideal practice is, of course, to process the sample as soon as it is collected. This appears impractical in many situations, but the decision to hold samples should still be made only on the basis of solid evidence that the practice will not unduly reduce the likelihood of detecting the organisms being sought.

As a general rule, rapid and profound chilling of samples, such as by direct immersion in ice or ice water, should be avoided. If there will be a delay of several hours before samples can be processed, still-air cooling of samples kept from contact with the coolant is preferable. An alternative that in many cases is even more effective is to begin enrichment at the sampling site.

For samples of plants, animals, plankton, or sediment, the appropriate collection procedures are somewhat intuitive. In most cases, samples such as these are homogenized, then plated or transferred to enrichment media. One possibility that should be considered is whether processing specific tissues or portions of samples rather than the whole would increase the sensitivity of the assay. Were vibrios to concentrate in certain organs or tissues, they might be more easily detected if the other parts of the sample, possibly harboring competitors, were discarded.

The sampling of water and sewage presents a somewhat different set of problems. Plating or enrichment of the sample as it is collected is often not sufficiently sensitive to detect low concentrations of vibrios. Pathogenic vibrios are often present infrequently and in low numbers. V. cholerae Ol is notable in this respect. Concentration techniques such as membrane filtration using celite have been used (Kaper et al. 1979) to combat the problem. Although the practice is effective, it is more involved than is desirable, particularly since samples must also be clarified by centrifugation prior to filtration.

A simple procedure that has proven highly effective in sewer surveillance for toxigenic V. cholerae Ol is the Moore swab, a 6-inch tuft of gauze attached to a wire and fixed in place in a flowing water source. This remains in place for up to several days, then is recovered and transferred to enrichment broth. The Moore swab appears to be a sensitive procedure for detecting V. cholerae in sewage (Barrett et al. 1979). There have, however, been no published comparisons with "grab sample" collection of sewage. The Moore swab has also been used in surface waters to isolate vibrios and appears to be effective, except when used in still waters.

Other disadvantages of the Moore swab are the failure to obtain a precise sampling time and the fact that, in some places, Moore swabs cannot be left in place without a high likelihood of their being removed before the investigator returns. An alternative is to use gauze filtration of collected water samples to improve the detection of V. cholerae.

We have recently described the use of such a simple filter in Bangladesh (Spira and Ahmed 1981). This filter was taken to ponds and rivers recently used by cholera victims. Ten liters of water were collected and poured through the gauze filter, a process which took about one minute. The gauze and additional water to bring the volume to 900 ml were transferred to enrichment broth as was a paired 900-ml water sample. The gauze filtration was significantly better in detecting V. cholerae El Tor than was water sampling. In pairs in which only one method was positive, the gauze yielded over four times more positives than did the water.

Another procedure that has recently been published is the use of columns of polystyrene beads coated with anti-bodies against the V. cholerae O1 antigen (Hranitzky et al. 1980). This sero-specific procedure is particularly designed to isolate O1 organisms from the population of non-O1 V. cholerae that tend to predominate in water samples. This is a novel approach that has potential applicability to the isolation of other pathogens, such as Salmonella or Shigella, as well.

Enrichment Procedures

The principles on which the commonly used enrichment media for Vibrio spp. are formulated include: a preference for alkaline conditions (pH 8.5-9.0), resistance to bile salts and sodium tellurite, and either the salt tolerance of the halophilic species or the ability to grow in media to which no NaCl has been added for V. cholerae and related organisms. Current enrichment procedures are reasonably effective in selecting Vibrio spp. over other common aquatic organisms, including Pseudomonas, Achromobacter, and Flavobacterium. The major problems from overgrowth usually occur with V. anguillarum and Aeromonas spp.

Of media used for enrichment, the one most generally recommended is alkaline peptone water (APW; Furniss et al. 1978). This contains 1% NaCl and is satisfactory for any of the pathogenic vibrios. Since overgrowth by halophilic vibrios can be a problem, the use of salt-free alkaline peptone when searching specifically for V. cholerae should be considered.

Alkaline bile peptone water, which contains 0.5% sodium taurocholate (ABPW), has proven to be an excellent enrichment for V. cholerae, but has not been extensively evaluated with other pathogenic vibrios. Glucose salt teepol broth (Cowan 1974), recommended for V. parahaemolyticus, does not appear to improve on APW for this organism and is substantially worse for other pathogenic vibrios. Salt colistin broth is another enrichment for V. parahaemolyticus which is not useful for some of the other pathogenic vibrios. There are other enrichments for V. parahaemolyticus, as well, such as arabinose-ethyl violet broth, that are valuable if one is searching specifically for this organism. There is no published evidence, however, that any of these is significantly better than APW. A gelatin-phosphate-sodium chloride broth has been suggested as a replacement for APW by Dr. H. Smith (personal communication). Since most Vibrio spp. are gelatinase-positive, a medium in which gelatin was the sole energy and nitrogen source is theoretically attractive. In practice, the presence of numerous other gelatinase-positive organisms in the aquatic environment presents a formidable obstacle to the effective use of this medium as an enrichment.

The temperature and length of enrichment culture used has varied between workers. Three common patterns for V. cholerae are plating after 6 and 18 hours at 37°C; plating after 6 hours at ambient temperature and again after an additional 12 hours at 37°C; and plating after 6 hours at 37°C, then subculturing and incubating for an additional 12 hours at 37°C. There has been no rigorous comparison of these regimens but, because V. cholerae grow rapidly and because they might be inhibited as the pH drops in older cultures, many workers advise plating after 6 hours of incubation if only one time is used.

A comparison of APW versus ABPW and of 6-hour versus 18-hour incubation at 37°C was made recently as part of the study of gauze filtration just discussed (Spira and Ahmed 1981). Lumping both sampling techniques and both media together and analyzing the time of enrichment suggests that 18-hour was substantially better than 6-hour enrichments. The longer enrichment time recovered 99% of all positives while 6-hour enrichment recovered only 55%. The situation is more complex, however. For water samples in which the microbial concentration is, presumably, low there is no difference between media, but there is a threefold improvement in isolation rate at 18 hours compared to 6 hours. When the starting concentration of vibrios and competitors is higher, as appears to be the case with the gauze filter samples, the difference between the two times is smaller. When APW was used, there was no difference seen between 6 and 18 hours. This appeared to be due to substantial overgrowth at the later time. Barrett et al. (1980) reported a similar lack of improvement over 6-hour enrichments using APW to enrich Moore Swabs used in sewer surveillance. When the more selective ABPW was used, however, a small but significant improvement in isolation rate was seen at 18 hours. In this medium, overgrowth was much less of a problem. This suggests that ABPW enrichment for 18 hours is the optimal choice for V. cholerae if only one enrichment is to be used. The 12 hours saved by doing a 6-hour enrichment is probably not going to be an important factor in many studies. In our experience, enrichment of samples is usually started during the afternoon of the day of collection. In such circumstances a 6-hour enrichment means a late evening plating, which is less convenient than plating after an overnight incubation.

Selective Plating

A wide variety of selective media have been designed for the isolation of V. cholerae and V. parahaemolyticus. Only one is commercially available at present, and, though it is not ideal for all vibrios, it is of sufficient utility to be the medium of choice for the routine laboratory. This medium is thiosulfate citrate bile salts sucrose (TCBS) agar. Most pathogenic vibrios will grow reasonably well on it, it is available from several commercial sources, and it does not require autoclaving. The selectivity of TCBS is based on high pH and the presence of bile salts. Sucrose is incorporated to differentiate between fermenters (e.g. V. cholerae) and nonfermenters (e.g. V. parahaemolyticus). Variation in selectivity between brands has been reported but did not appear in the recent study by Morris et al. (1979). The organisms involved were all fresh clinical isolates of V. cholerae biotype El Tor, however, and the experience with environmental samples and other Vibrio species may be substantially different. Given the high selectivity of TCBS, it is recommended that brand variation be assessed for the conditions and organisms actually involved before embarking on studies. Lot-to-lot variation has also been reported and should be monitored by a careful quality control routine.

If one is screening specifically for V. cholerae, taurocholate tellurite gelatine agar (TTGA; Monsur 1963) is actually a superior medium in some ways, to TCBS (Morris et al. 1979). TTGA is an alkaline gelatine agar containing 0.8% bile salts to which 0.0001% potassium tellurite is added. V. cholerae are able to reduce tellurite to nontoxic tellurium which accumulates as a black center in the colony and serves as an additional differential character to experienced workers. Both TTGA and TCBS are highly efficient in isolating V. cholerae from stool specimens. In my studies in Bangladesh I found the two media to be equal for environmental samples as well (unpublished data). One of TTGA's advantages is that certain important tests can be done directly from the plate. These include slide agglutination with V. cholerae O1 antiserum and the oxidase test. Neither is successful from TCBS because colonies are difficult to emulsify and because oxidase is inhibited. The disadvantages of TTGA--it needs to be autoclaved, it is not commercially available, and it requires careful titration of the tellurite to be successful--limit its use to moderately large laboratories with a substantial load of work with V. cholerae.

Differentiation of Vibrio spp.

The preliminary differentiation of vibrio-like organisms isolated from TCBS often involves traditional enteric media such as TSI, KIA, LIA and MIU. These are not the optimal methods for routine surveillance in which the spectrum of pathogenic vibrios are being sought. Preliminary differentiation on the following four characteristics is efficient and effective: salt requirement for growth, gelatinase production, sensitivity to 0/129 vibriostatic compound (2,4-diamino- 6,7-diisopropylpteridine; Shewan et al. 1954), and oxidase reaction. A combination of the following two plates is best: salt-free gelatine neopeptone agar (GNA; Smith and Goodner 1958) and gelatine agar (GA) with 1% NaCl. Quarter-plates of each agar are streaked with the isolated colony. Two 6-mm filter disks containing 10 or 150 mcgram of 0/129 vibriostatic compound are placed in each of the quadrants of the GA plate in the area where confluent growth would occur if the isolate were 0/129 resistant. 0/129 sensitivity has long been recognized as a property of vibrios and is extremely valuable in differentiating vibrios from other gram-negative rods, especially aeromonads. The degree of sensitivity is also useful in differentiating among Vibrio species.

After overnight incubation at 37°C, the isolates are scored for the ability to grow in the absence of added NaCl (i.e., on GNA), for gelatinase production, 0/129 sensitivity, and oxidase reaction. If V. cholerae O1 is suspected, a slide agglutination can also be performed from the GA plate.

The typical reactions of the pathogenic Vibrio species are shown in Table 1. Among the nonhalophiles, Enterobacteriaceae are differentiated by the oxidase test and by their resistance to 0/129. V. cholerae, V. mimicus, and Plesiomonas shigelloides can be presumptively differentiated by their colonial appearance on TCBS. Among the halophiles, which do not grow on GNA, V. metschnikovii is clearly distinguished from the rest by being oxidase-negative and 0/129 sensitive. V. vulnificus is oxidase-positive and is sensitive to 0/129. This differentiates it from V. fluvialis, V. alginolyticus, and V. parahaemolyticus, which all show reduced sensitivity. Colonial appearance on TCBS also yields clues to the presumptive identity of the isolate.

The confirmatory tests are shown in Table 2. V. cholerae O1 is, by definition, identified by its O antigen, but confirmatory biochemical tests are also useful. The Vibrio species are differentiated from P. shigelloides by gelatinase and arginine reaction. V. cholerae and V. mimicus are differentiated on the basis of sucrose fermentation, corn oil lipolysis, and Voges-Proskauer (VP) reaction.

Among the halophilic vibrios, V. metschnikovii is differentiated by its failure to produce oxidase or to reduce nitrate. Arginine, lysine, and ornithine reactions distinguish Vibrio parahaemolyticus, V. alginolyticus, and V. vulnificus from V. anguillarum and V. fluvialis. A battery of six tests then provides a minimum of three differential characters between each of these first three vibrios. The tests are: growth in 10% NaCl; lactose, sucrose, and arabinose fermentation; ONPG and VP. VP, growth on alanine, and resistance to novobiocin are useful in differentiating V. anguillarum and V. fluvialis.

Table 1. Presumptive Differential Scheme for _Vibrio_ spp.

GNA Growth[a]	Oxidase	O/129[b]	Typical Colony on TCBS[c]	Presumptive Isolate
+	+	S	Y, 2-3 mm	V. cholerae
			G, 2-3 mm	V. mimicus
			G, 1 mm	P. shigelloides
	0	R	Y, var.	Aeromonas spp.
	+	R	Y, < 1 mm	Enterobacteriaceae
0		S	Y, var.	V. anguillarum
		S	G, var.	V. vulnificus
		RS	Y, var.	V. fluvialis
		RS	Y, 2-5 mm	V. alginolyticus
		RS	G, 2-5 mm	V. parahaemolyticus
	0	S	Y, var.	V. metschnikovii

[a]Gelatine neo-peptone agar (i.e. growth in medium with no added NaCl).

[b]S = sensitive; zone around a 10-mcgram disk; RS = reduced sensitivity; no zone around 10-mcgram, zone around 150-mcgram disk; R = resistant, no zone around 150-mcgram disk.

[c]Y = yellow (Sucrose fermented); G = green (Sucrose not fermented or delayed). Typical size of colony after 24 hours given or listed as variable (var.).

Table 2.   Differential Tests for <u>Vibrio</u> spp.

Test	V. cholerae O1	V. cholerae non-O1	V. mimicus	P. shigelloides	V. parahaemolyticus	V. alginolyticus	V. vulnificus	V. anginolyticus	V. fluvialis	V. metschnikovii
O1 Agglutination	+	0	0	0						
Gelatinase	+	+	+	0						
Lipolysis										
(Corn oil)	+	+	0	0						
Kovacs Oxidase					+	+	+	+	+	0
NO$_3$ reduction					+	+	+	+	+	0
Arginine										
dihydrolase	0	0	0	+	0	0	0	+	+	+
Lysine										
Decarboxylase	+	+	+	+	+	+	+	0	0	V
Ornithine										
Decarboxylase	+	+	+	+	+	V	+	0	0	0
Growth-10% NaCl					0	+/0	0	0	0	0
Fermentation of										
Lactose					0	0	+ or (+)	0	0	0
Sucrose	+	+	0	0	0	+	0	+	+	+
Arabinose					+	0	0	V	+	0
ONPG					0	0	+	V	+	V
VP	+/0[a]	+	0	0	0	+	0	+	0	+
Growth on alanine						+		0	+	V
Novobiocin 5 ug										
resistance								0	+	

[a]Biovar difference: El Tor = +; Classical = 0.

Virulence Testing

The final step in the strategy for detecting pathogenic vibrios in the environment is to confirm that the isolates identified are, indeed, pathogenic. Identification of Vibrio species is not synonymous with identifying virulence potential, even for V. cholerae Ol. It is necessary, therefore, that tests for pathogenicity be part of the routine characterization of these organisms.

This is not to say that virulence testing should necessarily be made a part of every laboratory's routine. Most labs do not have the level of work or the interest to justify the substantial effort needed to establish carefully controlled repeatable biological assays for virulence factors. Antibody-based assays such as RIA and ELISA are more feasible and can be developed for well-characterized virulence antigens, of which precious few currently exist. Even here, however, careful control of conditions for production of the antigen and considered, knowledgeable evaluation of results are necessary if repeatability is to be achieved and an unacceptably high frequency of false positives and negatives is to be avoided. Particular caution must be used when extrapolating an assay developed for one group of organisms from a particular environment to other groups and other environments. There are frequent marginal reactions that call for considerable repetition and interpretation.

The future, however, is certainly bright: robust assays will eventually be developed. The molecular genetic approach, using radio- or enzyme-labelled DNA probes is a most exciting prospect. This ultimate in reductionist approaches to virulence testing has already proven itself with cholera toxin and with E. coli LT and ST (Moseley et al. 1980; Kaper et al. 1981). It remains to be simplified and standardized for more widespread use in routine testing of isolates. It also remains for us to identify the critical virulence factors in other pathogenic vibrios so that this approach can be applied to them, as well. For now, most routine characterization of virulence potential is focused on toxins. Cholera toxin is the single, definitely characterized virulence antigen in the cluster of nonhalophilic, arginine-negative vibrios. There are numerous routine assays and variations of assays for it including CHO or Y-1 adrenal cells tissue culture assays (Guerrant et al. 1974; Sack and Sack 1975); RIA; ELISA (Holmgren and Svennerholm 1973; Sack et al. 1980); RPHA; and DNA probes, currently based on the similarity between CT and E. coli LT, but which soon will be standardized using the actual genes for CT.

For those strains whose pathogenicity is not mediated by CT, there are no routine tests or, in most instances, no incriminated virulence antigens. One factor that may be incriminated in the near future is a cytotoxin from some of the non-Ol V. cholerae. It is currently being purified and appears to share a number of characteristics with the cytotoxin of V. vulnificus that has recently been reported by Kreger and Lockwood (1981).

The Kanagawa test for the thermostable hemolysin has proven of great value in identifying virulent V. parahae- molyticus. Though its relationship with virulence potential is still unclear, the production of this hemolysin is highly correlated with the ability of an organism to cause gastro- enteritis.

The final step in the characterization of pathogenic vibrios consists of assays that establish epidemiologic markers within clusters of isolates. One possible way of doing this is by serotyping. For V. cholerae/V. mimicus, there are over 80 recognized O groups. Unfortunately, two independent typing schemes are currently in existence, which serves to confuse the issue. The scheme described by Siebeling et al. in this volume appears to have the potential to supplant both of the former schemes and place the serogrouping of the non-Ol V. cholerae on a much sounder basis. There is, however, as yet no correlation between serogroup and pathogenicity except for V. cholerae Ol isolated from humans. For V. parahaemolyticus, 12 O and 56 K antigens are recognized. This system has proven to be epidemiologically useful; but, again, it has no intrinsic correlation with pathogenicity.

Another potential marker is vibriocine-typing. A limited system has been described for V. cholerae Ol, but it has been little developed and suffers from problems with interpretation and repeatability.

Phage typing has been far more successfully applied to V. cholerae O1. An expanded scheme employing 14 phages has been developed by Dr. John Lee at the Public Health Laboratory at Maidstone, England. This system has been used in a number of instances to provide important epidemiological information, most notably perhaps, the linking of the 1973 Texas and 1978 Louisiana cholera cases (Blake et al. 1980). There is also evidence that phage sensitivity pattern may also be a marker of pathogenicity (J.V. Lee, personal communication). This further suggests the use of this system in the study of V. cholerae O1 ecology and epidemiology.

A phage-typing scheme for non-O1 V. cholerae has been described but it is not well developed and is currently not in use.

Future prospects for the development of a wide range of epidemiologic markers appear good. Particularly promising are the analysis of restriction digest patterns and two-dimensional electrophoretic characterization of cell proteins to characterize isolates.

REFERENCES

T.J. Barrett, A. Blake, G.K. Morris, N.D. Puhr, H.B. Bradford, and J.G. Wells. 1980. Use of Moore swabs for isolating Vibrio cholerae from sewage. J. Clin. Microbiol. 11:385-388.

P.A. Blake, D.T. Allegra, J.D. Snyder, T.J. Barrett, L. McFarland, C.T. Caraway, J.C. Feeley, J.P. Craig, N.D. Puhr, and R.A. Feldman. 1980. Cholera--a possible endemic focus in the United States. N. Engl. J. Med. 302:305-309.

S.T. Cowan. 1974. Cowan and Steel's manual for the identification of medical bacteria. 2nd ed. University Press, Cambridge.

G.R. Fanning, B.R. Davis, J.M. Madden, H.B. Bradford, Jr., A.G. Steigerwalt, and D.J. Brenner. 1981.

Vibrio mimicus: a newly recognized cholera-like organisim. Abstr. Am. Soc. Microbiol. Page 50.

A.L. Furniss, J.V. Lee, and T.J. Donovan. 1978. The Vibrios. Public Health Laboratory Service. Monograph Series No. 11. Her Majesty's Stationery Office, London.

R.L. Guerrant, L.L. Brunton, T.C. Schnaitman, L.I. Rebhun, and A.G. Gilman. 1974. Cylic adenosine monophosphate and alteration of Chinese hamster ovary cell morphology: A rapid, sensitive in vitro assay for the enterotoxins of Vibrio cholerae and Escherichia coli. Infect. Immun. 10: 320-327.

J. Holmgren and A.-M. Svennerholm. 1973. Enzyme-linked immunosorbent assays for cholera serology. Infect. Immun. 7:759-763.

K.W. Hranitsky, A.D. Larson, D.W. Rangsdale, and R.J. Siebeling. 1980. Isolation of O1 serovars of Vibrio cholerae from water by serologically specific method. Science 210:1025-1026.

J. Kaper, H. Lockman, R.R. Colwell and S.W. Joseph, 1979. Ecology, serology, and entertoxin production of Vibrio cholerae in Chesapeake Bay. Appl. Environ. Microbiol. 37:91.

J.B. Kaper, S.L. Moseley, and S. Falkow. 1981. Molecular characterization of environmental and nontoxinigenic strains of Vibrio cholerae. Infect. Immun. 32:661-667.

A. Kreger and D. Lockwood. 1981. Detection of extracellular toxin(s) produced by Vibrio vulnificus. Infect. Immun. 33:583-589.

J.V. Lee, P. Shread, A.L. Furniss, and T.N. Bryant. 1981. Taxonomy and description of Vibrio fluvialis sp.

nov. (synonym group F vibrios, group EF6). J. Appl. Bacteriol. 50:73-94.

K.A. Monsur. 1963. Bacteriological diagnosis of cholera under field conditions. Bull. WHO 28:387-389.

G.K. Morris, M.H. Merson, I. Huq, A.K.M.B. Kibrya, and R. Black. 1979. Comparison of four plating media for isolating Vibrio cholerae. J. Clin. Microbiol. 9:79-83.

S.L. Moseley, I. Huq, A.R.M.A. Alim, M. So, M. Samadpour-Motalebi, and S. Falkow. 1980. Detection of entertoxigenic Escherichia coli by DNA colony hybridization. J. Infect. Dis. 142:892-898.

S.L. Mosely, and S. Falkow. 1980. Nucleotide sequence homology between the heat-labile enterotoxin gene of Escherichia coli and Vibrio cholera deoxyribonucleic acid. J. Bact. 144:444-446.

Oliver, J.D. 1981. Lethal cold stress of Vibrio vulnificus in oysters. Appl. Environ. Microbiol. 41:710-717.

Rogers, R.C., R.G.C.J. Cuffe, Y.M. Cossins, D.M. Murphy, and A.T.C. Bourke. 1980. The Queensland cholera incident of 1977. 2. The epidemiological investigation. Bull. W.H.O. 58:665-669.

Sack, D.A., and R.B. Sack. 1975. Test for enterogenic Escherichia coli using Y1 adrenal cells in miniculture. Infect. Immun. 11:35-40.

Sack, D.A., S. Huda, P.K.B. Neogi, R.R. Daniel, and W.M. Spira. 1980. Microtiter ganglioside enzyme-linked immunosorbent assay for vibrios and Escherichia coli heat-labile enterotoxins and anti-toxin. J. Clin. Microbiol. 11:35-40.

Smith, H.L., and K. Goodner. 1958. Detection of bacterial gelatinases by gelactic-agar plate methods. J. Bateriol. 76:662-665.

Spira, W.M., and Q.S. Ahmed. 1981. Gauze filtration and enrichment procedures for recovery of Vibrio cholerae from contaminated waters. Appl. Environ. Microbiol. 42:730-733.

Spira, W.M., A. Huq, Q.S. Ahmed, and Y.A. Saeed. 1981. Uptake of Vibrio cholerae biotype of el tor from contaminated water by water hyacinth (Eichornia crassipes). Appl. Environ. Microbiol. 42:550-554.

Chapter 18

METHODS FOR MONITORING VIBRIOS IN THE ENVIRONMENT

Nell C. Roberts and Ramon J. Seidler

Any adequate methodology today must consider stress, if not of the microbiologist, at least of the microorganism. Dr. Warren Litsky (1979) phrased it very well, "Gut critters are stressed in the environment, more stressed by isolation procedures." Environmentalists have traditionally employed methods developed by clinical microbiologists. Vibrio methodology is no exception. Here I will briefly review the methods used by the Sea Grant Vibrio Research Group.

The examination begins with a specimen which may be (1) clinical, (2) food, (3) sewage, or (4) environmental. All are inoculated into enrichment broths designed for specific Vibrio species.

Alkaline peptone (AP)--1% peptone, 1% salt, pH 8.5--is used for Vibrio cholerae. This is the oldest medium in use and still quite effective. For Vibrio parahaemolyticus, Horie's medium is used. Buchi's alkaline peptone (BAP) is used for Group F vibrios. Both are basic modifications of AP. Horie's medium (Horie et al. 1964) contains galactose as a specific enrichment for V. parahaemolyticus plus ethyl violet as an inhibitor and brom thymol blue as the pH indicator. Nishibuchi and co-investigators at Oregon State University (unpublished observations) increased the salt content of AP to 4% and added 5 mg/ml novobiocin. This formulation (BAP) is used for enrichment of Group F vibrios.

No specific enrichment procedure was used for lactose-positive (Lac$^+$) vibrios. Thiosulfate citrate bile salts sucrose (TCBS; Difco, Detroit, MI) plates from AP enrichment and membrane filters placed directly onto TCBS plates were screened for these organisms.

Clinical (Wachsmuth et al. 1980) and food (Food and Drug Administration) techniques recommend incubation of AP for 6 to 8 hours. The time limits overgrowth of V. cholerae by gut flora, not a bad idea at all when you consider the numbers of organisms present in feces. Kaper et al. (1979) recommend 18 to 24 hours incubation of AP to resuscitate vibrios stressed by sudden change of environments. We allow environmental specimens in enrichment broths to sit at room temperature (about 25°C) for several hours before placing them at 35°C for overnight incubation; (18 hours); thus allowing resuscitation of the vibrio and the microbiologist by sticking to office hours.

In the course of our examination the microbes have so far been subjected to thermal shock, extremes of pH, exposure to potentially lethal antibiotics, and a high carbohydrate diet. Things can't get much worse, but they do. After the prescribed incubation time, enrichment media are streaked to TCBS. This excellent but highly selective medium was developed in 1963 and is widely used in Vibrio work. Our research group required not less than 70% recovery of V. cholerae ATCC strains 14033 and 14035 as quantitated on trypticase soy agar. Only four of seven lots tested in my laboratory met this criteria.

Having successfully applied the law of survival of the fittest, stress now becomes minimized for the laboratory-adapted survivors. From this point, techniques are simple, straightforward, and designed to obtain maximum information from minimum effort and cost.

Colonies selected from TCBS are inoculated to gelatin agar containing 0% and 3% NaCl, and Kliglers iron agar (KIA) or Kaper's screening medium.

Oxidase tests are performed directly on gelatin plates. Agglutinations may also be done at this point if needed or following biochemical screening. We use antisera prepared by Ron Siebeling at Louisiana State University.

Oxidase-positive, gelatinase-positive isolates with alkaline slant, acid butt, and no hydrogen sulfide or gas are then selected for further minimal biochemical screening. This is the poor "bug's" last chance to make good. Failure to conform to the minimal characteristics listed in Table 1 mean the mandatory death sentence--the autoclave. Fame awaits those fortunate few that will be assigned strain numbers, preserved for posterity, and subjected to intensive probing and searching.

Methods do have limitations and do determine results. This may be manifested qualitatively and or quantitatively. The effect of length of incubation time of AP on recovery of V. cholerae was compared on 124 specimens (Moore swabs, 88; crabs, 77; shell oysters, 4; ice, 5). Six-hour incubation yielded 13 positive results. Eighteen-hour incubation yielded 18 positive results.

Combined qualitative/quantitative results of incubation times are illustrated in Table 2. Again 6-hour incubation produced fewer isolates than 18-hour incubation, but note that serovars recovered from the same portion enriched for 18 hours are different from those enriched for 6 hours.

Specificity of enrichment procedures is compared in Table 3. On 41 specimens (water, 7; sediment, 7; crabs, 4; crab feces, 2; oyster, 1; shrimp, 1; plankton 2; bird feces, 1; sewer grab samples, 11; Moore swabs from sewers, 5), we screened all TCBS plates for four vibrio groups. Toxigenic V. cholerae O1 Inaba from sewer grab samples were recovered from all four enrichment media. In general, there was a slight recovery advantage for each species in their respective enrichment medium.

Most probable number (MPN) examinations were done on environmental samples. Results of fecal coliform analyses showed typical number combinations; that is, positive results occurred more frequently in portions containing the greatest inoculum. Only 2 of 134 fecal coliform MPN's done by the Louisiana Department of Health and Human Resources team were "odd," 0-1-0 and 3-1-3, beginning with a 10-ml inoculum. The same team had different results with

Table 1. Biochemical Differentiation of Vibrio Isolates

Test or Substrate	V. cholerae	V. fluvialis	V. vulnificus	V. parahaemolyticus
Indole Production	+	V	+	+
Arginine Dihydrolase	-	+	-	-
Lysine Decarboxylase	+	-	+	+
Ornithine Decarboxylase	+	-	+	+
ONPG Hydrolysis	+	+	+	+
0% NaCl	+	-	-	-
7% NaCl	V	+	-	+
0/129 Sensitivity				
10 ug/ml	+	-	+	+
150 ug/ml	+	+	+	+
Sucrose Fermentation	+	+	-	-
Lactose Fermentation	-	-	+	-
Mannitol Fermentation	+	+	V	+
Mannose Fermentation	+	+	+	+
Arabinose Fermentation	-	+	-	V

Table 2. Effects of Method on Number and Serovars of
Vibrio cholerae Isolates Recovered

Type Samples	6-Hour Incubation	18-Hour Incubation
Water	5+/47 isolates HH:RR:Uk[a]	10+/45 G:H:J:AA:FF:GG:Uk
Sewer	No isolates	W
Sewer	M:R:CC:GG	H:M:Q:U
Sewer	No isolates	G:M:PP:RR

[a]Isolates serotyped by R.J. Siebeling et al. (this volume).

vibrios. Odd tube combinations such as 1-3-2, 0-1-3, 2-3-3
were seen in 16 of 149 V. cholerae MPN's, 13 of 68 V.
parahaemolyticus MPN's, 7 of 57 Lac+ MPN's, and 1 of 29
Group F MPN's. This same phenomenon was noted by the
teams in Maryland and Oregon. Beginning inocula for water
samples was either 1000 or 100 ml. High vibrio counts in
Louisiana waters may mean a competitive overgrowth in our
results but not in Maryland and Oregon waters. This
"Tower of Babel" phenomenon may simply mean that the
vibrios are present but turned off by our isolation
procedures.

To paraphase Walt Kelly, "It should be borne in mind
that at the time we were studying vibrios, vibrios had an
excellent opportunity to study us."

ACKNOWLEDGMENTS

We gratefully acknowledge the expert technical assistance of Connie Guillory, Kathy Johnson, Joyce Landor,

Table 3. Comparative Recovery of Vibrio Species From Four Enrichment Broths

Organism	AP[a]	Horie	PS[b]	BAP[c]
Vibrio cholerae	36	10	12	1
Vibrio parahaemolyticus	13	27	24	2
Vibrio vulnificus	17	8	9	0
Vibrio fluvialis	10	9	4	11
Negative[d]	5	8	10	24
Total	41	35	34	35

[a]Alkaline peptone broth (1% peptone, 1% NaCl, pH 8.5).
[b]Peptone saline (1% peptone, 3% NaCl, pH 8.5).
[c]BAP = Buchi's alkaline peptone (1% peptone, 4% NaCl, 5 mg/ml-novobiocin, pH 8.5).
[d]For specific Vibrio spp.

Billie Monsour, Willard Mahfouz, Opal Hair, Susan Searle, Allen Hebert, Mike Purpera, James Gillespie, and Betty Planchard. This work was supported in part by the Louisiana State University Sea Grant Program, and by the Oregon State University Sea Grant College Program, National Oceanic and Atmospheric Administration Office of Sea Grant, Department of Commerce, under Grants NA79AA-D-00128 and NA79AA-D-00106, project R/FSD8.

REFERENCES

Food and Drug Administration Bureau of Foods, Division of Microbiology. 1978. Bacteriological Analytical Manual, 1978. 5th ed. Association of Official Analytical Chemists, Washington, D.C.

Horie, S., K. Saheki, T. Kozima, M. Nava, and Y. Sekine. 1964. Distribution of Vibrio parahaemolyticus in plankton and fish in the open sea. Bull. Jpn. Soc. Sci. Fish. 30:786-791.

Kaper, J., H. Lockman, R.R. Colwell, and S.W. Joseph. 1979. Ecology, serology, and enterotoxin production of Vibrio cholerae in Chesapeake Bay. Appl. Environ. Microbiol. 37:91-103.

Litsky, W. 1979. Gut critters are stressed in the environment, more stressed by isolation procedures. Pages 345-347 in R.R. Colwell et al. (Eds.), Aquatic microbial ecology, proceedings of the conference. University of Maryland Sea Grant, College Park, Maryland.

Wachsmuth, I.K., G.K. Morris, and J.C. Feeley. 1980. Vibrio. Pages 226-234 in E.H. Lennette, A. Balows, W.J. Hausler Jr., and J.P. Truant (Eds.), Manual of clinical microbiology, 3rd ed. American Society for Microbiology, Washington, D.C.

Chapter 19

AN APPROACH TO ISOLATING DIFFERENT SEROVARS OF
VIBRIO CHOLERAE FROM ENVIRONMENTAL SAMPLES

A.D. Larson, Teresa Tyler, and R.J. Siebeling

The occurrence of cholera in Louisiana in 1978 provided an
impetus for elucidating the source(s) of Vibrio cholerae O1
organisms. Cholera has traditionally been viewed as a
disease which is spread from feces to mouth in a cycle
which does not involve the causative agent as a component
of the normal flora of the environment. It has been
proposed that V. cholerae, including the O1 group, is a
component of the microbial flora of brackish water. This
theory is supported by reports of the isolation of O1 Vibrio
from water and seafood which has not been polluted by
human wastes (Bashford et al. 1979; Colwell et al. 1981;
Desmarshelier and Reichelt 1981; Hood et al. 1981).

To date, the isolation of O1 and other serological types
of V. cholerae has been random in that no methods have
been developed by which a desired member of the genus
Vibrio can be isolated selectively. In this report we will
describe a procedure by which different serological types of
Vibrio can be isolated from environmental samples
providing, of course, that the desired type is present in
the sample. In addition, we will report results of our
efforts to isolate Vibrio cholerae O1 from seafood and
seafood-producing waters of Louisiana employing a selective
method.

277

METHODS

Hemolymph was collected from oysters by drilling a hole through the shell and removing hemolymph with a syringe and needle and 0.1 ml aliquots spread on thiosulfate citrate bile salts sucrose agar (TCBS; Difco, Detroit, MI) plates. The hole was then sealed with dental wax and the oysters placed in aerated seawater. Thus, hemolymph could be obtained at daily intervals employing the same hole. Oysters were shucked and homogenized for analysis in a Sorvall Omnimixer for 30 seconds at the maximum setting. Whole shrimp were homogenized before analysis in the same way as the oysters. Water samples were collected at intervals throughout the year. One-liter samples were collected by boat from five different areas of the body of water being sampled at a depth of 8 to 12 inches.

Analysis of homogenates and water for O1 serovars was done, using a modification of the serologically specific method we developed (Hranitzky et al. 1980) and the sloppy agar technique (Bhaskaran and Gorrill 1957). The modification we employed was the addition of 5 g of antibody-coated beads to a 500-ml filter flask. The samples were siphoned continuously into the bottom of the flask which was stirred with a magnetic mixer. The effluent was drained from the side arm as was the wash fluid. After washing with saline containing Tween 20, the beads were placed in alkaline peptone broth and incubated at 37°C for 16 to 24 hours. After incubation the culture was diluted such that 0.1 ml when spread on TCBS agar (Difco) plates would result in 30 to 50 colonies. Following colony development the colonies were replicated to brain heart infusion agar (BHIA; Difco, Detroit, MI) plates. After development of the colonies on BHIA, 10 ml of BHIA soft agar containing 0.1 ml of anti-O1 antiserum (prepared in rabbits with boiled cells of V. cholerae Inaba as antigen) was added to the plates. After a 30-minute incubation period at 37°C, the colonies which showed inhibition of motility were picked from the original TCBS plates and inoculated into Kliglers iron agar slants. Vibrio cholerae were identified by established techniques (Wachsmuth et al.

1980). The isolates were serologically identified by slide agglutination.

RESULTS AND DISCUSSION

The results of our analysis of seafood and seafood-producing waters are presented in Table 1. The most notable aspect of the data is that in no case did we isolate V. cholerae Ol. This was true in spite of the fact that in most of the water samples analyzed a significant number (see Table 1) of V. cholerae were present as determined by MPN. High numbers of V. cholerae were present even though the number of coliforms were low or absent. Except for the low temperatures of the water collected in late October from Vermilion Bay, the conditions for V. cholerae appeared ideal--salinity, alkaline pH, and temperatures near or at 30°C. In spite of the low water temperatures in late October, V. cholerae was still present in good number. The absence of V. cholerae Ol in water samples was reflected by their absence in seafood samples.

The method we employed in sample analysis proved to be successful when low numbers (40-100 viable cells) of V. cholerae Ol were added to samples of water or homogenized seafood. The antibody-coated beads favor concentration of Ol serovars even if nonspecific adsorption of non-Ol serovars occurs. However, such concentration is advantageous only if the ratio or growth rates of Ol to non-Ol organisms are near one or greater than one in the alkaline peptone water. We are not certain of this in all cases, but our strains of Inaba compete successfully with non-Ol V. cholerae in laboratory experiments in alkaline peptone broth.

The soft agar-antibody technique allowed us to identify quickly possible colonies of Ol serovars of V. cholerae. In addition, large numbers of colonies could be readily examined from each sample grown in alkaline peptone broth. We observed a number of colonies which showed characteristic lack of motility, but on careful serological analysis these were identified as non-Ol serovars. Therefore, the

Table 1. Results of Attempts to Isolate Vibrio cholerae O1

Collection Date	Sample and Source	Results	Description of Sample
3/01/81	Oyster, local supplier	Non-O1 isolates	Homogenates
4/01/81	Oyster, Pointe a La Hatche	Non-O1 isolates	Homogenates
4/22/81	Oyster, local supplier	No Vibrio	Homogenates & hemolymph
5/13/81	Oyster, local supplier	No Vibrio	Homogenates
5/19/81	Oyster, Point a La Hatche	No Vibrio	Homogenates, hemolymph & holding water
6/29/81	Oyster, Point a La Hatche	Non-O1 isolates	Homogenates, hemolymph & holding water
7/29/81	Water (5 x 1 L samples) Vermillion Bay	Non-O1 isolates	Salinity: 0.7-8.0 ppt Coliforms: 0 V. cholerae: 27-1600 +/100 ml Temperature: 29-30°C
8/11/81	Water (5 x 1 L samples) White Lake	Non-O1 isolates	Salinity: 1.1-2.0 ppt. pH: 7.2-7.4 Temperature: 30°C

280

Date	Sample	Isolates	Measurements
			Coliforms: 0
			V. cholerae: 17-540/100 ml
8/25/81	Water (5 x 1 L samples) Vermillion Bay	Non-O1 isolates	Salinity: 3.0-4.5 ppt
			pH: 7.6-8.0
			Temperature: 30°C
			Coliforms: 0
			V. cholerae: 27-1600 +/100 ml
9/11/81	Water (5/1 L samples) Baistaria Bay	Non-O1 isolates	Salinity: 20-31 ppt
			pH: 8.0-8.6
			Temperature: 30°C
			Coliforms: 0
			V. cholerae: 56-9200/100 ml
10/27/81	Water (5 x 1 L samples) Vermillion Bay	Non-O1 isolates	Salinity: 6.0-6.5 ppt
			pH: 7.6-7.8
			Temperature: 13-17°C
			Coliforms: 0
			V. cholerae > 1600

method is only as reliable as the quality of the antiserum employed.

It is somewhat puzzling that we did not isolate O1 organisms given the specificity of the antibody-coated beads and the number of colonies which were examined on the soft agar plates. The water samples contained many non-O1 V. cholerae. Possibly the presence of high numbers of non-O1 serovars does not necessarily indicate the presence of the O1 serovar. It may be that V. cholerae O1 has subtle environmental requirements which differ from those of the non-O1 serovars. Performing environmental studies on the different non-O1 serovars (some 80 in number) would be technologically difficult and perhaps beyond current capabilities. If our results reflect a genuine absence of O1 serovars in seafood and seafood-producing waters in Louisiana, then it is difficult to explain cases of cholera in Louisiana.

Many O1 environmental isolates have been shown to be nontoxigenic. We did not isolate any of these in our study; however, it has been our experience that unless antisera are carefully prepared and their specificities absolute, many isolates of V. cholerae can be erroneously classified as O1 organisms.

We think our methods can be employed for isolating many serologically different V. cholerae from environmental samples and possibly the methodology could be applied successfully to other bacteria in the environment. Future studies will be required to justify such an assumption.

ACKNOWLEDGMENTS

This research was supported by grants from the Louisiana Department of Health and Human Resources and the National Oceanic and Atmospheric Administration Office of Sea Grant, Department of Commerce, under grant number NA79AA-D-00128.

REFERENCES

Bashford, D.J., T.J. Donovan, A.L. Furniss, and J.V. Lee. 1979. Vibrio cholerae in Kent. Lancet i:436-437.

Bhaskaran, K., and R.H. Gorrill. 1957. A study of antigenic variation in Vibrio cholerae. J. Gen Microbiol. 16:721-729.

Colwell, R.R., R.J. Seidler, J. Kaper, S.W. Joseph, S. Garges, H. Lockman, H. Bradford, N. Roberts, E. Remmers, I. Huq, and A. Huq. 1981. Occurrence of Vibrio cholerae serotype O1 in Maryland and Louisiana Estuaries. Appl. Environ. Microbiol. 41:555-558.

Desmarshelier, P., and J.L. Reichelt. 1981. Phenotypic characterization of clinical and environmental isolates to Vibrio cholerae from Australia. Curr. Microbiol. 5:123-127.

Hood, M.A., G.E. Ness, and G.E. Rodrick. 1981. Isolation of Vibrio cholerae serotype O1 from eastern oyster, Crassostrea virginica. Appl. Environ. Microbiol. 41:559-560.

Hranitzky, K.W., A.D. Larson, D.W. Ragsdale, and R.J. Siebeling. 1980. Isolation of O1 serovars of Vibrio cholerae by serologically specific method. Science 210:1025-1026.

Wachsmuth, J.K., G.K. Morris, and J.C. Feeley. 1980. Vibrio. Pages 226-236 in E.H. Lennett, Jr. et al. (Eds.), Manual of clinical microbiology. American Society for Microbiology, Washington, D.C.

Chapter 20

IDENTIFICATION AND CLASSIFICATION
OF VIBRIONACEAE--AN OVERVIEW

Paul A. West and Rita R. Colwell

Species of the family Vibrionaceae can be isolated from
freshwater, estuarine, and seawater environments, as well
as from the alimentary tract of man and warm-blooded
animals. Some species are pathogenic for man and others
are pathogenic for marine vertebrates and invertebrates.
Several of the species that have been described to date
have not yet been found to cause disease and are probably
saprophytic in their natural environment. Typically, these
species comprise the commensal flora of fish and shellfish.
Some species may participate in the cycling of matter, i.e.
decomposition of organic matter.

The family Vibrionaceae described in the eighth edition
of Bergey's Manual of Determinative Bacteriology (Veron
1974), was created to include the genus Vibrio and related
genera, Aeromonas, Plesiomonas, Photobacterium, and
Lucibacterium, with the genus Beneckea (vide infra)
retained only as a genus of uncertain taxonomic position.
In the seventh edition of Bergey's Manual, the genus Vibrio
was assigned to the Spirillaceae, primarily on the basis of
curvature of the cell wall and negative Gram reaction
(Breed et al. 1957b). However, somatic curvature was not
confined to the genus Vibrio. Other genera, such as Pseudomonas and Spirillum, included species demonstrating
morphological similarities to Vibrio spp. The term "vibrio"
was, for many years, used as a vernacular name for any

bacterium demonstrating a single somatic curvature. A simple test, relying on the susceptibility of Vibrio species to the pteridine compound, designated vibriostatic agent 0/129 (2,4-diamino-6,7-diisopropylpteridine), was reported by Shewan et al. (1954) to differentiate Vibrio from Pseudomonas. Shewan (1963) later provided a scheme for differentiating certain genera of gram-negative bacteria, including Vibrio, using primarily morphology, 0/129 sensitivity, oxidase reaction, and mode of glucose utilization. The International Association of Microbiological Societies Subcommittee on the Taxonomy of Vibrios subsequently recommended a description for the genus Vibrio which distinguished Vibrio from Pseudomonas and related genera, based on the mode of the metabolism of glucose (Feeley 1966). As a result, a revised scheme for identification of vibrios and related organisms was published by Bain and Shewan (1968). Numerical taxonomic principles and molecular genetic studies, emerging in the sixties to become routine taxonomic methodologies, when applied to strains of Vibrio, Pseudomonas, and Spirillum confirmed that there existed sufficient dissimilarity among these genera to warrant separate family status (Leifson and Mandel 1969; Colwell 1970; Carney et al. 1975). Thus, the aggregate taxonomic properties of the genus Vibrio were not considered appropriate for inclusion of Vibrio within the Spirillaceae (Eddy and Carpenter 1964; Veron 1965, 1971). Accordingly, the family Vibrionaceae was created and a description provided in the eighth edition of Bergey's Manual (Veron 1974).

Major traits useful in differentiating the genera of the Vibrionaceae and other heterotrophic gram-negative, fermentative rods, notably those of the Enterobacteriaceae are listed in Table 1 and Figure 1. Members of the Pseudomonadaceae and Spirillaceae are not facultatively fermentative, when grown in glucose or other carbohydrate-containing media (Krieg and Smibert 1974; Buchanan and Gibbons 1974). Members of the Enterobacteriaceae are peritrichously flagellated when motile, and oxidase-negative (Cowan 1974b). In contrast, species assigned to the family Vibrionaceae have polar flagella (when grown in liquid media), and are oxidase-positive, with the following exceptions: Vibrio metschnikovii, Vibrio gazogenes, and

Table 1. Selected Features Distinguishing the Family Vibrionaceae from the Family Enterobacteriaceae and Separating Genera within the Vibrionaceae[a,b]

Feature	Genera of the Vibrionaceae				Genera of the Enterobacteriaceae
	Vibrio	Aeromonas	Plesiomonas	Photobacterium	
Flagellation on solid medium	Polar or mixed	Polar or none	Polar	Polar	Peritrichous or none
Cytochrome oxidase	+[c]	+	+	v	-
Gas from glucose	-[d]	v	-	v	v
Luminescence	v	-	-	+[e]	-
Sensitivity to O/129:					
10 µg/ml	v	-	+	v	-
150 µg/ml	+	-	+	+	-
Mol% G+C of the DNA	38-51	57-63	51	40-44	39-59

[a] Source of data: Shewan and Veron (1974), Lee et al. (1979), Baumann et al. (1980).
[b] + = Positive reaction for all strains. v = Reaction differs for strains and species in the genus.
  - = Negative reaction for all strains.
[c] V. metschnikovii and V. gazogenes are oxidase-negative.
[d] V. fluvialis biovar II and V. gazogenes produce gas.
[e] P. angustum is not luminescent.

287

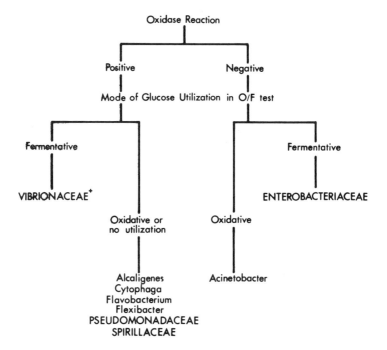

Figure 1. Scheme for screening some gram-negative asporogenous rods commonly encountered in natural aquatic environments. After Buchanan and Gibbons (1974). Note that V. metschnikovii, V. gazogenes, and Photobacterium phosphoreum are oxidase-negative.

Photobacterium phosphoreum, which are oxidase-negative, and Aeromonas salmonicida which is nonmotile.

Unfortunately, the burst of active research on the Vibrionaceae in the past decade has resulted in a confusion in nomenclature. In order to deal with these developments in an orderly fashion here, the following descriptions of each genus are given employing the names of genera and epithets for species as they appear in the eighth edition of Bergey's Manual of Determinative Bacteriology (Veron 1974). As appropriate, results of taxonomy studies and suggested nomenclatural alterations subsequent to the publication of the eighth edition of Bergey's Manual are also provided.

The genus Aeromonas

Members of the genus are widely distributed in fresh and brackish water and are ubiquitous as commensals of fish and amphibia (Hazen et al. 1978; Hazen 1979; Kaper et al. 1981). Aeromonas hydrophila has been identified as the causative agent of disease in animals (Shotts et al. 1972; Rigney et al. 1978) and it has also been associated with a variety of human diseases (Von Graevenitz and Mensch 1968; Davis et al. 1978). The nonmotile species, A. salmonicida, is responsible for disease in fish (McCarthy and Roberts 1980). Members of the genus Aeromonas are resistant to the vibriostatic agent 0/129 at 150 µg/ml and possess a mol% G+C in the range 57-63% (Table 1).

The taxonomy of the species of Aeromonas remains confused despite attempts to produce identification schemes employing phenotypic characteristics (Sakazaki and Balows 1981). Schemes based on the studies by Schubert (1967a; 1967b; 1968) were published in the eighth edition of Bergey's Manual (Schubert 1974). In the latter, nonnumerical taxonomic methods were employed and the anaerogenic aeromonads were classified as biovars of the aerogenic species. Accordingly, three subspecies (hydrophila, anaerogenes, and proteolytica) under A. hydrophila, two subspecies (punctata and caviae) under Aeromonas punctata and three subspecies (salmonicida, achromogenes, and masoucida) under A. salmonicida were published. In 1976, Popoff and Veron reported results of a numerical taxonomic study of motile Aeromonas strains. Species and subspecies of A. hydrophila and A. punctata could not be distinguished and were therefore united as one species, A. hydrophila, with biovars hydrophila and anaerogenes. A new species, Aeromonas sobria, was also described. The species A. hydrophila subsp. proteolytica was excluded from the genus based on mol% G+C content (50.9%), peritrichous flagellation on solid media, and the halophilic nature of its growth requirements. This species is presently included in the genus Vibrio (Baumann et al. 1980), but is doubtful as a valid member of the genus.

Features useful in the identification of Aeromonas spp. are listed in Table 2. Failure to hydrolyze arabinose and

Table 2. Features Useful in the Identification of Aeromonas spp. and Plesiomonas shigelloides[a]

Feature	A. hydrophila	A. sobria	A. salmonicida	P. shigelloides
Arginine dihydrolase	+	+	+	+
Lysine decarboxylase	v[b]	v	–	+
Ornithine decarboxylase	–	–	–	+
Sensitivity to O/129:				
10 µg/ml	–	–	–	+
150 uq/ml	–	–	–	+
Growth at 37°C	+	+	–	+
Motility	+	+	–	+
Acid from:				
L-arabinose	v	v	–	–
m-inositol	–	–	–	+
D-mannose	+	+	+	–
Sucrose	v	+	v	–
Production of:				
Amylase	+	+	+	–
Gelatinase	+	+	+	–
Lecithinase	+	+	+	–
Lipase (Tween 80)	+	+	+	–

	biovar hydrophila	biovar anaerogenes		
Growth in % NaCl:				
0	+	+	+	+
6	v	v	v	v
8	–	–	–	–
Esculin hydrolysis	+	v	v	–
Growth in KCN medium	+	v	–	–
Growth on:				
L-arginine	v	–	–	–
L-histidine	+	–	–	–
Gas from glucose	+	–	+	–
Voges-Proskauer reaction	+	v	–	–
Elastase production	+	–	–	–

[a]Source of data: Lee et al. (1979); Von Graevenitz (1980); West (1980); Sakazaki and Balows (1981).
[b]Different reactions among the species.

a positive Voges-Proskauer reaction are traits which differ among strains although Burke et al. (1982) have demonstrated a correlation of possession of both these traits with enterotoxigenic potential.

Further taxonomic investigation of the genus by Shaw and Hodder (1978), using analysis of lipopolysaccharide content of cell walls, revealed three distinct groups within 12 motile Aeromonas strains which corresponded to the taxonomic groups reported in the study of Popoff and Veron (1976). However, nucleic acid (DNA/DNA) homology studies differ in their support of the species groups of motile Aeromonas strains established on the basis of phenotypic characterization. Some workers have suggested that, for practical identification purposes, all motile Aeromonas strains be referred to as a single species, A. hydrophila (MacInnes et al. 1979). More recent studies have revealed that at least three species can be recognized, based on DNA/DNA homology data within motile Aeromonas strains (Popoff et al. 1981).

To confound the issue, a recently described species, Vibrio fluvialis (Lee et al. 1981), superficially resembles the aerogenic and anaerogenic biovars of A. hydrophila. Thus, it is possible that results of ecological studies, prior to publication of the description of V. fluvialis include overestimations of the incidence of A. hydrophila in aquatic environments, since V. fluvialis is found in similar habitats.

In taxonomic analyses of cultures expected to include Aeromonas spp., it is recommended that the following cultures be included as controls: A. hydrophila biovar hydrophila ATCC 7966; A. hydrophila biovar anaerogenes ATCC 15468; A. salmonicida ATCC 19261 or ATCC 14174; A. sobria Collection of the Institute Pasteur, Paris 75015, France, strain 7433.

The genus Plesiomonas

The genus Plesiomonas was proposed mainly because of the perplexing taxonomic position of this group of strains and an inability to allocate Plesiomonas shigelloides to any other genus because of its rather interesting and unique properties. P. shigelloides was identified as the C27 strain of Ferguson and Henderson (1947) and has in the past been placed in the genus Pseudomonas and, subsequently, Aeromonas (Habs and Schubert 1962), prior to its present generic designation.

P. shigelloides resembles species of the genus Vibrio in being oxidase-positive and sensitive to 0/129, but differs from Vibrio spp. in the restricted range of carbohydrates it is capable of fermenting, as well as in the absence of extracellular enzyme production (Schubert 1974; Von Graevenitz 1980). Table 2 lists characteristics useful in the identification of P. shigelloides. A serotyping scheme has also been reported for this species (Shimada and Sakazaki 1978).

Unfortunately the ecology of P. shigelloides and its role in human disease are, as yet, unclear, even though it has been implicated in diarrheal disease (Tsukamoto et al. 1978). The organism is often recovered on differential or selective plating media designed to isolate pathogenic members of the Enterobacteriaceae (Sakazaki and Balows 1981). The colonial appearance of P. shigelloides on deoxycholate-citrate agar is similar to that of colonies of Shigella spp. (Furniss 1979). In addition, many strains of P. shigelloides are agglutinated by Shigella sonnei phase 1 antiserum possibly because of the cross-reaction of a common somatic antigen (Whang et al. 1972), occasionally resulting in misidentification if only colonial appearance and serological reactions are employed. The oxidase test, using colonies grown on a nonselective medium without fermentable carbohydrates, should be used to prevent confusion in identification between P. shigelloides and Shigella strains.

Although P. shigelloides is a potential diarrheal agent, and therefore of medical interest, the ecology of this species has been largely neglected with the notable exception of studies done in Japan by Tsukamoto et al. (1978) and Arai et al. (1980). Suitable enrichment and selective plating media need to be developed for the isolation of P. shigelloides since the organism grows poorly, if at all, on thiosulphate citrate bile salts sucrose (TCBS) agar. Recommended control culture for taxonomic studies is ATCC 14029.

The genus Photobacterium

Bacteria possessing the ability to emit visible light are not rare in the aquatic environment, especially the marine environment. Common habitats include the water column, the surface and alimentary tract of marine animals and the luminous organ of some fish species (Baumann and Baumann 1977; Nealson and Hastings 1979; Orndorff and Colwell 1981).

Based on results of a phenotypic study of luminescent bacteria, Hendrie et al. (1970) recognized three genera: Vibrio, Photobacterium, and Lucibacterium. These groups were based on phenetic data without application of numerical taxonomy. Based on their data, the genus Photobacterium was concluded to contain two species. The recommended type strain was Photobacterium phosphoreum and a new species, Photobacterium mandapamensis, was described. One group of luminescent bacteria, Photobacterium fischeri, previously described in the seventh edition of Bergey's Manual (Breed et al. 1957a), was transferred to the genus Vibrio. The conclusions of this study were adopted when the description of the genus Photobacterium was prepared for the eighth edition of Bergey's Manual of Determinative Bacteriology (Hendrie and Shewan 1974a).

Since 1974, the genus Photobacterium has undergone several taxonomic and nomenclatural changes. The species P. mandapamensis was renamed Photobacterium leiognathi on the basis of priority of nomenclature (Reichelt and Baumann 1975) and the species Vibrio fischeri was returned to the genus. A group of nonluminescent bacteria, group B-2 of Baumann et al. (1971a), was recognized as a new species, Photobacterium angustum (Reichelt et al. 1976; Baumann and Baumann 1977). Phenotypic characterization of atypical P. fischeri strains resulted in the assignment of a new species, Photobacterium logei, to the genus Photobacterium (Bang et al. 1978b).

The genera Photobacterium and Vibrio cannot be readily distinguished by phenotypic characterization or analysis of phenetic data by numerical taxonomy (Baumann et al. 1980). Thus, comparisons of the properties of evolutionarily conserved information molecules in members of

Photobacterium and Vibrio have been performed and have provided greater insight into the taxonomic relationships of these genera. Extensive studies of the amino acid sequence of the glutamine synthetase and superoxide dismutase enzymes indicate evolutionary divergence between the genera Photobacterium and Vibrio (Baumann and Baumann 1980; Bang et al. 1981) and necessitated the transfer of P. fischeri and P. logei to the genus Vibrio and separation from other Photobacterium spp. (Baumann et al. 1980).

The genus Photobacterium currently comprises three closely related species; P. phosphoreum and P. leiognathi are luminescent while P. angustum does not demonstrate light emission (Baumann et al. 1980). All Photobacterium species described to date lack a sheath on polar flagella and fail to produce extracellular amylase. All species accumulate polyhydroxybutyrate intracellularly, when grown on D-glucose, but fail to utilize β-hydroxybutyrate when supplied in a minimal medium (Baumann et al. 1980). Some strains have an obligate requirement for organic growth factors, which can be overcome by addition of 0.01-0.05% yeast extract to the culture medium. Further revision of the genus Photobacterium may be indicated in the near future. Recommended control cultures are: P. phosphoreum ATCC 11040; P. leiognathi ATCC 25521; and P. angustum ATCC 25915.

The genus Lucibacterium

In a study of luminous marine bacteria, Hendrie et al. (1970) recognized a group of related isolates whose properties showed strong similarity to members of the genus Vibrio. However, possession of peritrichous, as well as polar, flagellation and insensitivity to 0/129 precluded the inclusion of these strains in the genus Vibrio in the judgment of these authors. The genus Lucibacterium was created to accommodate these strains and they were grouped within the single species Lucibacterium harveyi (Hendrie and Shewan 1974b). The creation of the genus Lucibacterium failed to recognize that a shift from polar flagellation in liquid medium to peritrichous-like flagellation on solid medium commonly occurs with marine Vibrio species (vide infra). Thus, these strains were transferred to the genus Beneckea by Reichelt et al. (1976), the latter having been described (vide infra) to include peritrichously-flagellated, marine Vibrio-like strains (Baumann et al. 1971a). These strains are now listed in the genus Vibrio following the abolition of the genus Beneckea (Baumann et al. 1980).

Vibrio harveyi is a marine bacterium commonly found in the water column and on fish in estuarine and marine environments. The species superficially resembles the human pathogen Vibrio parahaemolyticus and misidentification can occur if sole carbon source utilization studies are not performed. Features useful in the identification of V. harveyi are listed in Table 5. The recommended control culture for taxonomic studies or identification schemes is ATCC 14126.

The genus Beneckea

In addition to a single polar flagellum, some members of the Vibrionaceae are now known to produce peritrichous, or lateral, flagella under certain cultural conditions. Bacteria demonstrating this mode of flagellation were not included in the genus Vibrio when Baumann et al. (1971a) reported on their studies of the classification of oxidase-positive, facultatively anaerobic, chitin-digesting, gram-negative bacteria of marine origin. These strains were assigned to the genus Beneckea which had been redefined to accommodate them (Baumann et al. 1971a). However, members of the genus Beneckea resembled those in the genus Vibrio in several major physiological and biochemical properties, as well as Mol% G+C content of DNA. In addition, V. cholerae had previously been shown to be a chitin-digesting species (Dastidar and Narayanaswani 1968). Baumann et al. (1971a) did not assign their strains to Vibrio, since the definition of Vibrio at that time was restricted to polarly-flagellated organisms. Subsequent expansion of the genus Beneckea to include strains previously assigned to Vibrio created confusion, rather than clarification, of the taxonomy of the Vibrionaceae (Baumann et al. 1973), resulting, finally, in the abolition of the genus Beneckea.

In 1976, Reichelt et al. published a revised description of the genus Beneckea based on DNA/DNA hybridization and numerical taxonomic studies. Members of the genus Vibrio, including the type strain V. cholerae, were excluded from Beneckea on the basis of low DNA/DNA homology, although phenotypic characteristics and mol% G+C indicated considerable similarity between the two genera. In addition, exclusion of V. cholerae from Beneckea was based on the tenuous criterion of ecological habitat. The obligate requirement by Beneckea spp. for Na$^+$ for survival and growth was interpreted as reflecting their marine origin, whereas V. cholerae was considered a human intestinal inhabitant (Baumann and Baumann 1977).

The ecological studies described in this volume clearly indicate that habitat can not be used for separation of Beneckea and Vibrio since V. cholerae can be isolated from freshwater and brackish environments. For this reason, as well as phenotypic similarities, the validity of the taxonomic distinctions between Beneckea and Vibrio has been questioned.

The taxonomy of Beneckea and Vibrio has been reevaluated and clarified by study of the amino acid sequence homology and divergence in the enzymes glutamine synthetase (Baumann and Baumann 1980) and superoxide dismutase (Bang et al. 1981) as well as study of ribosomal ribonucleic acid homology (Baumann and Baumann 1976). None of these studies indicated that there was any objective and consistent division to be made between Vibrio, Beneckea, and some of the Photobacterium spp. Accordingly, all members of the genus Beneckea and some species previously assigned to Photobacterium have been placed in the genus Vibrio (Baumann et al. 1980).

The genus Allomonas

The genus Allomonas was created by Kalina et al. (1980a) to accommodate a phenotypically diverse group of 24 bacterial isolates from lake water, sewage liquor, and fecal samples. Allomonas strains were assigned to the family Vibrionaceae by these workers although their phenotypic characterization of strains of other related genera (Aeromonas, Plesiomonas, and Vibrio) suggests deficiencies in methodology. Nineteen strains were given species status as Allomonas enterica after analysis by numerical taxonomic techniques (Kalina et al. 1980b; Kalina 1980).

Strains of Allomonas gave more positive results in biochemical tests when NaCl was added to culture media. Most strains were arginine dihydrolase and ornithine decarboxylase-positive, but all failed to decarboxylate lysine. Strains were generally positive for the following characteristics: fermentation of arabinose and sucrose and production of lecithinase. The strains were, in general, negative for indole production, lactose fermentation, and methyl red reaction. An isolation medium for Allomonas spp. has been reported (Kalina 1981), but further phenotypic and genetic studies are required on more isolates to confirm the taxonomic status of Allomonas species.

The genus Vibrio

The genus contains organisms which are abundant in the aquatic environment, some of which can cause disease in man, as well as in marine vertebrates and invertebrates. The genus is the most extensively characterized, and medically important group of the Vibrionaceae yet the taxonomy of Vibrio is still in a considerable state of flux.

The amended description of Vibrio, following abolition of the genus Beneckea (Baumann et al. 1980), is as follows: "Cells generally single, straight or curved rods. When grown in liquid media, motile by sheathed polar flagella; monotrichous or multitrichous. On solid media may exhibit mixed flagellation with additional peritrichous unsheathed flagella of a shorter wavelength than the sheathed polar flagella. Gram negative. Do not form endospores or microcysts. Chemoorganotrophs: facultative anaerobes capable of respiratory and fermentative metabolism using D-glucose as the sole or principal source of carbon and energy. Molecular oxygen is a universal electron acceptor. Do not denitrify or fix molecular nitrogen. Growth stimulated by Na^+; most species will not grow in the absence of this ion. The G+C contents in the DNAs of the species range from 38 to 51 mol %."

Table 3 lists the species which have been assigned to the genus Vibrio by Baumann et al. (1980) together with their synonyms and more recent taxonomic history, where applicable, and the type strain designation.

Six species, Vibrio cholerae, Vibrio parahaemolyticus, Vibrio alginolyticus, Vibrio vulnificus, Vibrio fluvialis, and Vibrio metschnikovii, are potential pathogens of man and their taxonomy and identification warrants further discussion. Reviews of the clinical significance and disease syndromes associated with these species have been published by Barua and Burrows (1974) and Blake et al. (1980b).

1. Vibrio cholerae

V. cholerae is the causative agent of the disease cholera, characterized in its extreme form by severe watery diarrhea. Historically, epidemic strains of V. cholerae have been differentiated into hemolytic and nonhemolytic variants. For several decades, the hemolytic strains were treated as a separate species, Vibrio eltor, and regarded as nonpathogenic. However, in 1961, hemolytic strains were associated with a cholera outbreak in Indonesia which eventually developed into the seventh pandemic of the disease (Cvjetanovic and Barua 1972). Insufficient differences exist to justify separation at the species level of strains named V. cholerae and V. eltor (Hugh 1965; Citarella and Colwell 1970). Accordingly, the current definition of V. cholerae encompasses the classical (nonhemolytic) and El Tor (hemolytic) biovars (Shewan and Veron 1974).

Somatic (O) antigenic structure has fundamental importance in the classification and identification of this organism. The serovar of V. cholerae associated with epidemic cholera has been defined by its agglutination in specific polyvalent O1 antiserum (Gardner and Venkatraman

Table 3. Species of Vibrio with Their Synonyms, Taxonomic History and Recommended Type Strain[a]

Current Designation	Past Synonym(s)	Designation in Bergey's Manual, 8th ed. (1974)	Type Strain[b]
Vibrio alginolyticus	Beneckea alginolytica	V. parahaemolyticus biotype 2	ATCC 17749
V. anguillarum biovars I & II	B. anguillara biovars I & II	V. anguillarum	ATCC 19264
V. campbellii	B. campbellii	—	ATCC 25920
V. cholerae	—	V. cholerae biotypes cholerae, El Tor, and albensis	ATCC 14035
V. costicola	—	V. costicola	NCMB 701
V. fischeri	Photobacterium fischeri	V. fischeri	ATCC 7744
V. fluvialis biovars I & II	Group F vibrio, EF-6 group	—	NCTC 11327
V. gazogenes	B. gazogenes	—	ATCC 29988
V. harveyi	B. harveyi, B. neptuna	Lucibacterium harveyi	ATCC 14126
V. logei	P. logei	V. fischeri	ATCC 29985
V. marinus	—	V. fischeri	ATCC 15381
V. metschnikovii	V. proteus	V. cholerae biotype proteus	NCTC 8443
V. natriegens	B. natriegens, Pseudomonas natriegens	—	ATCC 14048
V. nereis	B. nereida	—	ATCC 25917
V. nigripulchritudo	B. nigripulchrituda	—	ATCC 27043
V. parahaemolyticus	B. parahaemolytica	V. parahaemolyticus biotype 1	ATCC 17802
V. pelagius biovars I & II	B. pelagia biovars I & II	—	ATCC 25916
V. proteolyticus	B. proteolytica	Aeromonas hydrophila subsp. proteolytica	ATCC 15338
V. splendidus biovars I & II	B. splendida biovars I & II	L. harveyi	ATCC 33125
V. vulnificus	B. vulnifica, L+ vibrio, Group C2	—	ATCC 27562

[a]After Baumann et al. (1980).
[b]ATCC: American Type Culture Collection, Rockville, Maryland 20852, USA; NCTC: National Collection of Type Cultures, Central Public Health Laboratory, Colindale, London NW9 5HT, England; NCMB: National Collection of Marine Bacteria, Torry Research Station, Aberdeen AB9 8DG, Scotland.

1935; Hugh and Feeley 1972). Interest has now shifted to those strains which are biochemically identical to V. cholerae O1 but do not possess the O1 somatic antigen. These strains are now collectively known as non-O1 V. cholerae having been referred to previously as nonagglutinable vibrios (NAGs), noncholera vibrios (NCVs), and V. enteritidis. The term "nonagglutinable" vibrios is a misnomer as all Vibrio strains are agglutinated in their homologous antiserum. The term originally referred to strains of V. cholerae not agglutinated by polyvalent O1 antiserum, but has become redundant as it was often used loosely for any Vibrio, Aeromonas, or even Enterobacteriaceae strains which failed to be agglutinated. The term "noncholera" vibrio has caused confusion, since it may be interpreted as any Vibrio species not associated with cholera. The alternative designation, Vibrio enteritidis (Finklestein 1973) has not been accepted by ecologists, taxonomists, or clinicians.

Data from numerical taxonomic (Sakazaki et al. 1967; Colwell 1970) enzyme analysis (Colwell et al. 1968; Hsieh and Liu 1970) and DNA/DNA hybridization studies (Citarella and Colwell 1970) have indicated a high degree of similarity between strains of V. cholerae O1 (classical and El Tor) and non-O1 V. cholerae. Accordingly, the species definition of V. cholerae currently encompasses O1 and non-O1 serovars (Hugh and Feeley 1972).

Laboratory procedures for the identification of V. cholerae have been described by Wachsmuth et al. (1980). Table 4 lists the characteristics useful for the identification of the biovars within the O1 serovar of V. cholerae. Features for the identification of O1 and non-O1 serovars of V. cholerae are listed in Table 5. Several historically important schemes have been developed to differentiate strains of O1 and non-O1 serovars for epidemiological and identification purposes.

Serology. Two schemes are currently available for the serotyping of non-O1 V. cholerae (Brenner et al. 1982). Differences between the system of Sakazaki (Sakazaki et al. 1970; Shimada and Sakazaki 1977) and the system of Smith (1979) lie in the methods of antiserum preparation and

Table 4. Reactions of biovars of Vibrio cholerae serovar O1[a]

	Biovar	
Feature	Classical	El Tor
Hemolysis of sheep erythrocytes	–	V[b]
Voges-Proskauer reaction	–	+
Chicken erythrocyte agglutination	–	+
Sensitivity to:		
Polymyxin B (50 i.u.)	+	–
Mukerjee classical phage IV	+	–
Mukerjee El Tor phage 5	–	+

[a]See Furniss et al. (1978), Furniss (1979), and Wachsmuth et al. (1980) for methods.
[b]Different reactions within the biovar.

numerical designation of serovars. A third system, based on lipopolysaccharide of the somatic antigen, is under development and discussed elsewhere in this volume (Siebeling et al.).

The O1 serovar of V. cholerae can be divided into subserovars Ogawa and Inaba by the use of absorbed sera. Rare strains which agglutinate in both Ogawa and Inaba monospecific antisera are designated as Hikojima subserovar (Furniss et al. 1978).

Phage Typing. Developments in the application of phages as an epidemiology typing system for the O1 serovar have been reviewed by Mukerjee (1978). A typing scheme has been described by Lee and Furniss (1981) and has proved useful in epidemiology studies, notably during the cholera outbreak in Louisiana in 1978 (Blake et al. 1980a). No scheme for phage typing non-O1 serovar strains has been tested in field conditions, following the preliminary studies of Sil et al. (1974).

Vibriocin Typing. A vibriocin typing scheme for V. cholerae was reported by Chakrabarty et al. (1970) following the pioneering studies on the factors controlling vibriocin production by Farkas-Himsley and Seyfried (1963). The efficacy and technical problems of vibriocin typing for use as an epidemiological and taxonomic method have been reviewed by Brandis (1978).

Biochemical Typing. A typing scheme for Vibrio species, including V. cholerae, was proposed by Heiberg (1936) on the basis of fermentation patterns with sucrose, D-mannose, and L-arabinose. Heiberg group I (sucrose and mannose, but not arabinose fermented) includes V. cholerae serovar O1. Strains of non-O1 V. cholerae have been assigned to Heiberg groups I, II (only sucrose fermented), and V (only mannose fermented). The scheme is not useful for biotyping V. cholerae from clinical or environmental samples since groups I and II do not remain distinct when strains were analyzed by numerical taxonomic techniques (West 1980; Kaper et al. 1983). However, Heiberg group V strains differ from those in groups I and II in being nonsucrose fermenters, giving a negative Voges-Proskauer reaction and not elaborating an extracellular amylase. Heiberg group V strains have been recently assigned species status, under the name Vibrio mimicus, following DNA/DNA homology studies (Davis et al. 1981).

Luminescence. In 1974, Shewan and Veron described a luminescent organism which was biochemically similar to V. cholerae and assigned the single strain extant at the time to the biotype albensis of V. cholerae. This unique strain was later given species status as Vibrio albensis (Hugh and Sakazaki 1975). Subsequent data from DNA/DNA homology studies (Reichelt et al. 1976) and comparison of the electrophoretic mobility of superoxide dismutases (Bang et al. 1978a) indicated high taxonomic similarity between the single strain of V. albensis and representatives of V. cholerae. Accordingly, luminescent strains are currently recognized

within the species V. cholerae (Baumann et al. 1980).
Since this redefinition of V. cholerae, it has become
apparent that luminescent non-O1 serovars are widely
distributed in the natural aquatic environment. Characterization of luminescent non-O1 serovars from brackish
water (West 1980) and freshwater (Desmarchelier and Reichelt 1981, 1982) have reinforced the taxonomic conclusions
that luminescence is a property of V. cholerae which may,
or may not, be expressed.

Enteropathogenic Potential. Spira and Daniel (1980)
identified several biotypes, on the basis of enteropathogenicity, within a set of non-O1 serovar V. cholerae from
Bangladesh and other global sources. No detailed phenotypic characterization was reported and, presently,
biotyping of V. cholerae by possession of virulence factors
has little taxonomic significance.

Pyrolysis Gas-Liquid Chromatography. Haddadin et al.
(1973) used the technique of pyrolysis gas-liquid chromatography to differentiate three biotypes (El Tor, classical
and "intermediate") in 45 strains of V. cholerae obtained
from different global areas. The method did not distinguish
between various Heiberg groups nor was it useful for
differentiating serovars. Nevertheless, the application of
analytical pyrolysis techniques may prove useful in epidemiological studies. High-resolution pyrolysis techniques
provide characteristic "fingerprints" of strains which could
be used to indicate possible common origins of outbreaks,
as well as routes of transmission of the disease. High cost
and lack of long-term reproducibility are problems which
need to be overcome before pyrolysis techniques can be
developed into routine laboratory methodologies (Gutteridge
and Norris 1979).

Electrophoretic Variation of Intracellular Enzymes.
Momen and Salles (1981) characterized the electrophoretic
variation of the enzymes malate dehydrogenase and glucose-
6-phosphate dehydrogenase in V. cholerae strains isolated
from a wide range of global sources. Six specific subgroups were detected which could not be correlated with

biovar type or geographical origin. However, the subgroup patterns could identify V. cholerae at the species level. The technique may prove useful in epidemiological studies of cholera outbreaks to determine sources and transmission routes of toxigenic strains.

Cell Lysate Characterization. Maiti et al. (1981) analyzed cell-free extracts of V. cholerae serovar O1 and "nonagglutinable" vibrios using polyacrylamide gel electrophoresis (PAGE) and infrared spectroscopy (IRS). The identification of the "nonagglutinable" vibrios was not presented and exemplifies the semantic confusion that can arise when this term is used. The studies indicated that PAGE and IRS could distinguish between V. cholerae O1 and the other isolates. Only PAGE yielded patterns useful in differentiating the classical and El Tor biovars of V. cholerae O1.

Inactivation of Cytochrome Activity by Triton X-100. A rapid visual test to detect V. cholerae O1 colonies was reported by Salles and Momen (1981). The test relies on detection of a shift in redox potential of the cytochrome system after treatment of cells with Triton X-100. The reaction was observed only with V. cholerae serovar O1 from human sources but was not correlated with toxin production. The underlying principles of the reaction are not known and the significance of this observation requires investigation.

2. Vibrio parahaemolyticus

Since its discovery and characterization, V. parahaemolyticus has been assigned to a variety of genera including Pasteurella, Pseudomonas, and Oceanomonas (Miyamoto et al. 1961). The organism was placed in the genus Vibrio by Shewan and Veron (1974) after the study by Sakazaki et al. (1963) had established a species description. The taxonomic history of this species has been reviewed by Fujino et al. (1974) and Joseph et al. (1982).

Strains of $\underline{V}$. parahaemolyticus implicated in gastro-enteritis appear as green (nonsucrose-fermenting) colonies on TCBS agar. However, sucrose-fermenting strains, otherwise phenotypically indistinguishable from nonsucrose-fermenting type and reference strains, are common in estuarine and coastal waters (Ayres and Barrow 1978; West and Colwell, unpublished data). The significance of sucrose-fermenting variants of $\underline{V}$. parahaemolyticus in seafood and cases of gastroenteritis is not known, since such isolates would usually be discarded without further characterization after isolation on TCBS agar.

Strains of $\underline{V}$. parahaemolyticus associated with gastro-enteritis produced a β-hemolysis of human erythrocytes, a reaction known as the Kanagawa phenomenon (Miyamoto et al. 1969). Hemolysis is best detected on Wagatsuma's agar, which contains mannitol to produce the optimum pH for hemolysis production (Cherwonogrodzky and Clark, 1981).

$\underline{V}$. parahaemolyticus can be serotyped on the basis of O and K antigens using commercially available diagnostic antisera (Toshiba Kagaku Kogyo Co. Ltd, Tokyo, Japan). Analyses of the chemical constituents of the 0-antigenic lipopolysaccaharides in $\underline{V}$. parahaemolyticus have indicated compositions unusual for gram-negative bacteria which may be taxonomically significant within the species as well as the genus Vibrio (Hisatsune et al. 1980a; 1982).

3. Vibrio alginolyticus

$\underline{V}$. alginolyticus is listed in the eighth edition of Bergey's Manual of Determinative Bacteriology as biotype 2 of $\underline{V}$. parahaemolyticus (Shewan and Veron 1974). In 1975, Hugh and Sakazaki recommended species status for the biotype 2 of $\underline{V}$. parahaemolyticus, in concordance with the earlier proposal of Sakazaki (1968).

Despite its specific epithet, members of this species do not digest alginic acid. The species is widely distributed in the marine environment and isolation from superficial lesions in man has been linked to a past history of exposure to seawater.

Strains of V. alginolyticus grow well on TCBS agar, as large yellow (sucrose-fermenting) colonies. Features characteristic of V. alginolyticus include pronounced swarming on nonselective solid media, positive Voges-Proskauer reaction, tolerance to 10% NaCl, and growth at 42°C (Larsen et al. 1981). Table 5 lists other useful and relevant identification test results.

4. Vibrio fluvialis

V. fluvialis has been recognized recently as an agent of diarrheal disease in man. Strains were previously referred to as Group F (Lee et al. 1981) and as EF-6 (Huq et al. 1980). Phenotypic characterizations of V. fluvialis suggest that two biovars exist. Biovar I is anaerogenic in glucose fermentation and is isolated frequently from diarrheal stools, whereas biovar II is aerogenic and is more commonly found in aquatic environments (Lee et al. 1981). Examination of the electrophoretic mobility of malate dehydrogenase has corroborated the designation of two biovars which was originally based on numerical taxonomic data (Momen and Salles 1981).

Other phenotypic characteristics useful in separating the biovars, as well as distinguishing the species from other members of the Vibrionaceae, have been published by Jensen et al. (1980). The taxonomic significance of the sugar composition of the cell wall lipopolysaccharide in V. fluvialis is under investigation (Hisatsune et al. 1980b).

V. fluvialis possesses an arginine dihydrolase system and superficially resembles other species of the Vibrionaceae, notably Vibrio anguillarum and A. hydrophila. Interpretation of early studies on the ecology of Aeromonas should be considered to be qualitative, rather than quantitative, since the recognition and definition of the species V. fluvialis. Overestimation of the incidence of Aeromonas in the environment may inadvertently have been reported as a consequence.

Table 5. Features Useful in the Identification of Species and Biovars within the Genus _Vibrio_, and Species within the Genus _Photobacterium_[a,b,c]

	_P_. angustum	_P_. leiognathi	_P_. phosphoreum
Cytochrome oxidase	+	v	-
Nitrate reduction	+	+	+
O/129 sensitivity:			
10 µg	-	+	+
150 µg	+	+	+
Swarming	-	-	-
Luminescence	-	+	+
Thornley's Arginine dihydrolase	+	+	+
Lysine decarboxylase	-	v	+
Ornithine decarboxylase	-	-	-
Growth at 42°C	-	-	-
Growth at % NaCl:			
0%	-	-	-
3%	+	+	+
6%	v	v	v
8%	v	v	v
10%	-	-	-
Voges-Proskauer reaction	-	+	+
Gas from glucose fermentation	-	-	+
Fermentation to acid:			
L-arabinose	-	-	-
m-inositol	-	-	-
D-mannose	+	+	+

Sucrose	−	−	v
Enzyme production:			
Alginase	−	−	−
Amylase	−	−	−
Chitinase	+	+	v
Gelatinase	−	−	+
Lipase	−	+	v
Utilization as sole source of carbon:			
γ-aminobutyrate	−	−	−
Cellobiose	−	−	−
L-citrulline	−	−	−
Ethanol	−	−	−
D-gluconate	+	+	+
D-glucuronate	v	−	−
L-leucine	−	−	−
Putrescine	−	−	−
Sucrose	−	−	v
D-xylose	−	−	+

Table 5. Continued

	V. alginolyticus	V. anguillarum biovar I	biovar II
Cytochrome oxidase	+	+	+
Nitrate reduction	+	+	−
O/129 sensitivity:			
10 μg	−	+	+
150 μg	+	+	+
Swarming	+	−	−
Luminescence	−	−	−
Thornley's Arginine dihydrolase	−	+	−
Lysine decarboxylase	+	−	−
Ornithine decarboxylase	+	−	−
Growth at 42°C	+	−	−
Growth at % NaCl:			
0%	−	v	−
3%	+	+	+
6%	+	+	+
8%	+	v	−
10%	+	−	−
Voges-Proskauer reaction	+	+	−
Gas from glucose fermentation	−	−	−
Fermentation to acid:			
L-arabinose	−	v	−
m-inositol	−	v	−
D-mannose	+	+	−

Sucrose	+	+	+
Enzyme production:			
Alginase	–	–	–
Amylase	–	+	+
Chitinase	–	+	+
Gelatinase	v	+	+
Lipase	+	+	+
Utilization as sole source of carbon:			
γ-aminobutyrate	–	–	–
Cellobiose	–	v	–
L-citrulline	–	–	–
Ethanol	–	–	v
D-gluconate	–	+	+
D-glucuronate	–	–	–
L-leucine	–	–	+
Putrescine	–	–	v
Sucrose	+	+	+
D-xylose	–	–	–

Table 5. Continued

	V. campbellii	V. cholerae	V. costicola
Cytochrome oxidase	+	+	+
Nitrate reduction	+	+	+
O/129 sensitivity:			
10 μg	-	+	-
150 μg	+	+	+
Swarming	-	-	-
Luminescence	-	v	-
Thornley's Arginine dihydrolase	-	-	+
Lysine decarboxylase	+	+	-
Ornithine decarboxylase	-	+	-
Growth at 42°C	-	+	-
Growth at % NaCl:			
0%	-	+	-
3%	+	+	+
6%	+	v	+
8%	v	-	+
10%	-	-	+
Voges-Proskauer reaction	-	+	+
Gas from glucose fermentation	-	-	-
Fermentation to acid:			
L-arabinose	-	-	-
m-inositol	-	-	-
D-mannose	+	v	+
Sucrose	-	+	+

Enzyme production:			
Alginase	−	−	−
Amylase	+	+	−
Chitinase	+	+	−
Gelatinase	+	+	+
Lipase	+	+	v
Utilization as sole source of carbon:			
γ-aminobutyrate	−	−	−
Cellobiose	v	−	−
L-citrulline	−	−	−
Ethanol	−	−	−
D-gluconate	−	+	−
D-glucuronate	−	−	−
L-leucine	−	−	−
Putrescine	−	−	−
Sucrose	−	+	+
D-xylose	−	−	−

Table 5. Continued

	V. fischeri	V. fluvialis biovar I	V. fluvialis biovar II	V. gazogenes
Cytochrome oxidase	+	+	+	−
Nitrate reduction	+	+	+	−
0/129 sensitivity:				
10 µg	+	−	−	+
150 µg	+	+	+	+
Swarming	−	−	−	−
Luminescence	+	−	−	−
Thornley's Arginine dihydrolase	−	+	+	−
Lysine decarboxylase	+	−	−	−
Ornithine decarboxylase	−	−	−	−
Growth at 42°C	−	−	−	+
Growth at % NaCl:				
0%	−	v	v	−
3%	+	+	+	+
6%	+	+	+	+
8%	+	v	v	−
10%	−	−	−	−
Voges-Proskauer reaction	−	−	−	−
Gas from glucose fermentation	−	−	+	+
Fermentation to acid:				
L-arabinose	−	+	+	+
m-inositol	−	−	−	−
D-mannose	+	+	+	+

314

	1	2	3	4
Sucrose	−	−	−	−
Enzyme production:				
Alginase	+	v	+	−
Amylase	−	+	+	v
Chitinase	+	+	+	−
Gelatinase	+	+	+	+
Lipase	−	+	+	−
Utilization as sole source of carbon:				
γ-aminobutyrate	+	+	v	+
Cellobiose	−	−	+	−
L-citrulline	−	−	+	−
Ethanol	−	+	+	−
D-gluconate	−	+	+	−
D-glucuronate	−	−	+	−
L-leucine	−	−	−	−
Putrescine	−	+	v	−
Sucrose	+	+	+	−
D-xylose	+	−	−	−

Table 5. Continued

	V. harveyi	V. logei	V. marinus	V. metschnikovii
Cytochrome oxidase	+	+	+	-
Nitrate reduction	+	+	+	-
0/129 sensitivity:				
10 µg	-	v	-	+
150 µg	+	+	+	+
Swarming	-	-	-	-
Luminescence	v	+	-	-
Thornley's Arginine dihydrolase	-	-	-	+
Lysine decarboxylase	+	+	+	v
Ornithine decarboxylase	+	-	-	-
Growth at 42°C	v	-	-	v
Growth at % NaCl:				
0%	-	-	-	v
3%	+	*	+	+
6%	+	*	-	+
8%	v	*	-	v
10%	v	*	-	-
Voges-Proskauer reaction	-	-	-	+
Gas from glucose fermentation	-	-	-	-
Fermentation to acid:				
L-arabinose	-	-	-	-
m-inositol	-	-	-	v
D-mannose	+	+	+	v

Sucrose	+	v	v	v
Enzyme production:				
Alginase	–	–	–	v
Amylase	+	–	–	+
Chitinase	+	+	+	+
Gelatinase	+	v	–	+
Lipase	+	+	v	+
Utilization as sole source of carbon:				
γ-aminobutyrate	–	–	–	–
Cellobiose	–	–	+	+
L-citrulline	–	–	–	v
Ethanol	–	–	–	–
D-gluconate	+	+	+	+
D-glucuronate	–	–	–	+
L-leucine	–	–	*	–
Putrescine	–	–	–	–
Sucrose	+	–	–	v
D-xylose	–	–	–	–

Table 5. Continued

	V. natriegens	V. nereis	V. nigripulchritudo
Cytochrome oxidase	+	+	+
Nitrate reduction	+	+	+
O/129 sensitivity:			
10 µg	-	-	-
150 µg	+	+	+
Swarming	-	-	-
Luminescence	-	-	-
Thornley's Arginine dihydrolase	-	+	-
Lysine decarboxylase	-	-	-
Ornithine decarboxylase	-	-	-
Growth at 42°C	v	v	-
Growth at % NaCl:			
0%	-	-	-
3%	+	+	+
6%	+	+	-
8%	v	v	-
10%	-	v	-
Voges-Proskauer reaction	-	-	-
Gas from glucose fermentation	-	-	-
Fermentation to acid:			
L-arabinose	+	-	-
m-inositol	v	-	v
D-mannose	-	-	-
Sucrose	+	+	-

Enzyme production:			
Alginase	−	−	−
Amylase	+	−	d
Chitinase	+	d	−
Gelatinase	+	d	+
Lipase	+	−	+
Utilization as sole source of carbon:			
γ-aminobutyrate	−	+	+
Cellobiose	+	−	d
L-citrulline	−	+	+
Ethanol	d	+	+
D-gluconate	d	+	+
D-glucuronate	+	−	d
L-leucine	−	+	d
Putrescine	−	+	+
Sucrose	−	+	+
D-xylose	−	−	−

Table 5. Continued

	V. parahae-molyticus	V. pelagius biovar I	V. pelagius biovar II	V. proteo-lyticus
Cytochrome oxidase	+	+	+	+
Nitrate reduction	+	+	+	+
0/129 sensitivity:				
10 µg	-	+	+	-
150 µg	+	+	+	+
Swarming	v	-	-	+
Luminescence	-	-	-	-
Thornley's Arginine dihydrolase	-	-	-	+
Lysine decarboxylase	+	-	-	+
Ornithine decarboxylase	+	-	-	-
Growth at 42°C	+	-	-	-
Growth at % NaCl:				
0%	-	-	-	+
3%	+	+	+	+
6%	+	+	+	+
8%	+	v	v	+
10%	-	-	-	-
Voges-Proskauer reaction	-	-	-	+
Gas from glucose fermentation	-	-	-	-
Fermentation to acid:				
L-arabinose	v	-	-	-
m-inositol	-	-	-	-
D-mannose	+	v	v	+

Characteristic				
Sucrose	−	+	+	−
Enzyme production:				
Alginase	−	+	+	−
Amylase	+	+	−	+
Chitinase	+	+	∇	+
Gelatinase	+	+	−	+
Lipase	+	+	+	+
Utilization as sole source of carbon:				
γ-aminobutyrate	−	+	−	−
Cellobiose	−	−	−	−
L-citrulline	−	+	+	−
Ethanol	−	−	∇	+
D-gluconate	+	+	+	+
D-glucuronate	−	−	−	∇
L-leucine	−	−	−	+
Putrescine	+	+	+	+
Sucrose	−	∇	+	−
D-xylose	−	−	−	−

321

Table 5. Continued

| | V. splendidus | | V. vulnificus |
	biovar I	biovar II	
Cytochrome oxidase	+	+	+
Nitrate reduction	+	+	+
0/129 sensitivity:			
10 µg	+	+	+
150 µg	+	+	+
Swarming	-	-	-
Luminescence	+	-	-
Thornley's Arginine dihydrolase	+	-	-
Lysine decarboxylase	-	-	+
Ornithine decarboxylase	-	-	+
Growth at 42°C	-	-	+
Growth at % NaCl:			
0%	-	-	-
3%	+	+	+
6%	v	v	+
8%	-	-	-
10%	-	-	-
Voges-Proskauer reaction	-	-	-
Gas from glucose fermentation	-	-	-
Fermentation to acid:			
L-arabinose	-	-	-
m-inositol	-	-	-
D-mannose	+	-	+

Sucrose	v	–	–
Enzyme production:			
Alginase	v	–	– +
Amylase	+	+	+ + +
Chitinase	+	+	+ + +
Gelatinase	+	+	+ + +
Lipase	+	+	+ +
Utilization as sole source of carbon:			
γ-aminobutyrate	–	–	–
Cellobiose	+	v	+
L-citrulline	+	–	–
Ethanol	–	–	–
D-gluconate	v	–	+
D-glucuronate	+	–	+
L-leucine	–	–	–
Putrescine	–	–	–
Sucrose	v	–	–
D-xylose	–	–	–

[a] Source of Data: Baumann et al. (1971a,b, 1973, 1978), Hendrie et al. (1971b), Reichelt and Baumann (1973), Reichelt et al. (1976), Bang et al. (1978a), Furniss et al. (1978), Harwood (1978), Lee et al. (1979), Jensen et al. (1980), West (1980), and West and Colwell, unpublished data.
[b] All strains are Gram-negative rods, motile and ferment glucose to produce acid.
[c] Symbols: +, positive trait for at least 90% of strains; –, negative trait for at least 90% of strains; v, differs for strains within the species; *, data not available.

5. Vibrio vulnificus

In 1976, Hollis and coworkers at the Centers for Disease Control reported the phenotypic characterization of 38 halophilic organisms for which no previous description could be found. These strains superficially resembled V. parahaemolyticus and V. alginolyticus but, unlike these species, fermented lactose and were referred to as lactose-positive (L+) vibrio. These L+ vibrio strains shared a low DNA/DNA homology with V. parahaemolyticus and V. alginolyticus (Clark and Steigerwalt 1977).

L+ vibrio strains were allocated to the genus Beneckea (Vibrio) with the species epithet vulnifica (Reichelt et al. 1976). In addition, strains previously designated as group C-2 (Baumann et al. 1973) were assigned to the B. vulnifica group. Proposals to transfer B. vulnifica to the genus Vibrio were discussed by Farmer (1979; 1980) prior to the amalgamation of Beneckea and Vibrio by Baumann et al. (1980). Tison and Seidler (1981) have reported the high degree of genetic relatedness of strains of V. vulnificus from clinical and environmental sources.

Two diagnostic features of strains of V. vulnificus are the fermentation of lactose and salicin. However, fermentation of lactose is often slow and/or weak in this species so hydrolysis of o-nitrophenyl-β-D-galactopyranoside (ONPG) has been used to detect β-galactosidase activity. Reichelt et al. (1976) and Baumann et al. (1981) reported that lactose fermentation may be due to the rapid, spontaneous emergence of lactose-fermenting mutants arising from lactose-nonfermenting wild types and have cautioned that lactose fermentation and ONPG hydrolysis may not be unequivocal diagnostic traits for this species.

6. Vibrio metschnikovii

V. metschnikovii has been retained within the genus Vibrio, despite its negative oxidase reaction and inability to reduce nitrate to nitrite. Shewan and Veron (1974) assigned organisms named V. metschnikovii and Vibrio proteus to biotype status within the species V. cholerae.

Results of a DNA homology study subsequently showed that V. metschnikovii was distinct from V. cholerae and other members of the genus (Reichelt et al. 1976). Based on extensive phenotypic characterization of V. metschnikovii and V. proteus it was later recommended that these species be combined as V. metschnikovii and that the species should be retained within the genus Vibrio (Lee et al. 1978).

Lack of oxidase activity in V. metschnikovii can be explained by the lack of cytochrome c suggesting divergence in evolution from other oxidase-positive members of the genus (West et al. 1978).

Features of Other Species
in the Genus Vibrio

In addition to the pathogenic species described above, Baumann et al. (1980) listed 14 species for the genus Vibrio as a result of the amalgamation of the genus Beneckea with Vibrio.

Vibrio anguillarum historically has included strains which cause disease in fish. However, many anaerogenic, Gram-negative, motile rods of marine origin that have been associated with fish kills have been identified as V. anguillarum on the basis of a few tests, principally arginine metabolism, 0/129 susceptibility, and salt tolerance range. As a result, the phenotypic description of the species has been expanded continuously when results of new studies are reported and has lost its diagnostic meaning (Evelyn 1971; Hendrie et al. 1971a; Roberts 1976). The study by Baumann et al. (1978) distinguished two biovars within the species. Characteristically, biovar I of the species is capable of utilizing a wider range of carbon compounds than biovar II.

Strains of Vibrio natriegens are common in coastal seawaters and characteristically utilize a wide range of diverse carbon compounds for growth (Baumann et al. 1971a). Other species which are distributed in the marine environment include: Vibrio campbellii, Vibrio harveyi, Vibrio nereis, Vibrio splendidus, and Vibrio pelagius

(Baumann et al. 1971a; Reichelt and Baumann 1973; Reichelt et al. 1976; Baumann et al. 1980).

Some strains from the marine environment produce pigmented colonies. Vibrio nigripulchritudo produces charcoal-colored colonies on minimal media (Baumann et al. 1971b). Colonies of Vibrio gazogenes appear red on marine agar (Difco) as a result of the production of the pigment prodigiosin (Harwood 1978). Strains of Vibrio logei and V. fischeri produce yellow-orange colonies on marine agar (Difco) containing 0.05% yeast extract. Interestingly, V. fischeri is often the sole bacterial species found in the luminous organ of some marine animals (Fitzgerald 1977; Nealson and Hastings 1979).

Strains of Vibrio costicola require at least 2% NaCl, and optimally 5%, for growth in laboratory media and are most commonly associated with salt-cured foodstuffs and brine reservoirs (Kushner 1978), and other hypersaline environments (Ventosa et al. 1982).

The remaining species, Vibrio proteolyticus (Merkel et al. 1964) and Vibrio marinus (Colwell and Morita 1964; Hendrie et al. 1971b) are, as yet, minimally characterized and require further studies of more wild strains to confirm the taxonomic status of these species.

Historical Notes

A group of gram-negative organisms showing somatic curvature, but neither oxidizing nor fermenting sugars, were previously referred to as the microaerophilic vibrios. The species of these microaerophilic vibrios, such as Vibrio fetus, Vibrio jejuni, and Vibrio sputorum, are now placed in the genus Campylobacter (Smibert 1978).

Wolin et al. (1961) described an obligately anaerobic, Gram-negative rod lacking the ability to ferment carbohydrates which was subsequently placed in the genus Vibrio, under the species name Vibrio succinogenes. The species has recently been transferred to the newly created genus Wolinella following phenotypic and DNA/DNA reassociation studies (Tanner et al. 1981).

Descriptions of genera published in the eighth edition of Bergey's Manual of Determinative Bacteriology employing "vibrio" as part of the genus epithet--for example, Succino-vibrio, Butyrivibrio, Desulfovibrio, and Bdellovibrio--have little or no taxonomic relationship with the genus Vibrio.

D'Aoust and Kushner (1972) placed a psychrophilic red-pigmented organism from the marine environment in the genus Vibrio as a new species, Vibrio psychroerythrus. The organism is different from pigmented members of V. gazogenes as described by Harwood (1978). The taxonomic status of V. psychroerythrus remains unclear (Reichelt et al. 1976).

IDENTIFICATION AND LABORATORY METHODS

Some of the phenotypic characterization tests employed by clinical laboratories for the Enterobacteriaceae can be applied to the Vibrionaceae. However, modifications in the salt concentration of media and incubation temperature are required (Baumann and Baumann 1981). These restrictions are outlined below, along with other recommended procedures. Figure 1 presents a schematic procedure for preliminary characterization of some gram-negative asporo-genous rods. A procedure for initial identification of members of the Vibrionaceae is presented in Figure 2. Table 5 gives the diagnostic reactions of species of the genus Vibrio, and of the genus Photobacterium. Additional identification traits are presented in the original, or emended, descriptions of these organisms.

In the following procedures, we have found that most strains grow well on a basal nutrient medium consisting of nutrient broth No. 2 (Oxoid) 25 g/l, NaCl 5 g/l and bacteriological grade agar 15 g/l. Some marine species, especially Photobacterium spp., prefer a basal medium of marine broth (Difco), gelled with agar, for growth since the nutrient and electrolyte content of this medium more closely approximates that of the marine environment.

Alginase. Add 20 g/l sodium alginate (Sigma Chemical Co.) to the ingredients of a suitable basal nutrient agar

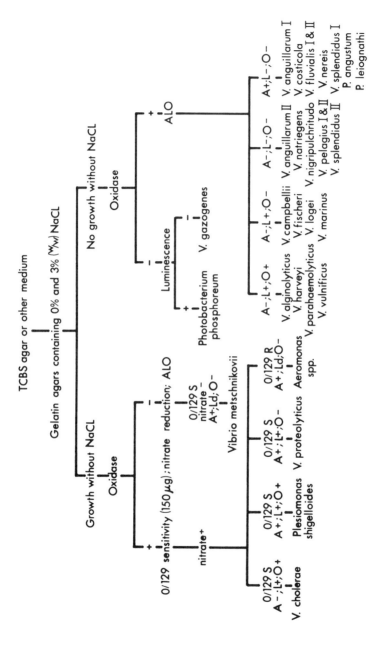

Figure 2. Scheme for preliminary identification of species of the Vibrionaceae where ALO: arginine dihydrolase, lysine decarboxylase, ornithine decarboxylase; O/129: 2,4-diamino-6,7-diisopropylpteridine phosphate (vibriostatic agent); S: sensitive, R: resistant, d: variable reaction among strains.

medium and dissolve by steaming to avoid charring of the medium. Sodium alginate should be used since alginic acid is not soluble in water. Sterilize by autoclaving. Pour plates while the medium is hot (60-70°C) because the viscosity increases as the medium cools. Dry the plates well before inoculation because this medium promotes swarming in some species. Plates are spot-inoculated and alginolytic activity is detected during incubation up to 14 days by observing a pitting and depression of the agar surface around the growth. Agar-digesting bacteria may give similar reactions and should be eliminated by an appropriate control plate containing no alginic acid.

Amylase. Spot-inoculate a basal nutrient agar plate containing 0.1% (w/v) soluble starch and incubate for 2 days. Flood with iodine solution to detect zones of clearing, indicative of a positive result (Cowan 1974a; MacFaddin 1980).

Antibiotic Sensitivity. This trait has little use in differentiating members of the Vibrionaceae, except for distinguishing biovars of V. cholerae Ol. Interpretation of zones of sensitivity, using disc diffusion techniques, should be modified by including appropriate controls if the basal nutrient agar contains sodium chloride and other electrolytes.

Arginine Dihydrolase. The method described by Thornley (1960) is used with the initial pH of the medium adjusted to 6.8 instead of 7.2. Results from this test correlate well with arginine decarboxylase medium results, although Baumann et al. (1971a) have recommended a chemical method for detecting arginine metabolism. Strains of Photobacterium spp. can produce alkaline products in Thornley's medium although none possess a constitutive arginine dihydrolase system when more sensitive analytical methods are used (Baumann et al. 1980).

Cell Morphology. Gram-staining should be performed using a culture grown on a solid medium. Strains may exhibit varying degrees of somatic curvature which has no

significance as a diagnostic feature. Old cultures of Vibrio
spp. often demonstrate highly pleomorphic forms including
rounding up of cells (Felter et al. 1969; Baker and Park
1975).

Chitinase. Chitin agar is prepared using a modification
of the method of Lingappa and Lockwood (1962). Crude,
unbleached chitin powder (Sigma Chemical Co.) is cleaned
by alternatively soaking for 24 hours in 1M NaOH and 1M
HCl five times. Wash four times with 95% ethanol and allow
to dry. Dissolve 20 g of cleaned chitin in 600 ml 50%
H_2SO_4 at room temperature with constant stirring. Filter
solution through glass wool. Precipitate chitin from solution
in 10 liters of ice-cold deionized water and add 10M NaOH
to bring pH to 7.0. Allow the suspension to stand for 24
hours then discard supernatant. Wash exhaustively in
deionized water and concentrate to a creamy paste by
centrifugation. Suspend the colloidal chitin paste in deionized water to a final concentration of 10% (w/v). Sterilize
by autoclaving. Suspension should be creamy-white and
can be stored indefinitely at 4°C. For use, 1 ml of colloidal chitin suspension is added to 9 ml molten bacteriological grade agar and poured as an overlay on a plate of
nutrient agar. Plates are spot-inoculated and incubated up
to 14 days to observe zones of clearing around growth
indicating chitin breakdown.

Colonial Morphology. Many members of the Vibrionaceae
show colonial variation on noninhibitory media. Most common variations are large-small, flat-pulvinate, opaque-
translucent, and smooth-rugose types. Variation may be so
pronounced as to suggest contamination of the culture, a
common complaint by workers newly exposed to Vibrionaceae
cultures and their idiosyncrasies. Accordingly, colonial
morphology has little use as a diagnostic or taxonomic trait
for the Vibrionaceae.

Decarboxylation of amino acids. Decarboxylation of
L-arginine, L-lysine, and L-ornithine represents important
diagnostic traits for identification of species within the
Vibrionaceae. Decarboxylation is detected by the method of

Møller (1955) using a liquid decarboxylase basal medium (Difco) overlaid with sterile paraffin oil. Inoculate tubes with a heavy inoculum taken from growth on solid media. Incubate for up to 14 days. An alkaline reaction indicates amine formation (MacFaddin 1980) and is recorded as a positive test.

Deoxyribonuclease. Spot-inoculate deoxyribonuclease agar (Oxoid). Incubate for 2 days or 7 days. Positive reactions appear as a clear zone around growth 2-5 minutes after flooding the plate with 1M HCl.

Electron Microscopy. Methods for examining the structure and arrangement of flagella in species of the Vibrionaceae by electron microscopy have been reported by Allen and Baumann (1971) and Belas and Colwell (1982). Sex pili were demonstrated in V. cholerae using negative staining with unbuffered 1% uranyl acetate by Bhaskaran et al. (1969). Ultrastructures of Vibrio spp. have been described by Kennedy et al. (1970).

Fermentation Reactions. Fermentation of carbon compounds is observed in semi-solid agar such as O/F basal medium (Difco) overlaid with sterile paraffin oil. All compounds should be added to cooled, molten agar base as filter-sterilized aqueous solutions to a final concentration of 1% (v/v). Incubate for up to 14 days before discarding results as negative. Gas production during fermentation is detected in liquid fermentation base media containing an inverted Durham tube.

Gelatinase. Detection of a change in composition of gelatin, rather than its liquefication, is observed using the methods of Smith and Goodner (1958). Gelatin agar consists of (g/l): peptone, 4; yeast extract, 1; gelatin, 15; NaCl, 10; and agar, 15. Plates are streaked and gelatinase activity is observed as a zone of opacity around growth. The use of acid mercuric chloride advocated in some methods is not recommended because of problems associated with disposal of the mercury reagent.

Growth on Single Carbon Sources for Nutritional Screening. The basal medium of Baumann et al. (1971a) is recommended for marine isolates but its electrolyte content is inhibitory for some brackish water, and most freshwater, isolates. For brackish water isolates, the medium employed by Lee et al. (1981) is recommended. It has a composition of (g/l): Solution A: NH_4Cl, 10; NH_4NO_3, 2; Na_2SO_4, 4; K_2HPO_4, 6; KH_2PO_4, 2; NaCl, 20. Solution B: $MgSO_4$ .7H_2O, 0.2; $MgCl_2$.6H_2O, 8; purified bacteriological agar, 30. Sterilize each solution separately by autoclaving. Cool to 50°C and mix thoroughly before addition of filter-sterilized aqueous solution of substrate to a final concentration of 0.1% (v/v). For freshwater isolates, NaCl and $MgCl_2$.6H_2O can be omitted. Plates are spot-inoculated and read according to the techniques described by Lee et al. (1978; 1981).

Incubation Temperatures. Most clinical human isolates grow at 35-37°C. Fish and environmental isolates should be incubated at 20-25°C, especially for primary isolation. Lower temperatures must be used for isolates from environments such as deep-sea trenches or polar regions. Growth at 42°C is tested in 1% (w/v) tryptone broth and 1% (w/v) NaCl with appropriate extra electrolytes if required for growth.

Indole Production. Detection of indole appears dependent on the method and medium used. For example, Lee et al. (1981) reported V. fluvialis as indole-negative when grown in tryptone broth and tested with Kovacs reagent. Seidler et al. (1980), however, were able to detect indole formation by V. fluvialis using an API-20E multitest system.

Lecithinase. Streak-inoculate a nutrient basal agar plate containing 10% (v/v) egg yolk emulsion (Oxoid). Examine daily for up to 7 days for a dense opaque zone around the inoculum.

Lipase. Lipolytic activity against Tween 80 (Sigma Chemical Co.) is detected on a medium containing (g/l): peptone, 10; NaCl, 10; $CaCl_2$.H_2O, 0.1; bacteriological agar, 20. Mix contents and adjust to pH 7.4. Sterilize by autoclaving and add Tween 80 to cool, molten medium to a final concentration of 1% (v/v). Streak-inoculate plates and examine daily up to 7 days for lipolytic activity indicated by dense opacity around the inoculum.

Luminescence. Several media have been developed to promote light emission by luminescent bacteria (Baumann and Baumann 1977; Nealson and Hastings 1979). A medium consisting of (g/l) nutrient broth No. 2 (Oxoid), 25; NaCl, 17.5; $MgCl_2.6H_2O$, 4; KCl, 1; bacteriological agar, 15, is suitable for many isolates of the Vibrionaceae. Streak plates to obtain discrete colonies and examine after 12, 18, and 24 hours incubation at 20-25°C. Luminescence is often lost on prolonged incubation. Examine plates in a completely dark room after vision has become dark-adapted for at least five minutes.

Maintenance of Cultures. Strains can be kept at least five years on appropriate nutrient agar stabs or slants covered with sterile paraffin oil and stored at room temperature in the dark. However, storage in liquid nitrogen or lyophilization is preferred to ensure viability and retention of phenetic and molecular genetic traits. A suspending medium used in this laboratory for storage of strains in liquid nitrogen consists of (g/l): tryptic soy broth (Difco), 30; NaCl, 5; and glycerol 8% (v/v). Additional electrolytes are added when required. Storage of Vibrionaceae strains by lyophilization has been reviewed by Furniss et al. (1978).
Working stocks of control strains can be kept on stabs of (g/l): peptone, 10; yeast extract, 1; NaCl, 10; bacteriological agar, 5. Use screw-cap vials to avoid desiccation of the medium. The effect of different storage strategies on the maintenance and stability of plasmids in members of the Vibrionaceae is not known.

Motility. Early stationary phase broth cultures should be examined for motility by hanging drop preparation and phase contrast or brightfield microscopy. The use of semi-solid stab media is not recommended as weakly motile strains cannot be detected. Cultures should be tested using a Craigie tube (Collins and Lyne 1976) and reexamined before being recorded as negative. The arrangement of flagella can be routinely determined by the modified silver-staining technique described by Gauthier et al. (1975). The method of Mayfield and Inniss (1977) can be used to determine motility and mode of flagellation on the same slide, although the method must be modified for marine isolates by the use of marine broth (Difco) or distilled water plus suitable electrolytes to form suspensions of bacteria. Other methods are described by Baumann et al. (1971a).

Nitrate Reduction. Cells are grown in nitrate broth (Difco) or an appropriate nitrite-free basal nutrient broth containing 0.1% (w/v) reagent grade potassium nitrate. The medium is dispensed almost to the brim of screw-cap vials to provide sufficient anaerobic conditions during incubation to enhance nitrate reduction. Formation of nitrite is detected using reagents A and B described by Crosby (1967). Solution A contains: sulfanilic acid 0.5 g, glacial acetic acid, 30 ml and deionized water 120 ml. Solution B contains: 0.2 g Cleve's acid (1-naphthylamine-7-sulfonic acid; Pfaltz and Bauer; Flushing, New York) dissolved in 120 ml deionized water overnight at 37°C and made up to 150 ml with glacial acetic acid. Store both solutions in brown glass bottles. Cleve's acid replaces the potentially carcinogenic compound α-naphthylamine used in previous methods. For use, add 1 ml each of Solution A and Solution B to 1 ml of broth culture. The presence of nitrite is indicated by development of a red color within 30 seconds. Cultures are tested after 1-day incubation and again after 5 days if negative. The zinc dust reduction procedure outlined by Cowan (1974a) and MacFaddin (1980) should be used to detect organisms which reduce nitrite.

0/129 Sensitivity. A variety of techniques have been described since the original method for detecting sensitivity to the vibriostatic agent 0/129 (2,4-diamino-6,7-diisopropyl pteridine) was reported by Shewan et al. (1954). Sprinkling crystals of compound 0/129 on inoculated agar plates is not recommended as the concentration cannot be determined. The availability of a water-soluble phosphate derivative of 0/129 (British Drug Houses Ltd.; Sigma Chemical Co.) has enabled minimum inhibitory concentrations of the agent for Vibrionaceae members to be determined. Furniss et al. (1978), reported that sensitivity to the phosphate derivative of 0/129 at concentrations of 150 µg/ml and 10 µg/ml are useful for identification purposes. For occasional use, prepare solutions of 7500 µg/ml and 500 µg/ml 0/129 in sterile deionized water. Do not autoclave or filter-sterilize but store at 4°C. Spot 20 µl of stock solution onto 6 mm diameter, sterile antibiotic assay discs (Whatman), dry in a desiccator at room temperature, and store at 4°C until required (Lee et al. 1979). For screening large numbers of isolates, incorporate the vibriostatic agent into basal nutrient agar medium and inoculate by automatic multipoint inoculation (West 1980). A control plate containing no 0/129 should be included. Concentration of inoculum greatly influences the interpretation of sensitivity so discs should be placed onto plates that have been inoculated to yield areas of discrete but confluent colonies after incubation. The procedure described by Lee et al. (1978) is recommended for inoculation of plates by multipoint inoculator.

ONPG Hydrolysis. The ability of bacteria to ferment lactose can be correlated with the presence of β-D-galactosidase (MacFaddin 1980). Lactose fermentation in the Vibrionaceae is often weak and delayed when determined in solid fermentation media so the fermenting ability is detected by hydrolysis of o-nitrophenyl-β-D-galactopyranoside (ONPG) by β-D-galactosidase. Strains are grown on basal nutrient agar containing 1% (w/v) lactose to induce β-D-galactosidase, which is then detected using the toluene modification method of ONPG hydrolysis described by Paik (1980).

Oxidase. The filter paper method described by Kovacs (1956) using tetramethyl-p-phenylenediame (TMPD) is recommended. Strains should be grown on a noninhibitory nutrient agar containing no carbohydrates to avoid inhibition of the reaction by acidic end products (Hunt et al.

1981). Baumann and Baumann (1977) have recommended toluene treatment of oxidase-negative cells to detect positive strains with an impermeability to TMPD. Do not use iron-based (Nichrome) loops or needles to remove colonies from plates (MacFaddin 1980).

Poly β-hydroxybutyrate Accumulation. Intracellular accumulation of this storage polymer can be detected using the method of Reichelt and Baumann (1973).

Quality Control Procedures. Regular quality control testing of identification media is recommended to ensure each batch has sufficient electrolytes to support growth. Recommended control cultures for diagnostic traits have been published by Furniss et al. (1978). Appropriate control cultures are particularly useful for interpretation of growth on single carbon source utilization media.

Rapid Multitest Systems. Commercial multitest kits using units of biochemical tests in microcuples have been used extensively in clinical laboratories for the rapid identi-fication of Enterobacteriaceae members. The use of these kits, prepared according to the manufacturers' instructions, to characterize Vibrionaceae members from the marine environment can result in misidentification (Davis and Sizemore 1981). It appears that such misidentification occurs because marine isolates grow suboptimally in the recommended suspending fluid which does not contain sufficient sodium chloride and other electrolytes. The studies of Sanyal (1981) support this conclusion, since only non-marine isolates showed good growth and correlation with conventional tests in one commercial kit. It is necessary to modify the electrolyte composition of suspending fluids in some commercial kits for use with marine and estuarine species (MacDonell et al. 1982). We do not recommend the use of commercial kits designed for use with the Entero-bacteriaceae unless several independent tests such as oxidase, salt tolerance, 0/129 sensitivity, and growth on sole carbon sources are performed as well.

Salt Content of the Media. The sodium chloride concentration in all media should be raised to 1% where indicated. Most Vibrionaceae members will grow optimally at this concentration although some Aeromonas strains and P. shigelloides grow better in media containing 0.5% NaCl. Some marine isolates may require an additional 1% NaCl as well as 0.4% $MgCl_2$.$6H_2O$ and 0.1% KCl based on the studies of MacLeod (1965), Leifson (1970), and Reichelt and Baumann (1974).

Salt Tolerance. Growth at concentrations of NaCl up to 10% (w/v) is tested by observing growth in 1% (w/v) tryptone broth containing varying amounts of analytical grade NaCl. Broths should be autoclaved in tubes sealed tightly with screw caps to avoid changes in NaCl concentration due to evaporation. Tubes are inoculated with 20 μl of a mid-logorithmic phase culture in tryptone broth containing 1% NaCl. Do not incubate longer than 2 days. Growth or lack of growth is detected visually. Different brands of tryptone contain varying amounts of contaminating Na^+ which interfere with the growth range, especially at the upper and lower limits of tolerance (Singleton et al. 1982). Tryptone from Oxoid Ltd. has given consistently good results in our laboratory.

Salt Requirement. The ability to grow in the absence of sodium chloride is an important preliminary diagnostic feature for the Vibrionaceae members (Figure 2). The use of gelatin agar with and without NaCl is convenient as strains can be stored on this medium until completion of characterization tests as well as tested for gelatinase activity and oxidase reaction. The use of cysteine-lactose-electrolyte-deficient (CLED) agar (Oxoid Ltd.) has been suggested since contaminating concentrations of Na^+ are very low (Lee et al. 1979). More recent studies have indicated that V. cholerae has an absolute requirement for Na^+ (Singleton et al. 1982). However, most commercial media components contain sufficient contaminating amounts of this ion for V. cholerae to grow without addition of NaCl.

String Test. Smith (1970) reported a presumptive test for V. cholerae in which colonies were picked from agar plates and emulsified in a loopful of 0.5% sodium deoxycholate in saline. A positive string test was recorded if a mucus-like "string" was observed between the slide and the loop when the two are gently separated to a distance of about 3 cm. Chatterjee and Neogy (1972) have demonstrated positive reactions with Aeromonas strains and, accordingly, this test is not recommended for use in identification schemes for Vibrionaceae members.

Swarming. Pour plates of basal nutrient agar and allow to set but not dry. Divide the medium into quadrants by cutting gutters in the agar at least 1 cm wide. Remove excess moisture from the gutter trenches with sterile cotton swabs. Inoculate each quadrant with a streak or spot of culture and examine plates daily up to 2 days for spreading over the entire surface.

Voges-Proskauer Reaction. Several methods have been described for detection of acetoin from glucose fermentation. The methods of Baumann et al. (1971a), Lee et al. (1979), and Cowan (1974a) have been used. Incubation time, rather than type of method, and temperature influence the production of acetoin.

Coda

The taxonomic position of several unnamed strains characterized by Baumann and coworkers is still unclear despite the resemblance of these strains to members of the Vibrionaceae (Baumann and Baumann 1977).

Baross et al. (1978) reported the isolation of agar-digesting Vibrio spp. from shellfish taken from the near shore areas of Oregon. Strains of agar-digesting Vibrio spp. and V. parahaemolyticus were lysed by a set of bacteriophages suggesting taxonomic relatedness between the species. Agar digestion is a rare trait within the Vibrionaceae and further characterization of strains with this property is required.

Five new species and one biovar have been assigned to the genus Vibrio since the amended description of the genus by Baumann et al. (1980).

Strains of V. cholerae atypical in several biochemical reactions, including negative sucrose fermentation, have been placed in a separate species, Vibrio mimicus, on the basis of DNA/DNA reassociation studies (Davis et al. 1981). The type strain is ATCC 33653. Whether V. mimicus warrants separate species status is open to question.

A series of arginine dihydrolase-positive Vibrio strains has been isolated from lesions on damselfish (Chromis punctipinnis) as well as from extraintestinal infections of humans. The organisms do not resemble other members of the genus Vibrio by DNA/DNA relatedness yet have been alloted to the species Vibrio damsela (Love et al. 1981).

Extensive characterization of the two biovars of V. anguillarum indicates considerable phenotypic, molecular genetic, and serological differences. The species name Vibrio ordalii has been proposed for those strains currently designated as biovar II of V. anguillarum (Schiewe et al. 1981).

The species name Vibrio hollisae has been proposed for a collection of strains isolated from human diarrheal stools. Characteristically, these strains fail to decarboxylate L-arginine, L-lysine, and L-ornithine; do not produce gelatinase and deoxyribonuclease; and ferment only a limited range of carbohydrates (Hickman et al. 1982; Morris et al. 1982).

Organisms pathogenic for cultured eels in Japan have been named Vibrio anguillicida after phenotypic and molecular characterization (Nishibuchi et al. 1979). Subsequent study of DNA/DNA relatedness indicates that V. anguillicida and V. vulnificus belong to the same species. The name V. vulnificus has been retained and eel pathogens are given biovar status as V. vulnificus biogroup 2 (Tison et al. 1982).

Guerinot and Patriquin (1981) described two nitrogen-fixing strains isolated from the gastrointestinal tract of sea urchins. These strains were placed in the genus Vibrio pending further characterization. Phenotypic and molecular comparison of these strains with similar isolates from inland waters in England, and other members of the genus Vibrio, support the inclusion of nitrogen-fixing strains as a new species, Vibrio diazotrophicus, in the genus (Guerinot et al. 1982). Inclusion of these strains in the genus Vibrio requires a redefinition of the genus since the description by Shewan and Veron (1974) and by Baumann et al. (1980) excludes strains which fix molecular nitrogen.

CONCLUSION

The family Vibrionaceae contains genera and species whose taxonomy is still in a state of flux, despite nearly a decade of extensive phenotypic and molecular genetic characterization. There is no doubt that several decisive advances in the taxonomic understanding of this group of organisms have resulted from the dovetailing of the disciplines of aquatic microbial ecology and bacterial taxonomy and will continue to do so in the next decade.

This volume, taken as a whole, indicates the medical and economic significance of members of the genus Vibrio. Accordingly, it is necessary to identify these strains with confidence before assigning significance to their isolation from the marine environment, seafood, or clinical samples. Amalgamation of Beneckea with Vibrio has created a genus containing at least 20 species with the taxonomic position of several newly described species awaiting inclusion in the genus. Herein, we have attempted to provide a practical review of the classification and identification of Vibrionaceae strains for clinical and environmental laboratories and have provided information useful in carrying out selected tests for identification and classification.

To the taxonomic purist, the collection of diverse strains in the genus Vibrio seems unlikely to be reasonably accommodated by a single genus description. However, studies on evolutionarily conserved information molecules suggest the contrary. More recent studies on the amino acid divergence in alkaline phosphatase (Woolkalis and Baumann 1981) and oligonucleotide cataloguing of 16S ribosomal RNA (Fox et al. 1980) are now providing insights into the phylogenic characteristics of genera in the

Vibrionaceae. Unique sequences in 5S ribosomal RNA of barophilic Vibrio spp. have been reported (Deming 1981; Deming et al. 1983).

ACKNOWLEDGMENTS

We thank M.T. MacDonell for translation of Allomonas references. This work was supported by funding from NIH grant 5-R-22-AI-14242 and NSF grant DEB-77-14646.

REFERENCES

Allen, R.D., and P. Baumann. 1971. Structure and arrangement of flagella in species of the genus Beneckea and Photobacterium fischeri. J. Bacteriol. 107:295-302.

Arai, T., N. Ikejima, T. Itoh, S. Sakai, T. Shimada, and R. Sakazaki. 1980. A survey of Plesiomonas shigelleoides from aquatic environments, domestic animals, pets and humans. J. Hyg. (Cambridge) 84:203-211.

Ayres, P.A., and G.I. Barrow. 1978. The distribution of Vibrio parahaemolyticus in British coastal waters: report of a collaborative study 1975-76. J. Hyg. (Cambridge) 80:281-294.

Bain, N., and J.M. Shewan. 1968. Identification of Aeromonas, Vibrio and related organisms. Pages 79-84 in B.M. Gibbs and D.A. Shapton (Eds.), Identification methods for microbiologists, Part B. Society for Applied Bacteriology Technical Series No. 2. Academic, London.

Baker, D.A., and R.W.A. Park. 1975. Changes in mor- phology and cell wall structure that occur during growth of Vibrio sp. NCTC 4716 in batch culture. J. Gen. Microbiol. 86:12-28.

Bang, S.S., M.J. Woolkalis, and P. Baumann. 1978a. Electrophoretic mobilities of superoxide dismutases from species of Photobacterium, Beneckea, Vibrio, and selected terrestrial enterobacteria. Curr. Microbiol. 1:371-376.

Bang, S.S., P. Baumann, and K.H. Nealson. 1978b. Phenotypic characterization of Photobacterium logei (sp. nov.), a species related to P. fischeri. Curr. Microbiol. 1:285-288.

Bang, S.S., L. Baumann, M.J. Woolkalis, and P. Baumann. 1981. Evolutionary relationships in Vibrio and Photobacterium as determined by immunological studies of superoxide dismutase. Arch. Microbiol. 130:111-120.

Baross, J.A., J. Liston, and R.Y. Morita. 1978. Ecological relationship between Vibrio parahaemolyticus and agar-digesting vibrios as evidenced by bacteriophage susceptibility patterns. Appl. Environ. Microbiol. 36:500-505.

Barua, D., and W. Burrows (Eds.). 1974. Cholera. W.B. Saunders Co., Philadelphia.

Baumann, L., and P. Baumann. 1976. Study of the relationship among marine and terrestrial enterobacteria by means of in vitro DNA/ribosomal RNA hybridization. Microbios L. 3:11-20.

Baumann, L., and P. Baumann. 1980. Immunological relationships of glutamine synthetases from marine and terrestrial enterobacteria. Curr. Microbiol. 3:191-196.

Baumann, P., L. Baumann, and M. Mandel. 1971a. Taxonomy of marine bacteria: The genus Beneckea. J. Bacteriol. 107:268-294.

Baumann, P., L. Baumann, M. Mandel, and R.D. Allen. 1971b. Taxonomy of marine bacteria: Beneckea nigrapulchrituda sp. n. J. Bacteriol. 108:1380-1383.

Baumann, P., L. Baumann, J.L. Reichelt. 1973. Taxonomy of marine bacteria: Beneckea parahaemolytica and Beneckea alginolytica. J. Bacteriol. 113:1144-1155.

Baumann, P., and L. Baumann. 1977. Biology of the marine enterobacteria: genera Beneckea and Photobacterium. Ann. R. Microbiol. 31:39-61.

Baumann, P., S.S. Bang, and L. Baumann. 1978. Phenotypic characterization of Beneckea anguillara biotypes I and II. Curr. Microbiol. 1:85-88.

Baumann, P., L. Baumann, S.S. Bang, and M.J. Woolkalis. 1980. Reevaluation of the taxonomy of Vibrio, Beneckea, and Photobacterium: abolition of the genus Beneckea. Curr. Microbiol. 4:127-132.

Baumann, P., L. Baumann, and B.G. Hall. 1981. Lactose utilization by Vibrio vulnificus. Curr. Microbiol. 6:131-135.

Baumann, P. and L. Baumann. 1981. The marine gram-negative Eubacteria: Genera Photobacterium, Beneckea, Alteromonas, Pseudomonas, and Alcaligenes. Pages 1302-1331 in M. P. Starr, H. Stolp, H. G. Truper, A. Balows, and H. G. Schlegel (Eds.), The Prokaryotes: A Handbook on habitats, isolation, and identification of bacteria. Springer-Verlag, Berlin.

Belas, M.R., and R.R. Colwell. 1982. Scanning electron microscope observation of the swarming phenomenon of Vibrio parahaemolyticus. J. Bacteriol. 150:956-959.

Bhaskaran, K., P.Y. Dyer, and G.E. Rogers. 1969. Sex pili in Vibrio cholerae. Aust. J. Exper. Biol. Med. Sci. 47:647-650.

Blake, P.A., D.T. Allegra, J.D. Snyder, T.J. Barrett, L. McFarland, C.T. Caraway, J.C. Feeley, J.P. Craig, J.V. Lee, N.D. Puhr, and R.A. Feldman. 1980a.

Cholera--a possible endemic focus in the United States. N. Engl. J. Med. 302:305-309.

Blake, P.A., R.E. Weaver, and D.G. Hollis. 1980b. Diseases of humans (other than cholera) caused by vibrios. Ann. R. Microbiol. 34:341-367.

Brandis, H. 1978. Vibriocin typing. Pages 117-126 in T. Bergan, and J.R. Norris (Eds.), Methods in microbiology No. 12. Academic, New York.

Breed, R.S., E.G.D. Murray, and N.R. Smith (Eds.). 1957a. Genus V. Photobacterium. Pages 193-197 in Bergey's manual of determinative bacteriology, 7th ed. The Williams & Wilkins Co., Baltimore.

Breed, R.S., E.G.D. Murray, and N.R. Smith (Eds.). 1957b. Family VII. Spirillaceae. Pages 228-261 in Bergey's manual of determinative bacteriology, 7th ed. The Williams & Wilkins Co., Baltimore.

Brenner, D.J., B.R. Davis, Y. Kudoh, M. Ohashi, R. Sakazaki, T. Shimada, and H.L. Smith. 1982. Serological comparison of two collections of Vibrio cholerae non O1. J. Clin. Microbiol. 16:319-323.

Buchanan, R.E. and N.E. Gibbons (Eds.). 1974. Family I. Pseudomonadaceae. Pages 217-253 in Bergey's manual of determinative bacteriology, 8th ed. The Williams & Wilkins Co., Baltimore.

Burke, V., J. Robinson, H.M. Atkinson, and M. Gracey. 1982. Biochemical characteristics of enterotoxigenic Aeromonas spp. J. Clin. Microbiol. 15:48-52.

Carney, J.F., L. Wan, T.E. Lovelace, and R.R. Colwell. 1975. Numerical taxonomy study of Vibrio and Spirillum spp. Int. J. Sys. Bacteriol. 25:38-46.

Chakrabarty, A.N., S. Adhya, J. Basu, and S.G. Dastidar. 1970. Bacteriocin typing of Vibrio cholerae. Infect. Immun. 1:293-299.

Chatterjee, B.D., and K.N. Neogy. 1972. Studies on Aeromonas and Plesiomonas species isolated from cases of choleraic diarrhoea. Ind. J. Med. Res. 60:520-524.

Cherwonogrodzky, J.W., and A.G. Clark. 1981. Effect of pH on the production of the Kanagawa hemolysin by Vibrio parahaemolyticus. Infect. Immun. 34:115-119.

Clark, W.A., and A.G. Steigerwalt. 1977. Deoxyribonucleic acid reassociation experiments with a halophilic, lactose-fermenting Vibrio isolated from blood culture. Int. J. Sys. Bacteriol. 27:194-199.

Citarella, R.V., and R.R. Colwell. 1970. Polyphasic taxonomy of the genus Vibrio: polynucleotide sequence relationships among selected Vibrio species. J. Bacteriol. 104:434-442.

Collins, C.H., and P.M. Lyne. 1976. Microbiological methods. 4th ed. Butterworths, London.

Colwell, R.R. 1970. Polyphasic taxonomy of the genus Vibrio: numerical taxonomy of Vibrio cholerae, Vibrio parahaemolyticus, and related Vibrio species. J. Bacteriol. 104:410-433.

Colwell, R.R., and R.Y. Morita. 1964. Reisolation and emendation of description of Vibrio marinus (Russell) Ford. J. Bacteriol. 88:831-837.

Colwell, R.R., V.I. Adeyemo, and H.H. Kirtland. 1968. Esterases and DNA base composition analysis of Vibrio cholerae and related vibrios. J. Appl. Bacteriol. 31:323-335.

Cowan, S.T. 1974a. Cowan and Steel's manual for the identification of medical bacteria. 2nd edition. University Press, Cambridge.

Cowan, S.T. 1974b. Family I. Enterobacteriaceae. Pages 290-340 in R.E. Buchanan and N.E. Gibbons (Eds.), Bergey's manual of determinative bacteriology, 8th ed. The Williams & Wilkins Co., Baltimore.

Crosby, N.T. 1967. The determination of nitrite in water using Cleve's acid, 1-naphthylamine-7-sulphonic acid. Proc. Soc. for Water Treatment and Examination. 16:51-55.

Cvjetanovic, B. and D. Barua. 1972. The seventh pandemic of cholera. Nature 239:137-138.

D'Aoust, J.Y., and D.J. Kushner. 1972. Vibrio psychroerythrus sp. n. classification of the psychrophilic marine bacterium NRC 1004. J. Bacteriol. 111:340-342.

Dastidar, S.G., and A. Narayanaswani. 1968. The occurrence of chitinase in vibrios. Ind. J. Med. Res. 56:654-658.

Davis, B.R., G.R. Fanning, J.M. Madden, A.G. Steigerwalt, H.B. Bradford, H.L. Smith, and D.J. Brenner. 1981. Characterization of biochemically atypical Vibrio cholerae strains and designation of a new pathogenic species, Vibrio mimicus. J. Clin. Microbiol. 14:631-639.

Davis, J.W., and R.K. Sizemore. 1981. Nonselectivity of Rimler-Shotts medium for Aeromonas hydrophila in estuarine environments. Appl. Environ. Microbiol. 42:544-545.

Davis, W.A., J.G. Kane, and V.F. Garagus. 1978. Human Aeromonas infections: a review of the literature and a case report of endocarditis. Medicine (Baltimore) 57:267-277.

Deming, J.W. 1981. Ecology of deep-sea barophilic bacteria. Ph.D. Thesis, University of Maryland, College Park, USA.

Deming, J.W., K. Leurhsen, G. Fox, H. Hada, and R.R. Colwell. 1983. Unique 5S ribosomal RNA sequences in deep-sea barophilic *Vibrio* spp. J. Bacteriol.: in preparation.

Desmarchelier, P.M., and J.L. Reichelt. 1981. Phenotypic characterization of clinical and environmental isolates of *Vibrio cholerae* from Australia. Curr. Microbiol. 5:123-127.

Desmarchelier, P.M., and J.L. Reichelt. 1982. Genetic relationships among clinical and environmental isolates of *Vibrio cholerae* from Australia. Curr. Microbiol. 7:53-57.

Eddy, B.P., and K.P. Carpenter. 1964. Further studies on *Aeromonas*. II. Taxonomy of *Aeromonas* and C27 strains. J. Appl. Bacteriol. 27:96-109.

Evelyn, T.P.T. 1971. First records of vibriosis in Pacific salmon cultured in Canada, and taxonomic status of the responsibile bacterium, *Vibrio anguillarum*. J. Fisheries Research Board of Canada 28:517-525.

Farkas-Himsley, H., and P.L. Seyfried. 1963. Lethal biosynthesis of a bacteriocin, vibriocin, by *V. comma*. I. Conditions affecting its production and detection. Can. J. Microbiol. 9:329-338.

Farmer, J.J. 1979. *Vibrio* ("*Beneckea*") *vulnificus*: the bacterium associated with sepsis, septicaemia, and the sea. Lancet 2:903.

Farmer, J.J. 1980. Revival of the name Vibrio vulnificus. Int. J. Sys. Bacteriol. 30:656.

Feeley, J.C. 1966. Minutes of the IAMS subcommittee on taxonomy of vibrios. Int. J. Sys. Bacteriol. 16:135-142.

Felter, R.A., R.R. Colwell, and G.B. Chapman. 1969. Morphology and round body formation in Vibrio marinus. J. Bacteriol. 99:326-335.

Ferguson, W.W., and N.D. Henderson. 1947. Description of strain C27: a motile organism with the major antigen of Shigella sonnei phase I. J. Bacteriol. 54:179-181.

Finkelstein, R.A. 1973. Cholera. CRC Crit. R. Microb. 2:553-623.

Fitzgerald, J.M. 1977. Classification of luminous bacteria from the light organ of the Australian Pinecone fish, Cleidopus gloriamaris. Arch. Microbiol. 112:153-156.

Fox, G.E., E. Stackebrant, R.B. Hespell, J. Gibson, J. Maniloff, T.A. Dyer, R.S. Wolfe, W.E. Balch, R.S. Tanner, L.J. Magrum, L.B. Zablem, R. Blakemore, R. Gupta, L. Bonen, B.J. Lewis, D.A. Stahl, K.R. Luehrsen K.N. Chen, and C.R. Woese. 1980. The phylogeny of prokaryotes. Science 209:457-463.

Fujino, T., G. Sakaguchi, R. Sakazaki, and Y. Takeda. 1974. (Eds.). International symposium on Vibrio parahaemolyticus. Saikon Publishing Co., Tokyo.

Furniss, A.L., J.V. Lee, and T.J. Donovan. 1978. The Vibrios. Public Health Laboratory Service Monograph Series No. 11. Her Majesty's Stationery Office, London.

Furniss, A.L. 1979. Identification of human vibrios. Pages 143-150 in F.A. Skinner and D.W. Lovelock (Eds.), Identification methods for microbiologists.

Society for Applied Bacteriology Technical Series No. 14. Academic, London.

Gardner, A.D., and K.V. Venkatraman. 1935. The antigens of the cholera group of vibrios. J. Hyg. (Cambridge) 35:262-282.

Gauthier, M.J., J.M. Shewan, D.M. Gibson, and J.V. Lee. 1975. Taxonomic position and seasonal variations in marine neritic environment of some gram-negative antibiotic-producing bacteria. J. Gen. Microbiol. 87:211-218.

Gibson, D.M., M.S. Hendrie, N.C. Houston, and G. Hobbs. 1977. The identification of some gram negative heterotrophic aquatic bacteria. Pages 135-159 in F.A. Skinner, and J.M. Shewan (Eds.), Aquatic microbiology. Society for Applied Bacteriology Symposium series No. 6. Academic, London.

Guerinot, M.L., and D.G. Patriquin. 1981. N_2-fixing vibrios isolated from the gastrointestinal tract of sea urchins. Can. J. Microbiol. 27:311-317.

Guerinot, M.L., P.A. West, J.V. Lee, and R.R. Colwell. 1982. Vibrio diazotrophicus sp. nov., a marine N_2-fixing bacterium. Int. J. Sys. Bacteriol. 32:350-357.

Gutteridge, C.S., and J.R. Norris. 1979. The application of pyrolysis techniques to the identification of micro-organisms. J. Appl. Bacteriol. 47:5-43.

Habs, H., and R.H.W. Schubert. 1962. Uber die biochemischen merkmale und die taxonomische stellung von Pseudomonas shigelloides (Bader). Zentralbl. Bakterol. Parasitenkd. Infektionsk. Hyg. Abt. 1 Orig. 186:316-327.

Haddadin, J.M., R.M. Stirland, N.W. Preston, and P. Collard. 1973. Identification of Vibrio cholerae by pyrolysis gas-liquid chromatography. Appl. Microbiol. 25:40-43.

Harwood, C.S. 1978. Beneckea gazogenes sp. nov., a red, facultatively anaerobic, marine bacterium. Curr. Microbiol. 1:233-238.

Hazen, T.C., C.B. Fliermans, R.P. Hirsch, and G.W. Esch. 1978. Prevalence and distribution of Aeromonas hydrophila in the United States. Appl. Environ. Microbiol. 36:731-738.

Hazen, T.C. 1979. Ecology of Aeromonas hydrophila in a South Carolina cooling reservoir. Microb. Ecol. 5:179-195.

Heiberg, B. 1936. The biochemical reactions of vibrios. J. Hyg. (Cambridge) 36:114-117.

Hendrie, M.S., W. Hodgkiss, and J.M. Shewan. 1970. The identification, taxonomy and classification of luminous bacteria. J. Gen. Microbiol. 64:151-169.

Hendrie, M.S., W. Hodgkiss, and J.M. Shewan. 1971a. Proposal that the species Vibrio anguillarum Bergman 1909, Vibrio piscium David 1927, and Vibrio ichthyodermis (Wells and Zobell) Shewan, Hobbs, and Hodgkiss, 1960 be combined as a single species, Vibrio anguillarum. Int. J. Sys. Bacteriol. 21:64-68.

Hendrie, M.S., W. Hodgkiss, and J.M. Shewan. 1971b. Proposal that Vibrio marinus (Russell 1891) Ford 1927 be amalgamated with Vibrio fischeri (Beijerinck 1889) Lehmann and Neumann 1896. Int. J. Sys. Bacteriol. 21:217-221.

Hendrie, M.S., and J.M. Shewan. 1974a. Genus IV. Photobacterium. Pages 349-351 in R.E. Buchanan and N.E. Gibbons (Eds.), Bergey's manual of determinative bacteriology, 8th ed. The Williams & Wilkins Co., Baltimore.

Hendrie, M.S., and J.M. Shewan. 1974b. Genus V. Lucibacterium. Pages 351-352 in R.E. Buchanan and N.E. Gibbons (Eds.), Bergey's manual of determinative bacteriology, 8th ed. The Williams & Wilkins Co., Baltimore.

Hickman, F.W., J.J. Farmer, D.G. Hollis, G.R. Fanning, A.G. Steigerwalt, R.E. Weaver, and D.J. Brenner. 1982. Identification of Vibrio hollisae sp. nov. from patients with diarrhea. J. Clin. Microbiol. 15:395-401.

Hisatsune, K., A. Kiuye, S. Kondo, and K. Takeya. 1980a. Chemical composition of O-antigenic lipopolysaccharides isolated from Vibrio parahaemolyticus. Pages 166-184 in Proc. 15th U.S.-Japan cooperative medical science program joint conference on cholera, Bethesda, Maryland, 1979. N.I.H. Publication 80-2003.

Hisatsune, K., S. Kondo, T. Iguchi, and K. Takeya. 1980b. Comparative study on sugar composition of 0-antigenic lipopolysaccharides isolated from Vibrio cholerae, group F vibrios, Aeromonas, V. metschnikovii and V. proteus. Pages 148-165 in Proc. 15th U.S.-Japan cooperative medical science program joint conference on cholera, Bethesda, Maryland, 1979. N.I.H. Publication 80-2003.

Hisatsune, K., S. Kondo, T. Iguchi, M. Machida, S. Asou, M. Inaguma, and F. Yamamoto. 1982. Sugar composition of lipopolysaccharides of Family Vibrionaceae. Absence of 2-keto-3-deoxyoctonate (KDO) except in Vibrio parahaemolyticus O6. Microbiol. Immunol. 26:649-664.

Hollis, D.G., R.E. Weaver, C.N. Baker, and C. Thornsberry. 1976. Halophilic Vibrio species isolated from blood cultures. J. Clin. Microbiol. 3:425-431.

Hsieh, H.C., and P.V. Liu. 1970. Serological identities of proteases and alkaline phosphatases of the so-called nonagglutinable (NAG) vibrios and those of Vibrio cholerae. J. Infect. Dis. 121:251-259.

Hugh, R. 1965. A comparison of Vibrio cholerae Pacini and Vibrio eltor Primbram. Int. Bull. Bacteriol. Nomencl. and Taxon. 15:61-68.

Hugh, R., and J.C. Feeley. 1972. Report (1966-1970) of the subcommittee on taxonomy of vibrios to the International Committee on Nomenclature of Bacteria. Int. J. Sys. Bacteriol. 22:123.

Hugh, R., and R. Sakazaki. 1975. Minutes of the International Committee on Systematic Bacteriology subcommittee on the taxonomy of vibrios. Int. J. Sys. Bacteriol. 25:389-391.

Hunt, L.K., T.L. Overman, and R.B. Otero. 1981. Role of pH in oxidase variability of Aeromonas hydrophila. J. Clin. Microbiol. 13:1054-1059.

Huq, M.I., A.K.M.J. Alam, D.J. Brenner, and G.K. Morris. 1980. Isolation of Vibrio-like group, EF-6, from patients with diarrhea. J. Clin. Microbiol. 11:621-624.

Jensen, M.J., P. Baumann, M.Mandel, and J.V. Lee. 1980. Characterization of facultatively anaerobic marine bacteria belonging to group F of Lee, Donovan, and Furniss. Curr. Microbiol. 3:373-376.

Joseph, S.W., R.R. Colwell, and J.B. Kaper. 1982. Vibrio parahaemolyticus and related halophilic vibrios. CRC Crit. R. Microb. 10:77-124.

Kalina, G.P. 1980. Allomonas, a new group of micro-organisms of the family Vibrionaceae. Communication II. Determination of the differentiating significance of individual Allomonas characteristics on the basis of statistical analysis. Zh. Mikrobiol. Epidemiol. Immunobiol. 57(7):13-18.

Kalina, G.P., A.G. Somova, L.S. Podosinnikova, and T.I. Grafova. 1980a. Allomonas, a new group of micro-organisms of the family Vibrionaceae. Communication I. Methods of study and preliminary results of differentiating Allomonas from Aeromonas and Vibrio. Zh. Mikrobiol. Epidemiol. Immunobiol. 57(1):40-46.

Kalina, G.P., V.A. Nikonova, T.I. Grafova, L.S. Podosinnikova, A.G. Somova, and M.I. Lapenkov. 1980b. Allomonas, a new group of microorganisms of the family Vibrionaceae. Communication III. Taxonomic analysis of similarity between Allomonas and other genera of the family. Zh. Mikrobiol. Epidemiol. Immunobiol. 57(8):16-21.

Kalina, G.P. 1981. Allomonas, a new group of micro-organisms of the family Vibrionaceae. Communication IV. Culture media for the isolation, counting and simplified identification of Allomonas. Zh. Mikrobiol. Epidemiol. Immunobiol. 58(6):32-36.

Kaper, J.B., H. Lockman, R.R. Colwell, and S.W. Joseph. 1981. Aeromonas hydrophila: ecology and toxigenicity of isolates from an estuary. J. Appl. Bacteriol. 50:359-377.

Kaper, J.B., H. Lockman, E.F. Remmers, K. Kristensen, and R.R. Colwell. 1983. Numerical taxonomy of Vibrio spp. isolated from estuarine environments. Int. J. Sys. Bacteriol. In press.

Kennedy, S.F., R.R. Colwell, and G.B. Chapman. 1970. Ultrastructure of a marine psychrophilic Vibrio. Can. J. Microbiol. 16:1027-1031.

Kovacs, N. 1956. Identification of Pseudomonas pyocyanea by the oxidase reaction. Nature 178:703.

Krieg, N.R., and R.M. Smibert. 1974. Family I. Spirillaceae. Pages 196-216 in R.E. Buchanan and N.E. Gibbons (Eds.), Bergey's manual of determinative bacteriology, 8th ed. The Williams & Wilkins Co., Baltimore.

Kushner, D.J. 1978. Life in high salt and solute concentrations: halophic bacteria. Pages 317-368 in D.J. Kushner (Ed.), Microbial life in extreme environments. Academic, New York.

Larsen, J.L., A.F. Farid, and I. Dalsgaard. 1981. A comprehensive study of environmental and human pathogenic Vibrio alginolyticus strains. Zentralbl. Bakteriol. Mikrobiol. Hyg. Abt. 1 Orig. A. 251:213-222.

Lee, J.V., T.J. Donovan, and A.L. Furniss. 1978. Characterization, taxonomy and emended description of Vibrio metschnikovii. Int. J. Sys. Bacteriol. 28:99-111.

Lee, J.V., M.S. Hendrie, and J.M. Shewan. 1979. Identification of Aeromonas, Vibrio and related organisms. Pages 151-166 in F.A. Skinner and D.W. Lovelock (Eds.), Identification methods for microbiologists. Society for Applied Bacteriology Technical Series No. 14. Academic, London.

Lee, J.V., and A.L. Furniss. 1981. The phage-typing of V. cholerae serovar O1. Pages 119-122 in T. Holme, J. Holmgren, M.H. Merson and R. Mollby (Eds.), Acute enteric infections in children: New prospects for treatment and prevention. Elsevier, Amsterdam.

Lee, J.V., P. Shread, A.L. Furniss, and T.N. Bryant. 1981. Taxonomy and description of Vibrio fluvialis sp. nov. (synonym group F Vibrios, group EF6). J. Appl. Bacteriol. 50:73-94.

Leifson, E. 1970. Motile marine bacteria IV. Ionic relationships of marine and terrestrial bacteria. Zentralbl. Bakteriol. Parasitenk. Infektionsk. Hyg. Abt. 2. 125:170-206.

Leifson, E., and M. Mandel. 1969. Motile marine bacteria. II. DNA base composition. Int. J. Sys. Bacteriol. 19:127-137.

Lingappa, Y., and J.L. Lockwood. 1962. Chitin media for selective isolation and culture of Actinomycetes. Phytopathology 52:317-323.

Love, M., D. Teebken-Fisher, J.E. Hose, J.J. Farmer, F.W. Hickman, and G.R. Fanning. 1981. Vibrio damsela, a marine bacterium, causes skin ulcers on the damselfish Chromis punctipinnis. Science 214:1139-1140.

McCarthy, D.H., and R.J. Roberts. 1980. Furunuculosis of fish--the present state of our knowledge. Adv. Aquatic Microb. 2:293-341.

MacDonell, M.T., F.L. Singleton, and M.A. Hood. 1982. Diluent composition for use of API20E in characterizing marine and estuarine bacteria. Appl. Environ. Microbiol. 44:423-427

MacFaddin, J.F. 1980. Biochemical tests for identification of medical bacteria. 2nd edition. The Williams & Wilkins Co., Baltimore.

MacInnes, J.I., T.J. Trust, and J.H. Crosa. 1979. Deoxyribonucleic acid relationships among members of the genus Aeromonas. Can. J. Microbiol. 25:579-586.

MacLeod, R.A. 1965. The question of the existence of specific marine bacteria. Bacteriol. R. 29:9-23.

Maiti, M., P. Sur, and S.N. Chatterjee. 1981. Poly-acrylamide gel electrophoresis and infrared spectroscopy of vibrio biotypes. Can. J. Microbiol. 27:1048-1052.

Mayfield, C.I., and W.E. Inniss. 1977. A rapid, simple method for staining bacterial flagella. Can. J. Microbiol. 23:1311-1313.

Merkel, J.R., E.D. Traganza, B.B. Mukherjee, T.B. Griffin, and J.M. Prescott. 1964. Proteolytic activity and general characteristics of a marine bacterium, Aeromonas proteolytica sp. n. J. Bacteriol. 87:1227-1233.

Miyamoto, Y., K. Nakamura, and K. Takizawa. 1961. Pathogenic halophiles. Proposals of a new genus "Oceanomonas" and of the amended species names. Jap. J. Microbiol. 5:477-486.

Miyamoto, Y., T. Kato, Y. Obara, S. Akiyama, K. Takizawa, and S. Yamai. 1969. In vitro hemolytic characteristic of Vibrio parahaemolyticus: its close correlation with human pathogenicity. J. Bacteriol. 100:1147-1149.

Møller, V. 1955. Simplified tests for some amino acid decarboxylases and for the arginine dihydrolase system. Acta Pathologica et Microbiologica Scandinavica 36:158-172.

Momen, H., and C.A. Salles. 1981. An electrophoretic analysis of variation in the Glucose-6-Phosphate dehydrogenase and Malate dehydrogenase of Vibrio cholerae, Vibrio parahaemolyticus and Vibrio fluvialis. J. Appl. Bacteriol. 51:425-432.

Morris, J.G., H. Miller, R. Wilson, C. Tacket, D.G. Hollis, F. Hickman, R.E. Weaver, and P.A. Blake. 1982. Illness caused by Vibrio damsela and Vibrio hollisae. Lancet 1:1294-1297.

Mukerjee, S. 1978. Principles and practice of typing *Vibrio* cholerae. Pages 51-115 in T. Bergan and J.R. Norris (Eds.), Methods in microbiology No. 12. Academic, New York.

Nealson, K.H., and Hastings, J.W. 1979. Bacterial bioluminesence: its control and ecological significance. Microb. R. 43:496-518.

Nishibuchi, M., K. Muroga, R.J. Seidler, and J.L. Fryer. 1979. Pathogenic *Vibrio* isolated from cultured eels. IV. Deoxyribonucleic acid studies. Bull. Jap. Soc. Sci. Fish. 45:1469-1473.

Orndorff, S.A., and R.R. Colwell. 1980. Distribution and identification of luminous bacteria from the Saragasso Sea. Appl. Environ. Microbiol. 39:983-987.

Paik, G. 1980. Reagents, stains, and miscellaneous test procedures. Pages 1000-1024 in E. H. Lennette, A. Balows, W.J. Hausler, and J.P. Truant (Eds.), Manual of clinical microbiology, 3rd ed. American Society for Microbiology, Washington, D.C.

Popoff, M., and M. Veron. 1976. A taxonomic study of the *Aeromonas* hydrophila--Aeromonas *punctata* group. J. Gen. Microbiol. 94:11-22.

Popoff, M.Y., C. Coynault, M. Kiredjian, and M. Lemelin. 1981. Polynucleotide sequence relatedness among motile *Aeromonas* species. Curr. Microbiol. 5:109-114.

Reichelt, J.L., and P. Baumann. 1973. Taxonomy of the marine, luminous bacteria. Arch. Microbiol. 94:283-330.

Reichelt, J.L., and P. Baumann. 1974. Effect of sodium chloride on growth of heterotrophic marine bacteria. Arch. Microbiol. 97:329-345.

Reichelt, J.L., and P. Baumann. 1975. *Photobacterium mandapamensis* Hendrie et al., a later subjective synonym of Photobacterium leiognathi Boisvert et al. Int. J. Sys. Bact. 25:208-209.

Reichelt, J.L., P. Baumann, and L. Baumann. 1976. Study of genetic relationships among marine species of the genera Beneckea and Photobacterium by means of in vitro DNA/DNA hybridization. Arch. Microbiol. 110:101-120.

Rigney, M.M., J.W. Zilinksy, and M.A. Rouf. 1978. Pathogenicity of Aeromonas hydrophila in red leg disease in frogs. Curr. Microbiol. 1:175-179.

Roberts, R.J. 1976. Bacterial diseases of farmed fishes. Pages 55-62 in F.A. Skinner and J.G. Carr (Eds.), Microbiology in agriculture, fisheries and food. Society for Applied Bacteriology Symposium Series No. 4. Academic, London.

Sakazaki, R. 1968. Proposal of Vibrio alginolyticus for the biotype 2 of Vibrio parahaemolyticus. Jap. J. Med. Sci. Biol. 21:359-362.

Sakazaki, R., and A. Balows. 1981. The genera Vibrio, Plesiomonas, and Aeromonas. Pages 1272-1301 in M.P. Starr, H. Stolp, H.G. Truper, A. Balows, and H.G. Schlegel (Eds.), The Prokaryotes: A handbook on habitats, isolation, and identification of bacteria. Springer-Verlag, Berlin.

Sakazaki, R., S. Iwanami, and H. Fukumi. 1963. Studies on the enteropathogenic, facultatively halophilic bacteria, Vibrio parahaemolyticus. I. Morphological, cultural and biochemical properties and its taxonomic position. Jap. J. Med. Sci. Biol. 16:161-188.

Sakazaki, R., C.Z. Gomez, and M. Sebald. 1967. Taxonomic studies of the so-called NAG vibrios. Jap. J. Med. Sci. Biol. 20:265-280.

Sakazaki, R., K. Tamura, C.Z. Gomez, and R. Sen. 1970. Serological studies on the cholera group of vibrios. Jap. J. Med. Sci. Biol. 23:13-20.

Salles, C.A., and H. Momen. 1981. A rapid visual test to characterize cholera vibrios. J. Appl. Bacteriol. 51:433-437.

Sanyal, S.C. 1981. Evaluation of a test-kit (oxi-ferm system) for identification of vibrios. Zentralbl. Bakteriol. Mikrobiol. Hyg. Abt. 1 Orig. A. 251:70-78.

Schiewe, M.H., T.J. Trust, and J.H. Crosa. 1981. Vibrio ordalii sp. nov.--a causative agent of vibriosis in fish. Curr. Microbiol. 6:343-348.

Schubert, R.H.W. 1967a. The taxonomy and nomenclature of the genus Aeromonas Kluyver and Van Niel 1936. I. Suggestions on the taxonomy and nomenclature of the aerogenic Aeromonas species. Int. J. Sys. Bacteriol. 17:23-37.

Schubert, R.H.W. 1967b. The taxonomy and nomenclature of the genus Aeromonas Kluyver and Van Niel 1936. II. Suggestions on the taxonomy and nomenclature of the anaerogenic aeromonads. Int. J. Sys. Bacteriol. 17:273-279.

Schubert, R.H.W. 1968. The taxonomy and nomenclature of the genus Aeromonas Kluyver and Van Niel 1936. III. Suggestions on the definition of the genus Aeromonas Kluyver and Van Niel 1936. Int. J. Sys. Bacteriol. 18:1-7.

Schubert, R.H.W. 1974. Genus II. Aeromonas. Pages 345-348 in R.E. Buchanan and N.E. Gibbons (Eds.), Bergey's manual of determinative bacteriology, 8th ed., The Williams & Wilkins Co., Baltimore.

Seidler, R.J., D.A. Allen, R.R. Colwell, S.W. Joseph, and O.P. Daily. 1980. Biochemical characteristics and virulence of environmental Group F bacteria isolated in the United States. Appl. Environ. Microbiol. 40:715-720.

Shaw, D.H., and H.J. Hodder. 1978. Lipopolysaccharides of the motile aeromonads; core oligosaccharide analysis as an aid to taxonomic classification. Can. J. Microbiol. 24:864-868.

Shewan, J.M. 1963. The differentiation of certain genera of Gram negative bacteria frequently encountered in marine environments. Pages 499-521 in C.H. Oppenheimer (Ed.), Symposium on marine microbiology. C.C. Thomas, Springfield, Illinois.

Shewan, J.M., W. Hodgkiss, and J. Liston. 1954. A method for the rapid differentiation of certain nonpathogenic, asporogenous bacilli. Nature 173:208-209.

Shewan, J.M., and M. Veron. 1974. Genus I. Vibrio. Pages 340-345 in R.E. Buchanan and N.E. Gibbons (Eds.), Bergey's manual of determinative bacteriology, 8th ed. The Williams & Wilkins Co., Baltimore.

Shimada, T., and R. Sakazaki. 1977. Additional serovars and inter-0 antigenic relationships of Vibrio cholerae. Jap. J. Med. Sci. Biol. 30:275-277.

Shimada, T., and R. Sakazaki. 1978. On the serology of Plesiomonas shigelloides. Jap. J. Med. Sci. Biol. 31:135-142.

Shotts, E.B., J.L. Gaines, L. Martin, and A.K. Prestwood. 1972. Aeromonas induced deaths among fish and reptiles in an eutrophic inland lake. J. Am. Vet. Med. Assn. 161:603-607.

Sil, J., N.K. Dutta, S.C. Sanyal, and S. Mukerjee. 1974. Bacteriophage typing of Vibrio cholerae other than O serotype I. Ind. J. Med. Res. 62:15-21.

Singleton, F.L., R. Attwell, S. Jangi, and R.R. Colwell. 1982. Effects of temperature and salinity on Vibrio cholerae growth. Appl. Environ. Microbiol. 44:1047-1058.

Smibert, R.M. 1978. The genus Campylobacter. Ann. R. Microbiol. 32:673-709.

Smith, H.L. 1970. A presumptive test for vibrios: the "string" test. Bull. WHO 42:817-818.

Smith, H.L. 1979. Serotyping of non-cholera vibrios. J. Clin. Microbiol. 10:85-90.

Smith, H.L., and K. Goodner. 1958. Detection of bacterial gelatinases by gelatin-agar plate methods. J. Bacteriol. 76:662-665.

Spira, W.M., and R.R. Daniel. 1980. Biotype clusters formed on the basis of virulence characteristics in non-O1 group 1 Vibrio cholerae. Pages 440-458 in Proc. 15th U.S.-Japan cooperative medical science program joint conference on cholera, 1979. N.I.H. publication 80-2003.

Tanner, A.C.R., S. Badger, C.H. Lai, M.A. Listgarten, R.A. Visconti, and S.S. Socransky. 1981. Wolinella gen. nov., Wolinella succinogenes (Vibrio succinogenes Wolin et al.) comb. nov., and description of Bacteriodes gracilis sp. nov., Wolinella recta sp. nov., Campylobacter concisus sp. nov., and Eikenella corrodens from humans with periodontal disease. Int. J. Sys. Bacteriol. 31:432-445.

Thornley, M.J. 1960. The differentiation of Pseudomonas from other gram-negative bacteria on the basis of arginine metabolism. J. Appl. Bacteriol. 23:37-52.

Tison, D.L., and R.J. Seidler. 1981. Genetic relatedness of clinical and environmental isolates of lactose-positive Vibrio vulnificus. Curr. Microbiol. 6:181-184.

Tison, D.L., M. Nishibuchi, J. Greenwood, and R.J. Seidler. 1982. Vibrio vulnificus biogroup 2: new biogroup pathogenic for eels. Appl. Environ. Microbiol. 44:640-646.

Tsukamoto, T., K. Kinoshita, T. Shimada, and R. Sakazaki. 1978. Two epidemics of diarrhoeal disease possibly caused by Plesiomonas shigelloides. J. Hyg. (Cambridge) 80:275-280.

Ventosa, A., E. Quesada, F. Rodriguez-Valera, F. Ruiz-Berraquero, and A. Ramos-Cormenzana. 1982. Numerical taxonomy of moderately halophilic gram-negative rods. J. Gen. Microbiol. 128:1959-1968.

Veron, M. 1965. La position taxonomique des Vibrio et de certaines bacteries comparables. Comptes Rendues de L'Academie des Sciences, Paris 261:5243-5246.

Veron, M. 1971. Classification et definition du bacille du cholera. Medicine Tropicale 31:31-39.

Veron, M. 1974. Family II. Vibrionaceae. Pages 340-352 in R.E. Buchanan and N.E. Gibbons (Eds.), Bergey's manual of determinative bacteriology, 8th ed. The Williams & Wilkins Co., Baltimore.

Von Graevenitz, A., and A.H. Mensch. 1968. The genus Aeromonas in human bacteriology. Report of 30 cases and review of the literature. N. Engl. J. Med. 278:245-249.

Von Graevenitz, A. 1980. Chapter 17. Aeromonas and Plesiomonas. Pages 220-225 in E.H. Lennette, A. Balows, W.J. Hausler, and J.P. Truant. Manual of clinical microbiology, 3rd ed. American Society of Microbiology, Washington, D.C.

Wachsmuth, I.K., G.K. Morris, and J.C. Feeley. 1980. Chapter 18. Vibrio. Pages 226-234 in E.H. Lennette, A. Balows, W.J. Hausler, and J.P. Truant. Manual of clinical microbiology, 3rd ed., American Society for Microbiology, Washington, D.C.

West, P.A., R.M. Daniel, C.J. Knowles, and J.V. Lee. 1978. Tetramethyl-p-phenylenediamine (TMPD) oxidase activity and cytochrome distribution in the genus Vibrio. FEMS Microbiology Letters 4:339-342.

West, P.A. 1980. Ecology and taxonomy of the genus Vibrio. Ph.D. Thesis, University of Kent at Canterbury, England.

Whang, H.Y., M.E. Heller, and E. Neter. 1972. Production by Aeromonas of common enterobacterial antigen and its possible taxonomic significance. J. Bacteriol. 110:161-164.

Wolin, M.J., E.A. Wolin, and N.J. Jacobs. 1961. Cytochrome-producing anaerobic vibrio, Vibrio succinogenes sp. n. J. Bacteriol. 81:911-917.

Woolkalis, M.J., and P. Baumann. 1981. Evolution of alkaline phosphatase in marine species of Vibrio. J. Bacteriol. 147:36-45.

Ecology

Chapter 21

ECOLOGY OF PATHOGENIC VIBRIOS
IN CHESAPEAKE BAY

Rita R. Colwell, Paul A. West, David Maneval,
Elaine F. Remmers, Elisa L. Elliot,
and Nancy E. Carlson

Our program on the microbial ecology of Chesapeake Bay was initiated in 1964 at Georgetown University, and has been continued and extended at the University of Maryland since 1972. With the inception of the program, analyses of seasonal and regional differences in the microflora and autecology studies, notably of Vibrio spp., have been undertaken. During the first three years of this research now extending over nearly two decades, two areas of Chesapeake Bay were intensively studied. Samples of water, sediment, and oysters were collected at six-week intervals from Marumsco Bar, near Crisfield, Maryland, on the lower Eastern Shore and from Eastern Bay, on the upper Eastern Shore of Maryland. Marumsco Bar suffers annual mortalities of its shellfish population and is no longer a highly commercially productive area for oysters, whereas Eastern Bay remains a thriving oyster harvesting area. Results of the initial studies showed that although the total microbial populations in the water column, sediment, and oysters are roughly the same, the generic composition of the associated bacterial communities showed Vibrio spp. to be present in significantly greater numbers in the Marumsco Bar sites (Lovelace et al. 1968; Krantz et al. 1969). Several of these

Vibrio spp. were subsequently found to be pathogenic for bivalve larvae (Tubiash at al. 1970).

Vibrio parahaemolyticus

In 1969, the discovery of V. parahaemolyticus in Chesapeake Bay was reported (Krantz et al. 1969), notably in association with dead and dying blue crabs. V. parahaemolyticus had been recognized as one of the most important causative agents of food poisoning in Japan for at least a decade (Colwell 1974). As a result of the discovery of V. parahaemolyticus in Chesapeake Bay, outbreaks of food poisoning were predicted. The first fully documented outbreaks of food-associated gastroenteritis did not occur in Maryland, however, until August 1971 (Molenda et al. 1972). The epidemiological data implicated steamed crabs served at two unrelated picnics, and a crab salad served at a medical institution.

The isolates from the Maryland food poisoning out-breaks, cultures from moribund and dead Chesapeake Bay blue crabs, and V. parahaemolyticus isolated from samples of water, sediment, blue crabs, oysters, and clams collected in several areas of Chesapeake Bay were subjected to numerical taxonomic, deoxyribonucleic acid (DNA) base composition, serologic, isozymic, gas chromatographic, bacteriophage sensitivity, and DNA/DNA reassociation analyses. Results confirmed the identification and classification of V. parahaemolyticus and permitted establishment of genetic relationships of the Chesapeake Bay strains with isolates from victims of food poisoning in Japan and from samples taken in geographically diverse areas of the United States (Colwell 1970; Colwell et al. 1973; Staley and Colwell 1973).

The ecology of V. parahaemolyticus in Chesapeake Bay was further examined with the first autecology studies carried out in the Rhode River, a sub-estuary of Chesa-peake Bay. Incidence of V. parahaemolyticus was found to be correlated with water temperature and the organism was not detected in the water column during the winter months. However, it could be isolated from sediment, even during the winter months (November–March) but only in very small numbers. During April through early June, sediment in the shallow sub-estuaries of the Rhode River is mixed with the water column by the wind, tide, and water movement resulting from runoff from the land at shallow sites. It now is recognized that V. parahaemolyticus can survive the winter, being released into the water column at neap tides to attach to plankton, thereupon proliferating after initiation of the association with plankton (Kaneko and Colwell 1973, 1975a, 1975b, 1978). Interestingly, absorption of V. parahaemolyticus onto plankton or chitin-containing materials occurs with higher efficiency under conditions of estuarine salinity (Kaneko and Colwell 1975a). The absorption kinetics of the attachment of V. parahaemolyticus to chitin have recently been reported (Belas and Colwell 1982).

When the water temperature rises to 19°C, V. parahaemolyticus is easily detected in the water column, with release of the bacteria resulting during and after growth on plankton, along with continued release of the bacteria from sediment. Peaks in bacterial counts occur during June, July, and August, with maximum counts recorded at ca. 10^7 to 10^8/g net wet weight of plankton. The maximum numbers of V. parahaemolyticus occur in the summer months on plankton, in the water column, and in sediment. During the summer, V. parahaemolyticus associated with proliferating plankton populations are involved in mineralization of the plankton, eventually breaking down and disintegrating the plankton, following a plankton bloom (Kaneko and Colwell 1978).

Distribution of V. parahaemolyticus in the Chesapeake Bay most probably is a function of the total organic content of the water, which is higher than that of the open sea. In 1971, studies of the distribution of V. parahaemolyticus in the ocean were done, using water, sediment, and plankton samples collected during cruises aboard the R/V EASTWARD. A series of stations along four tracklines, from the coast of South Carolina and Georgia to 72 miles offshore, to the edge of the continental shelf were sampled. The results showed that V. parahaemolyticus could not be isolated from seawater or sediment in the open ocean. Even samples taken at stations as close to shore as four miles did not yield V. parahaemolyticus. These data, combined with results of studies examining the optimum salinity, pH, and other parameters for attachment of V. parahaemolyticus to zooplankton lead us to the conclusion that this organism is an estuarine bacterium and it does not compete successfully in the high salinity, low temperature, low nutrient, and high hydrostatic pressure environment of the deep ocean (Colwell and Kaneko 1974; Schwarz and Colwell 1974). It is now generally accepted that the distribution of V. parahaemolyticus is predominantly in coastal and estuarine regions, especially at the mouth of the rivers. Interestingly, no correlation between Escherichia coli and V. parahaemolyticus counts has been observed in the Chesapeake Bay (Kaneko and Colwell 1973).

The broader implications of the life history, taxonomy, physiology and pathogenic properties of Vibrio parahaemolyticus, recently reviewed by Joseph et al. (1982), are that this organism serves primarily an ecological function in the overall process of the Chesapeake Bay ecosystem. The pathogenic potential of V. parahaemolyticus, unfortunate from the anthropocentric point of view, must be considered in its pragmatic aspects, particularly in the processing of seafood for human consumption.

Temperatures below 10°C inhibit or reduce the growth of V. parahaemolyticus. However, some strains of V. parahaemolyticus may grow at 5°C under laboratory conditions, after very long periods of incubation (Kaneko and Colwell 1978). The number of V. parahaemolyticus in samples collected during the winter are at barely detectable concentrations, except in the case of sediment samples. Yet even in sediment samples, the number of V. parahaemolyticus is extremely low in the winter (Kaneko and Colwell 1978). Divalent ions such as Ca^{++} and Mg^{++} may act to protect V. parahaemolyticus against the effects of low temperatures, that is, at temperatures < 5°C, permitting survival at low temperatures. Whether V. parahaemolyticus undergoes a "nonrecoverability" state as has recently been discovered for Vibrio cholerae (Xu et al. 1983; vide infra) remains to be determined.

Studies of the distribution of V. parahaemolyticus in the Upper Chesapeake Bay, carried out from December 1973 through December 1974 and again in May and June 1975, showed that the frequency of occurrence of V. parahaemolyticus was highest at stations in the lower regions of the Upper Chesapeake Bay. The occurrence of V. parahaemolyticus in sediment samples and suspended sediment samples collected during upper Bay studies in the areas of lower salinity, was attributed to tidal transport. The percentage of samples containing V. parahaemolyticus increased from 0% at Conowingo Dam, to 20% in water and sediment samples collected at stations of ca. 12 ppt. in the middle region of the Chesapeake Bay. From concurrently measured fecal coliform densities and the relatively low fecal streptococci ratios obtained, it was found that V. parahaemolyticus is not associated with domestic sewage contamination in Chesapeake Bay, a result reaffirming the autochthonous nature of V. parahaemolyticus in the estuarine environment (Sayler et al. 1976).

Studies have further demonstrated that the hemolymph of normal, healthy Chesapeake Bay blue crabs, is not sterile but harbors V. parahaemolyticus (Colwell et al. 1975; Sizemore et al. 1975; Tubiash et al. 1975). Thus, the association of V. parahaemolyticus with crustaceans appears to be significant, both ecologically and from the public health standpoint.

One of the hypotheses arising from studies of V. parahaemolyticus in Chesapeake Bay is that the autochthonous, or "normal," microbial flora of bodies of water, such as the Chesapeake Bay, are subjected to competition and genetic exchange, when allochthonous bacterial populations enter the water. Extrachromosomal material, that is, plasmids, offer a mechanism whereby the autochthonous bacterial flora can be altered. Multiple drug resistance factors, heavy metal tolerance, and factors operative in pathogenicity can be transferred via this genetic mode. Strains of V. parahaemolyticus have been examined for plasmid DNA and multiple plasmid species of cryptic function have been observed (Guerry and Colwell 1977). More importantly, strains of V. parahaemolyticus were found to be capable of receiving and stably maintaining plasmids conjugally transferred from E. coli (Guerry and Colwell 1977).

Recent studies of pathogenic vibrios in Chesapeake Bay from June 1979 to August 1981 confirmed the ubiquitous distribution of V. parahaemolyticus in waters whose range of salinity was 8-20 ppt. Seasonality was confirmed and a more frequent isolation of this organism from plankton homogenates, crabs, and sediment than from the water column was observed (Table 1). Counts of V. parahaemolyticus obtained during the most recent studies were in the range of 0.3-300 bacteria per gram of sediment or liter of water.

Oysters collected in August 1981 from 18 different oyster fishing areas in the Chesapeake Bay all contained V. parahaemolyticus when 50-gram samples of oyster meat were homogenized and examined bacteriologically. Current studies of the bacteriological quality of commercially processed Chesapeake Bay crabs and oysters indicate a remarkably high quality of these products, based on V. parahaemolyticus and other indicator bacterial counts (Elliot and Colwell, unpublished data). See Table 2.

Table 1. Summary of Isolation of Vibrio parahaemolyticus from Chesapeake Bay (June 1979-August 1981)

- Ubiquitous in regions of 8-20 ppt.; seasonality observed for isolation rate

- More frequently isolated from plankton homogenates, crabs, and sediment than from the water column

- Counts in the range 0.3-300 cells per gram of sediment or liter of water

- Oysters taken in August 1981 from 18 different bars in the bay all contained Vibrio parahaemolyticus in 50 grams of meat homogenate

---

Table 2. Bacteria in Processed Crab and Oyster Samples

Sample[a]	Halophilic Vibrio spp.[b] (MPN/g or ml)	Vibrio cholerae[b] (MPN/g)	Fecal Coliforms[c] (MPN/g)	Total Aerobic Count[d] (Bacteria/g or ml)
Oyster Samples				
Live	590(180-2000)[e]	< 0.02	34(10-110)	3.6×10^4
Shucked	84(25-280)	< 0.02	5.4(1.6-18.0)	4.8×10^5
Shucked and Washed	280(85-920)	< 0.02	7.6(2.3-25.0)	1.2×10^5
Crab Samples				
Whole Live	660(200- $\geq$ 2400)	< 0.02	< 0.2	$> 3.0 \times 10^6$
Whole Cooked	< 0.02	< 0.02	< 0.2	8.3×10^3
Picked Meat	108(33-360)	< 0.02	< 0.2	8.4×10^4
Pasteurized Meat	< 0.2	< 0.02	< 0.2	$< 3.0 \times 10^3$

[a]Dates for samples: oyster (December 1981), pasteurized crab meat (March 1982), other crab samples (May 1982).

[b]Samples were homogenized and diluted with phosphate-buffered saline (7.2g NaCl, 1.48g Na_2HPO_4, 0.43g KH_2PO_4 per 1, pH 7.2) MPN enrichment broth for halophilic Vibrio spp. was alkaline peptone broth (10g peptone, 30g NaCl per 1, pH 8.5). Vibrio spp. identified included V. parahaemolyticus, V. fluvialis, V. alginolyticus, and V. anguillarum. Enrichment broth for Vibrio cholerae was alkaline peptone broth (no NaCl added). Enrichment was followed by selective isolation on TCBS agar (Oxoid) and identification using biochemical tests.

[c]Fecal coliforms enumerated according to the FDA Bacteriological Analytical Manual (1980, revision).

[d]Total Aerobic Count on Plate Count Agar (Difco) with 1% NaCl (w/v) after 7 days at 25°C.

[e]95% confidence intervals.

Vibrio cholerae

Studies on the taxonomy, molecular genetics, and ecology of V. cholerae have been underway in our laboratory since 1963 and these include isozymic, DNA base composition, gas chromatographic, DNA/DNA reassociation, and numerical taxonomic analyses (Colwell and Yuter 1965; Colwell et al. 1968; Citarella and Colwell 1970; Colwell 1970; Staley and Colwell 1973). In the fall of 1976 and spring 1977, strains of V. cholerae (non-O1 serovar) were first isolated at several locations in Chesapeake Bay (Colwell et al. 1977). Since then non-O1 V. cholerae has been routinely isolated and in 1977, V. cholerae serovar O1 was recovered from a water sample collected in Chesapeake Bay (Colwell et al. 1981).

The ecology of V. cholerae in the Chesapeake Bay has proven to be interesting and, in some respects, is similar in distribution to V. parahaemolyticus, but differs in several important characteristics. Vibrio cholerae can be isolated from both domestic sewage polluted and unpolluted areas of the Chesapeake Bay. In contrast to Salmonella spp., which are allochthonous pathogens, V. cholerae, like V. parahaemolyticus is an autochthonous species of the estuarine ecosystem. The occurrence of V. cholerae is not correlated with other microbial indicators of fecal pollution. In fact, the converse is true. Kaper et al. (1979) did not isolate V. cholerae during the summer of 1977 at the heavily polluted site, Jones Falls in Baltimore Harbor. Yet, the initial isolation of V. cholerae was made at Jones Falls in Baltimore Harbor during October 1976 (Colwell et al. 1977). Jones Falls, a station where the salinity of the water usually is less than 5 ppt., frequently demonstrates almost anoxic water conditions, with a dissolved oxygen content of as low as 0.1 mg/liter. Under such conditions many allochthonous bacterial species can be isolated, viz., 240,000 total coliforms/100 ml, 46,000 fecal coliforms/100 ml, and total viable, heterotrophic counts of 1.1×10^7/ml (Kaper et al. 1979). To establish the autochthonous nature of V. cholerae in Chesapeake Bay, a pollution gradient of water samples was examined to determine association, if any, with microbial indicators of pollution. Salmonella spp. were isolated only from samples collected in the highly polluted Baltimore Harbor, where significant numbers of fecal coliforms were also isolated. Results of a correlation matrix calculation indicated that the presence of Salmonella spp. was clearly associated with large numbers of fecal coliforms (P < 0.01), but no correlation between incidence of fecal coliforms and V. cholerae could be detected (Kaper et al. 1979).

Unlike V. parahaemolyticus (Kaneko and Colwell 1978) an unequivocal seasonal incidence of V. cholerae in Chesapeake Bay has not been observed, at least by the monitoring methods presently available. The newly developed technique of immune-fluorescence-epifluorescence direct microscopy enumeration may prove helpful in answering this question (Xu et al. 1983). Recent studies have confirmed that V. cholerae is present in low concentrations (ca. 1 to 46 cells/liter) throughout the year in Chesapeake Bay (Table 3). Data obtained during transect cruises in

Table 3. Summary of Isolation of Vibrio cholerae from Chesapeake Bay (June 1979-August 1981)

- No O1 serotype has been isolated

- Isolations are more frequent when water temperature > 17°C when the organism is often recovered from plankton samples as well

- Highest count to date--46 cells/L water

- No isolation from oyster meat but two isolations from crab meat and surface swabs of crabs

- Approximately 10% of isolates from the bay are bioluminescent--abolition of Vibrio albensis?

Chesapeake Bay, accomplished in June 1979 and in August 1981, are summarized in Tables 4 and 5. From the data accumulated to date, the salinity range for isolation of V. cholerae from Chesapeake Bay is concluded to be ca. 2 to 20 ppt.

Salinity has proven a fascinating parameter with respect to the ecology of V. cholerae. A requirement for NaCl for growth of V. cholerae alluded to in the volume published by Pollitzer (1959), but a definitive study showing an absolute requirement for NaCl has only recently been done (Singleton et al. 1982b), in which selected concentrations of NaCl or $MgCl_2$, the major salts of seawater, were employed and growth after incubation for 4 days at 25°C was measured. It was observed that when the concentrations of $MgCl_2$ were varied, little or no effect was observed on total or culturable cell counts. However, the effect evidenced when the NaCl concentration was altered was dramatic. Both total direct and culturable cell counts followed a similar pattern, with maximum population sizes occurring at optimum salinity and minimum population sizes at lower or higher NaCl concentrations. Uptake of ^{14}C-amino acids by V. cholerae at different concentrations of NaCl or $MgCl_2$ showed that heterotrophic activity was also affected. Maximum uptake of amino acid mixture occurred in the presence of intermediate, or control, $MgCl_2$ concentration, that is, 7.74 g/l. When the $MgCl_2$ concentration was increased or decreased, uptake decreased. A similar uptake pattern was observed when different NaCl concentrations were used. With increasing or decreasing NaCl concentration, compared to intermediate concentrations (approximating estuarine salinities), uptake decreased. These data suggested that V. cholerae has a preference for the estuarine environment, rather than for fresh water or open sea water.

The influence of Na^+ on growth and metabolism was also studied. In a chemically defined basal salts medium containing no added Na^+, growth was not observed. In fact, as the NaCl concentration was decreased from 0.3 M to 0.1 M, the population size of V. cholerae decreased. Maximum heterotrophic uptake occurred when 0.1 M NaCl and 0.2 M KCl were added to the chemically defined medium. LiCl

Table 4. Isolation of _Vibrio cholerae_ from Chesapeake Bay during June 1979.

| Site | Water Temperature (°C) | Salinity (ppt.) | Isolation of _V. cholerae_ | |
			Top Water (MPN cells/L)	Plankton
Tolchester Beach	21.7	2.4	5.3	Present
Magothey River	21.4	4.6	3.5	Absent
Chester River	21.0	5.4	3.6	Absent
Eastern Bay	22.5	7.8	46.0	Present Absent
Cook Point	21.6	8.3	0.7	Present Absent
Patuxent River	21.1	9.2	15.0	Present
Smith Point	22.6	10.2	Absent	Absent
Rappahannock River	22.5	12.4	12.0	Present
York River	21.7	16.0	24.0	Present
Cape Henry	21.2	20.0	4.3	Present

Table 5. Isolation of Vibrio cholerae from Chesapeake Bay oyster bar sites during August 1981.[a]

Oyster Bar Location	Water Temperature (°C)	Salinity (ppt.)	Isolation of V. cholerae		
			Top Water (MPN cells/L)	Plankton (MPN cells/g)	Crabs[b]
Swan Point	25.0	11.9	0.6	Absent	Absent
James River	25.8	12.9	Absent	Absent	Absent
Tolley Point	24.8	13.4	0.9	4.5	Absent
Cobb Island	25.3	14.7	0.3	Absent	Carapace swab positive
Eastern Bay	26.0	14.8	0.3	Absent	Absent
Choptank River	26.4	15.3	0.3	Absent	Absent
Broome Island, Patuxent River	26.4	15.4	Absent	Absent	Absent
Sharkfin Shoal	23.3	16.4	Absent	Absent	Absent
Little Deal Island	25.1	18.2	Absent	Absent	Absent

[a]V. cholerae not isolated from oyster meat homogenates.
[b]Crab feces, hemolymph, carapace swab samples.

could not replace the NaCl requirement and KCl was sparing only to ca. 0.1 M NaCl, but the requirement for Na$^+$ was absolute (Colwell et al. 1983).

The influence of salinity on survival of V. cholerae incubated at 10°C is unequivocal, based on results of recent studies in our laboratory (Singleton et al. 1982a, 1982b). V. cholerae can survive up to 42 days at a salinity of 25 ppt., but not at 5 ppt. In the latter case, the bacteria were not detected by culture methods at 4 days. Thus, in Chesapeake Bay, where V. cholerae is now known to be present, the distribution of the organism may be explained by its "overwintering" in waters of optimum salinity for V. cholerae.

The effect of temperature on the distribution of V. cholerae in Chesapeake Bay has also proven to be significant. Isolation of non-O1 V. cholerae from Chesapeake Bay since May 1979, relative to environmental temperature, is shown in Figure 1. Clearly isolations of V. cholerae are more frequent when the water temperature is greater than 17°C. Effects of temperature on viability of V. cholerae are discussed elsewhere in this volume.

In studies of the association of V. cholerae with the biota of the Chesapeake Bay, there have been no isolations to date from oyster meat, but two isolations from crab meat and from surface swabs of crabs have been made. From data given in Table 2, it can be concluded that commercially processed Chesapeake Bay seafood does not offer a threat of transmission of V. cholerae.

The association of V. cholerae with zooplanktonic biota has proved interesting. Huq et al. (1983) found that strains of V. cholerae, both O1 and non-O1 serovars, attach to the surfaces of live copepods maintained in natural water samples collected from the Chesapeake Bay. The specificity of attachment to the oral region and egg sac of the copepod, and the extension of the survival of V. cholerae in water in the presence of live copepods, offer clues to the ecological niche and/or role(s) of V. cholerae in the environment. Zooplankton offer an environmental reservoir of V. cholerae.

It is interesting to consider that there may be an interaction of V. cholerae with crustaceans, perhaps a

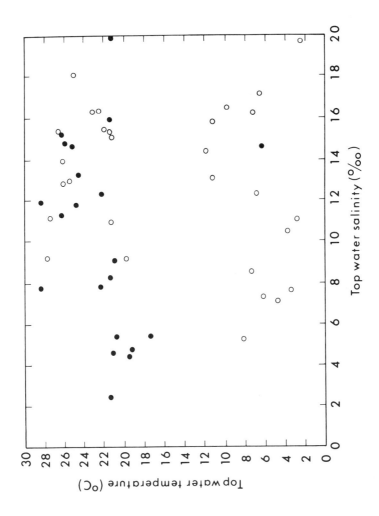

Figure 1. Effect of salinity and water temperature on the isolation of non-O1 Vibrio cholerae from Chesapeake Bay since May 1979. ● non-O1 V. cholerae isolated; ○ non-O1 V. cholerae not isolated.

commensal relationship. It has been suggested that the enterotoxin of V. cholerae may function in salt tolerance and/or osmoregulation (Colwell et al. 1981). V. cholerae may, in fact, sequester Na$^+$ from its commensal host for growth. When cholera toxin binds to the cell receptor of human intestinal epithelial cells, adenylate cyclase activity increases, which increases the level of cyclic 3', 5'-adenosine monophosphate (cAMP). The increase in cAMP activity results in an efflux of Na$^+$ and other electrolytes from epithelial cells, along with quantities of water, producing the symptoms of cholera (van Heyningen 1977). Cholera toxin acting on epithelial cells of crustacea would provide a mechanism for V. cholerae to obtain sufficient quantities of Na$^+$ from its host when the salinity of the environment falls below that required for survival and growth. It is also possible that V., cholerae may interact with its host in osmoregulation, enabling the wide salinity range of migration characteristics of its hosts including zooplankton species.

A recent discovery, based on data gathered on the effect of temperature and salinity interactions influencing the survival and distribution of V. cholerae in Chesapeake Bay, is the "non-recoverability" phenomenon occurring when either temperatures or salinities, below or above that optimum for V. cholerae, occur. Results of our studies to date show that V. cholerae remains active, that is, viable but non-recoverable under certain regimes of temperature and salinity. Plating methods for estimating survival of V. cholerae, thus, do not provide a valid estimate of the viable populations of V. cholerae in natural waters. These results were obtained by combining the techniques of immune-fluorescent staining and the acridine orange direct microscopy, utilizing epifluorescent microscopy. We have observed that at the time when V. cholerae "dies off," such as when it is subjected to low temperatures (< 10°C) and/or reduced salinity (ca. < 10 ppt.), the organism undergoes a "nonrecoverable" stage of existence. Results of direct microscopy indicate that the number of cells does not decline yet the plate counts drop (Xu et al. 1983). When conditions are again optimum for growth, the bacterial cells return to a "recoverable" stage, i.e. will grow on laboratory media. This observation may explain the distribution of V. cholerae in the environment, as well as the sporadic occurrence of both V. cholerae in aquatic environments and outbreaks of cholera.

Other Pathogenic Vibrios

Other pathogenic vibrios isolated from Chesapeake Bay include Vibrio vulnificus, Vibrio fluvialis, and Vibrio mimicus. However, ecological studies of these organisms are hindered by the present lack of suitable isolation media and methods, as well as difficulties in species identification. Vibrio vulnificus has only rarely been isolated from Chesapeake Bay water, sediment, plankton, oysters, and crabs. It has been isolated from water samples in the salinity range of 5-20 ppt. The highest counts to date are 230 cells/liter of water, 9 cells/cc sediment slurry and 2.3 cells/gram of oyster meat. It has only rarely been isolated from plankton or crabs.

SUMMARY

The ecology of Vibrio spp. continues under investigation. The results to date have provided fascinating insight into the ecology, systematics, epidemiology, and pathogenicity of these organisms. Clearly, the majority of the vibrios, both pathogenic and nonpathogenic, either require, or are enhanced in growth by the presence of, salt. The occurrence of vibrios in estuarine and marine waters suggests the autochthonous nature of these species is estuarine and/or marine. Fortuitously, the vibrios provide an extraordinarily interesting interface for microbial ecology, epidemiology, and pathogenic microbiology. It is clear that unless the ecology of the vibrios is fully understood, complete control of disease caused by these microorganisms will not be possible.

REFERENCES

Belas, M.R., and R.R. Colwell. 1982. Absorption kinetics of laterally and polarly flagellated Vibrio. J. Bacteriol. 151:1568-1580.

Citarella, R.V., and R.R. Colwell. 1970. Polyphasic taxonomy of the genus Vibrio: polynucleotide sequence relationships among selected Vibrio species. J. Bacteriol. 104: 434-442.

Colwell, R.R. 1970. Polyphasic taxonomy of the genus Vibrio: numerical taxonomy of Vibrio cholerae, Vibrio parahaemolyticus, and related Vibrio species. J. Bacteriol. 104:410-433.

Colwell, R.R. 1974. Occurrence and biology of Vibrio parahaemolyticus. Pages 230-240 in D. Schlesinger (Ed.), Microbiology--1974. American Society for Microbiology, Washington, D.C.

Colwell, R.R., and Kaneko, T. 1974. Ecological studies of Vibrio parahaemolyticus. Pages 536-545 in R.R. Colwell and R.Y. Morita (Eds.), Effect of the ocean environments on microbial activities. University Park Press, Baltimore.

Colwell, R.R., and M. Yuter. 1965. Adansonian analysis and deoxyribonucleic acid base composition studies of Vibrio cholerae and el tor vibrios. Bacteriol. Proc., p. 18.

Colwell, R.R., V.I. Adeyemo, and H.H. Kirtland. 1968. Esterases and DNA base composition analysis of Vibrio cholerae and related vibrios. J. Appl. Bacteriol. 31:323-335.

Colwell, R.R., J. Kaper, and S.W. Joseph. 1977. Vibrio cholerae, Vibrio parahaemolyticus and other vibrios: occurrence and distribution in Chesapeake Bay. Science 198:394-396.

Colwell, R.R., T.E. Lovelace, L. Wan, T. Kaneko, T. Staley, P.K. Chen, and H. Tubiash. 1973. Vibrio parahaemolyticus--isolation, identification, classification and ecology. J. Milk and Food Tech. 36:202-231.

Colwell, R.R., T.C. Wicks, and H.S. Tubiash. 1975. A comparative study of the bacterial flora of the haemolymph of Callinectes sapidus. Marine Fisheries R. 37:29-33.

Colwell, R.R., R. Seidler, J. Kaper, S. Joseph, S. Garges, H. Lockman, D. Maneval, H. Bradford, N. Roberts, E. Remmers, I. Huq, and A. Huq. 1981. Occurrence of Vibrio cholerae O-group 1 in Maryland and Louisiana estuaries. Appl. Environ. Microbiol. 41:5555-558.

Colwell, R.R., F.L. Singleton, A. Huq, H-S. Xu, and N. Roberts. 1983. Ecology of Vibrio cholerae, Vibrio parahaemolyticus, and related vibrios in the natural environment. Proc. International Symposium on Bacterial Diarrheal Disease, Osaka University, Japan. Marcel-Dekker, New York: In press.

Food and Drug Administration. 1978. Bacteriological Analytical Manual for Foods. 5th ed., 1980 rev. Assoc. Offic. Anal. Chemists, Washington, D.C.

Guerry, P., and R.R. Colwell. 1977. Isolation of cryptic plasmid deoxyribonucleic acid from Kanagawa positive strains of Vibrio parahaemolyticus. Infect. Immun. 16:328-334.

Huq, A., E.B. Small, P.A. West, M.I. Huq, R. Rahman, and R.R. Colwell. 1983. Ecological relationships between Vibrio cholerae and planktonic crustacean copepods. Appl. Environ. Microbiol. 45:275-283.

Joseph, S.W., R.R. Colwell, and J.B. Kaper. 1982. Vibrio parahaemolyticus and related halophilic vibrios. CRC Crit. R. Microbiol. 10:77-124.

Kaneko, T., and R.R. Colwell. 1973. Ecology of Vibrio parahaemolyticus in Chesapeake Bay. J. Bacteriol. 113:24-32.

Kaneko, T., and R.R. Colwell. 1975a. Absorption of Vibrio parahaemolyticus onto chitin and copepods. Appl. Microbiol. 29:269-274.

Kaneko, T., and R.R. Colwell. 1975b. Incidence of Vibrio parahaemolyticus in Chesapeake Bay. Appl. Microbiol. 30:251-257.

Kaneko, T., and R.R. Colwell. 1978. The annual cycle of Vibrio parahaemolyticus in Chesapeake Bay. Microb. Ecol. 4:135-155.

Kaper, J., H. Lockman, R.R. Colwell, and S.W. Joseph. 1979. Ecology, serology, and enterotoxin production of Vibrio cholerae in Chesapeake Bay. Appl. Environ. Microb. 37:91-103.

Krantz, G.E., R.R. Colwell, and E. Lovelace. 1969. Vibrio parahaemolyticus from the blue crab Callinectes sapidus in Chesapeake Bay. Science 164:1286-1287.

Lovelace, T.E., H. Tubiash, and R.R. Colwell. 1968. Quantitative and qualitative commensal bacterial flora of Crassostrea virginica in Chesapeake Bay. Proc. Nat. Shellfisheries Assn. 58:82-87.

Molenda, J.R., W.G. Johnson, M. Fishbein, B. Wentz, I.J. Mehlman, and T.A. Dadisman. 1972. Vibrio parahaemolyticus gastroenteritis in Maryland: laboratory aspects. Appl. Microbiol. 24:444-448.

Pollitzer, R. 1959. Cholera. World Health Organization, Geneva.

Sayler, G.S., J.D. Nelson, A. Justice, and R.R. Colwell. 1976. Incidence of Salmonella spp., Clostridium botulinum, and Vibrio parahaemolyticus in an estuary. Appl. Microbiol. 31:723-730.

Schwarz, J.R., and R.R. Colwell. 1974. Effect of hydrostatic pressure on growth and viability of Vibrio parahaemolyticus. Appl. Microbiol. 28:977-981.

Singleton, F.L., R.W. Attwell, M.S. Jangi, and R.R. Colwell. 1982a. Influence of salinity and organic nutrient concentration on survival and growth of Vibrio cholerae in aquatic microcosms. Appl. Environ. Microbiol. 43:1080-1085.

Singleton, F.L., R. Attwell, S. Jangi, and R.R. Colwell. 1982b. Effects of temperature and salinity on Vibrio cholerae growth. Appl. Environ. Microb. 44:1047-1058.

Sizemore, R.K., R.R. Colwell, H.S. Tubiash, and T.E. Lovelace. 1975. Bacterial flora of the hemolymph of the blue crab Callinectes sapidus: numerical taxonomy. Appl. Microbiol. 29:393-399.

Staley, T.E., and R.R. Colwell. 1973. Polynucleotide sequence relationships among Japanese and American strains of Vibrio parahaemolyticus. J. Bacteriol. 114:916-927.

Tubiash, H., R.R. Colwell, and R. Sakazaki. 1970. Marine vibrios associated with bacillary neurosis, a disease of larval and juvenile bivalve mollusks. J. Bacteriol. 103:271-272.

Tubiash, H.S., R.K. Sizemore, and R.R. Colwell. 1975. Bacterial flora in the hemolymph of the blue crab, Callinectes sapidus: most probable numbers. Appl. Microbiol. 29:388-392.

van Heyningen, S. 1977. Cholera toxin. Biological R. 52:509-549.

Xu, H-S., N. Roberts, F.L. Singleton, R.W. Attwell, D.J. Grimes, and R.R. Colwell. 1983. Extended survival of non-culturable *Escherichia coli* and *Vibrio cholerae* in saltwater microcosms. Microb. Ecol.: in press.

CHAPTER 22

ECOLOGY OF <u>VIBRIO</u> <u>CHOLERAE</u> IN LOUISIANA COASTAL AREAS

Nell C. Roberts, Henry B. Bradford, Jr.
and Joan R. Barbay

To understand the ecology of <u>Vibrio</u> <u>cholerae</u>, one must first understand the region in question. Our studies have been confined to the coastal areas from the Pearl River on the east over 1,700 miles of coast line to the Sabine River on the west and bordered on the north by I-10. Collection points are shown in Figure 1.

The Louisiana coastal area is divided into three distinct areas: the eastern coastal plain marked with Lakes Maurepas and Ponchatrain; the Mississippi alluvial plain containing the swamplands, that is, the Atchafalaya basin and swamp; and the West Gulf coastal plain consisting of the marshes or "wet prairies" marked with land islands called chenieres. Average yearly precipitation ranges from 64 inches at New Orleans to 58 inches in the western section. Winters are mild and short. First freezes occur in late November or early December and last freezes occur from mid February to early March (Calhoun 1979).

From January 1980 through July 1981, 418 water, sediment, seafood, and sewer samples were processed. Methods were essentially those used by Kaper et al. (1979). A total of 1,756 <u>V</u>. <u>cholerae</u> isolates were presumptively identified (this volume). Results are summarized in Figure 1. The upper figure is the minimum most probable number

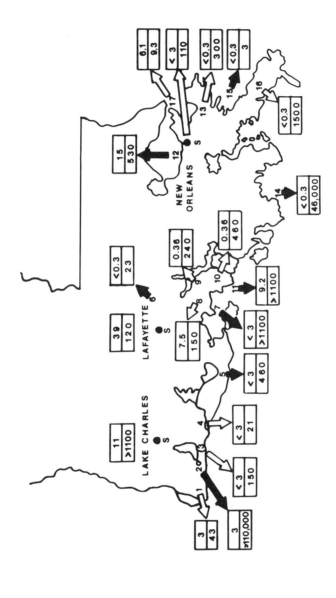

Figure 1. Vibrio cholerae distribution, Louisiana, 1980. Collection stations are designated by number except for the sewer locations at Lafayette, Lake Charles, and New Orleans which are designated with the letter S. Arrows point to boxes containing the Vibrio cholerae MPN per liter of water for that station. Upper figures are minimum and lower figures are maximum MPN per liter. Black arrows mark shallow (1 meter or less in depth) water areas.

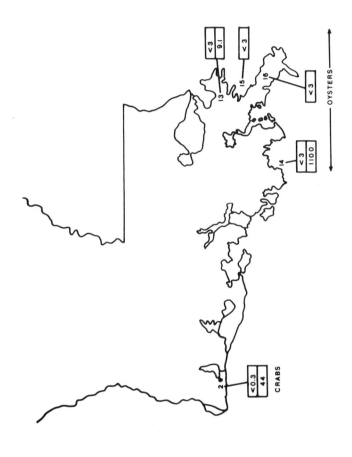

Figure 2. Distribution of Vibrio cholerae from crabs collected at Station 2 and oysters from Stations 13, 14, 15, and 16. Upper figures are minimum and lower figures are maximum MPNs per gram of sample.

391

(MPN) and the lower figure the maximum MPN per liter of water. MPN's of V. cholerae ranged from < 3 to > 110,000/liter of water. Sediment MPN's ranged from < 3 to > 110,000/g.

Factors determining the numbers of vibrios present (this volume) are as complex as the environment itself. Although we can readily measure water temperature, pH, dissolved oxygen, and salinity, these simple observations fail to convey the dynamic impact upon the microbial community of local climate and hydrography. Water depths in marshland areas and landlocked salt water bays are greatly affected by winds and tides. Black arrows in Figure 1 denote shallow (1 meter or less in depth) water areas. Incoming tides supported by a south wind yield maximum water depths. When cold fronts pass through the coastal plains, the strong north winds supported by an outgoing tide will drop water depths several feet and expose areas normally covered by water. Nutrient levels are high in marsh waters. Plankton counts are high and natural vegetation affords many shelters for the smaller members of the food chain. Highest V. cholerae counts are noted in these areas when copepods are found in the plankton populations. The strong currents and water flow of the deep rivers have the net effect of reducing numbers of microorganisms as compared to the more stagnant waters of marsh and swamp areas. Although station 15 has a shallow depth this is an open water area.

Figure 2 shows the distribution of V. cholerae in seafoods. Stations 13, 14, and 16 are restricted oyster harvesting areas and station 15 is an approved area. National Shellfish Sanitation Program guidelines are based upon fecal coliform (FC) counts (Wilt 1977). At Cocodrie, Station 14, V. cholerae varies independently of FC levels (Figure 3). Data from the first three sampling periods show that while FC's exceeded V. cholerae in the water column, oysters contained more V. cholerae than FC's. During the fourth and fifth sampling periods, V. cholerae increased dramatically in both the water column and in the oysters, but the FC's remained at low stable levels.

Crabs were collected in the traditional Louisiana way—using bait, line, and hand net. MPN's were performed on

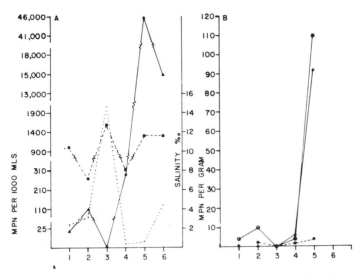

Figure 3. Bacteriological and salinity parameters at Cocodrie (Station 14) from (A) water and (B) sediment and oysters. Vibrio cholerae ▲——▲; fecal coliforms ■---■; salinity ·······; Vibrio cholerae oyster ○——○.

pools of aseptically dissected body tissue and the individual animal feces were tested for vibrios.

Crabs from Mud Lake (Figure 1, Station 2) were implicated during the 1978 cholera outbreak. It is readily accessible to the public and is a popular crabbing location. First Bayou drains a large marshy area to the west of Mud Lake. Parts of this marsh are in the Sabine Migratory Waterfowl Refuge. There are no human dwellings in this area but a large cattle herd is pastured in this marsh. Mud Lake, which drains into the Gulf of Mexico by Mud Pass, contains fresh water during wet, rainy seasons but becomes brackish and salty during prolonged dry spells. The depth of the lake varies from 18 inches to 2 or 3 feet.

Figure 4 shows results of monitoring Mud Lake from January 1980 to July 1981. The high V. cholerae counts in June 1980 are shown as 11,000 and 110,000/liter, but these values exceeded the MPN dilutions and are probably greater than 110,000/liter. Temperature and salinity values appeared to correlate. V. cholerae numbers dropped from 1,100/liter in January 1980, to 4.3/liter two weeks later

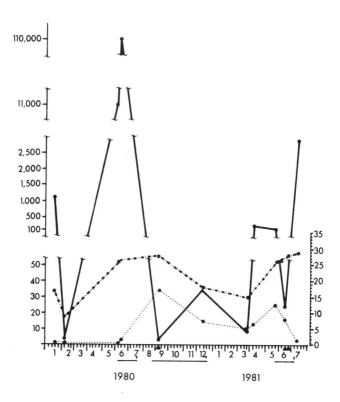

Figure 4. _Vibrio cholerae_ MPN's Mud Lake (Station 2) with environmental parameters; _Vibrio cholerae_ ———— ; temperature –·–·– ; salinity ··········· ; ▲ below base line are dates of isolation of _Vibrio cholerae_ O1 from Lake Charles sewer. ————' shrimping season.

following a severe cold front. _V. cholerae_ numbers rose with temperature when salinities were < 1 ppt but dropped dramatically at a temperature of 28°C when salinity was 15 ppt. However, when temperatures in July of 1981 exceeded 28°C, _V. cholerae_ numbers were again high with low salinities. FC and _V. cholerae_ fluctuated independently at this station.

The source of FC's at Mud Lake is probably the large animal population. Cow feces were examined several times in 1981 but no _V. cholerae_ were found. Bird feces were collected and examined on two occasions. On the first occasion, June 1981, non-O1 V. cholerae were recovered. On the second occasion, July 1981, no V. cholerae were found but Vibrio parahaemolyticus and lactose-positive vibrios were recovered. Schlater et al. (1981) and Lee et al. (1981) have noted V. cholerae in birds.

Lines across the bottom of Figure 4 mark the shrimping seasons during this period. Young shrimp spawned in the Gulf migrate to the marsh areas when salinities are high. Here they feed on the abundant food supply in a sheltered environment. In the springs of 1978 and 1981, environmental conditions resulted in large harvests of shrimp (Lake Charles American Press, 16 August 1981).

The triangles below the horizontal axis (Figure 4) in September 1980 and June 1981 denote the occurrence of toxigenic V. cholerae O1 Inaba in the 18th Street sewer plant in Lake Charles (Figure 1). This sewer was not routinely monitored during this study prior to September 1980. V. cholerae are not always found in sewers. Lowest numbers occurred during the winter months. Highest counts (11,000/liter) occurred during June 1981. This particular sewer treatment plant serves all three hospitals in Lake Charles.

V. cholerae isolates were serotyped at the Lake Charles Regional Laboratory using antisera prepared by Dr. R.J. Siebeling, Louisiana State University. Details of antisera preparation have been described (this volume).

Distribution of V. cholerae non-O1 serovars are widespread throughout the state. From the water and sediment 45 different serovars were isolated; 32 were isolated from seafood; 40 from sewage; and 17 from human disease. All but 1 serovar found in human disease was also found in sewage.

Serovar distribution for Mud Lake is shown in Figure 5. Although the data are somewhat difficult to interpret because of variability in available samples and unidentifiable serovars, several interesting observations were noted. In January and February, crabs were not available, and non-O1 V. cholerae were detected in sediments collected in January. However, V. cholerae MPN's in January were 1,100/liter, and the strains isolated included 5 identifiable serovars: C, G, J, M, and Q. In February, 2 serovars were identified from sediment and water as H and J, respectively. On June 2, 18 different serovars were identified of which 3 (J, M, and U) were common to water, crabs, and sediment; 3 (K, Q, and AA) to water and crabs; and 1 (V) to crabs and sediment. On June 9, sediments were not collected but V. cholerae MPN's in water were high; that is > 110,000/liter. Of the 17 different serovars identified, J, U, and Y were the most common in water and crabs. On September 8, V. cholerae was not detected in sediments and only 3 serovars were identified; 1 in water, and 2 in crabs. In December, 8 serovars were found with FF being common to both water and crabs.

Certain serovars were more abundantly isolated throughout the year than others. For example, serovar J was found in five of the six water samples examined. Seasonally, the most abundant distribution of serovars occurred in June. During this month, 26 of the known 27 serovars were identified, and there were no serovars which were unidentified. Although there may be other distinct seasonal patterns of serovar distribution in the environment than indicated by Figure 5, the unknown serovars must be identified in order to make this determination.

The public health significance of these autochthonous V. cholerae are unknown. Studies are in progress to assess their potential as human pathogens. However, the increasing recognition of human vibrio disease and the sporadic occurrence of high numbers of non-O1 V. cholerae in sewage indicate that caution must be applied in interpreting these organisms as innocuous local residents.

SUMMARY

V. cholerae occur naturally in the Louisiana coastal environment. Numbers are determined by nutrient level, temperature, salinity, and hydrography and fluctuate independently from FC. V. cholerae are found sporadically in coastal community sewers with the highest MPN's in

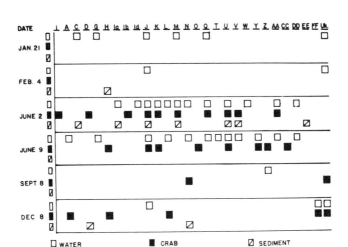

Figure 5. Vibrio cholerae serovar distribution at Mud Lake (Station 2), 1980.

warmer months. All but one serovar found in human diseases was also found in sewage.

ACKNOWLEDGMENT

We gratefully acknowledge the expert technical assistance of Connie Guillory, Kathy Johnson, Joyce Landor, Billie Monsour, Willard Mahfouz, Opal Hair, Susan Searle, Allen Hebert, Mike Purpera, James Gillespie, and Betty Planchard. This work was supported in part by National Oceanic and Atmospheric Administration Office of Sea Grant, Department of Commerce, under Grant NA 79AA-D-00128.

REFERENCES

Calhoun, J. (Ed.) 1979. Louisiana Almanac 1979-1980. 30th ed. Pelican Publishing Co., Gretna, Louisiana.

Kaper, J., H. Lockman, R.R. Colwell, and S.W. Joseph. 1979. Ecology, serology, and enterotoxin production of Vibrio cholerae in Chesapeake Bay. Appl. Environ. Microbiol. 37:91-103.

Lee, J.V., D.J. Bashford, T.J. Donovan, A.L. Furniss, and P.A. West. 1981. The incidence of Vibrio cholerae in water, animals and birds in Kent, England. J. Appl. Bacteriol. 52:281-291.

Schlater, L.K., B.O. Blackburn, R. Harrington, D.J. Draper, J. Van Wagner, and B.R. Davis. 1981. A non-1 Vibrio cholerae isolated from a goose. Avian Diseases. 25:199-201.

Wilt, D.S., (Ed.). Proc. 10th National Shellfish Sanitation Workshop, June 29 and 30, 1977. U.S.D.H.E.W., P.H.S., F.D.A., Shellfish Sanitation Branch.

Chapter 23

THE ECOLOGY OF <u>VIBRIO CHOLERAE</u> IN TWO FLORIDA ESTUARIES

Mary A. Hood, G.E. Ness, G.E. Rodrick,
and N.J. Blake

As part of a collaborative effort between Sea Grant-funded investigators at Louisiana State University, Louisiana State Public Health, the University of Maryland, Oregon State University, the University of West Florida, and the University of South Florida, to examine the ecology of <u>Vibrio</u> <u>cholerae</u> in U.S. coastal environments, a study was conducted to determine the distribution of <u>V</u>. <u>cholerae</u> in two Florida estuaries. The two estuaries that were chosen for study represented two economically important bays in Florida. Apalachicola Bay, located in a relatively undeveloped area of the state, is a drowned river estuary typical of the Gulf Coast estuaries. It is the state's largest commercial oyster harvesting area. In 1980 approximately six million pounds of oysters at a market value of over six million dollars were harvested from Apalachicola Bay. Tampa Bay, although heavily impacted by urban development, supports, in addition to oysters, an active clam industry. Approximately 120 thousand pounds of clams were harvested from Tampa Bay in 1980. From an ecological standpoint, Tampa Bay is also unique in that it is one of the most southernly located estuaries in the country and has a relatively high temperature regime.

DISTRIBUTION STUDIES

Oysters (<u>Crassostrea</u> <u>virginica</u>) and clams (<u>Mercenaria</u> <u>compechiensis</u>) were collected approximately bimonthly from six sites in the estuaries representing a variety of water qualities from April 1980 through August 1981. Additional samples of blue crabs (<u>Callinectes</u> <u>sapidus</u>), sediment, water, plankton, other crabs, mussels, and a macro-filamentous algae commonly attached to oyster reefs were collected at three-month intervals. Physical/chemical parameters of temperature, salinity, dissolved oxygen, total suspended particles, and volatile suspended particles were also determined. Isolation and enumeration of <u>V. cholerae</u> using the techniques described by Kaper et al. (1979) and Hood et al. (1981) revealed that <u>V. cholerae</u> non-O1 strains were present in 45% of all oyster samples, 67% of all blue crabs, 50% of the waters, and 30% of the sediments. Although investigations by the Food and Drug Administration (Twedt et al. 1981) have reported that 14% of oysters collected from Gulf Coast and Atlantic Coast waters contained <u>V. cholerae</u>, the oysters were all of market quality having low fecal coliform levels of less than 230/100g tissue.

Strong linear correlations between levels of <u>V. cholerae</u> and fecal coliforms were not observed in our studies. However, there was a relationship between the classification of sites from which the shellfish were harvested and the mean levels of <u>V. cholerae</u>. Prohibited shellfish harvesting waters contained the highest mean levels of <u>V. cholerae</u>, conditionally approved shellfish harvesting waters contained intermediate levels, and approved waters contained the lowest mean levels of <u>V. cholerae</u>.

Strong linear correlations between <u>V. cholerae</u> levels and the selected physical/chemical parameters were not observed, although salinity and temperature were relevant to the distribution of the organism. The bacterium was most abundant when salinities were 10 ppt to 25 ppt (Table 1). In vitro growth responses of 97 environmental isolates to a range of salinities provided further support to the findings that estuarine salinities of 10 ppt to 25 ppt were

Table 1. Effect of Salinity on the Distribution and Growth of Vibrio cholerae

Salinity (ppt)	In situ Mean Concentrations in Shellfish (number/g)	In vitro Growth Response of 97 Isolates (% of optimum mean growth)
0-5	0	20-30
5-10	0.07	30-55
11-15	0.05	55-90
16-20	0.50	90-100
21-25	4.1	85-90
26-30	0.1	60-85
31-35	0.02	55-60

optimum for the organism. Seasonally, the organism was most abundant in later summer and early fall (Figure 1).

V. cholerae serotype non-O1 strains were the most abundant isolates, while strains of serotype O1 were isolated from only one sample of oysters collected during April 1980. Other studies (Colwell et al. 1981; Kaper et al. 1979) have also reported the relative scarcity of serotype O1 in the environment. Serotyping of the non-O1 isolates by Dr. R.J. Siebeling revealed that seven isolates from oysters and waters were serovar DD, three were BB, and two were CC and Q. The remaining serovars of which one isolate each was represented included Id, JJ, N, O, E, U, X, T, M, LL, K, Z, and (multiple antigens) Y/NN, Id/W/V/J/P, Q/Y, Y/NN, and Id/CC.

Dissection studies of shellfish revealed that V. cholerae was concentrated in the digestive tract of the oyster and throughout the body of the blue crab. V. cholerae was most abundant in the oyster when large numbers of diatoms, dinoflagelates, and detrital particles were observed in the digestive tract. Although V. cholerae was not

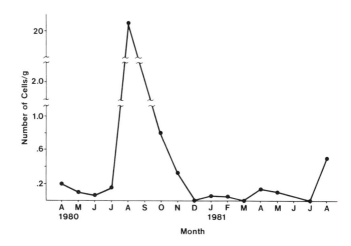

Figure 1. Seasonal distribution of <u>Vibrio</u> <u>cholerae</u> in oysters collected from Apalachicola and Tampa Bay.

isolated from plankton collected from Apalachicola Bay, it is commonly isolated from Chesapeake Bay plankton by workers in Dr. Rita Colwell's laboratory. The presence of the bacterium when there was an abundance of plankton and other particles, coupled with the knowledge that the organism readily attaches to chitin and other materials, suggests that <u>V</u>. <u>cholerae</u> may be concentrated as a result of the oyster feeding on certain plankton to which the bacterium is attached.

In contrast to the oyster, <u>V</u>. <u>cholerae</u> was isolated from the gills, the surface of the exoskeleton, the digestive tract, and the chitinous internal structures of the blue crab. The feeding habits and movements of the blue crab may explain in part why <u>V</u>. <u>cholerae</u> was found throughout the body of the animal. The blue crab is a scavenger, feeding along the surface of the sediment. Large amounts of water pass over the extended gills as the animal moves about. With exposure to such large quantities of water and the fact that the gills are lined with a chitinous membrane, it would seem that the gills would be a likely place to find the bacterium.

SURVIVAL STRATEGY

In addition to the distribution studies discussed here, other information suggests that V. cholerae is an indigenous resident of the estuary. It has been shown that V. cholerae survives quite well in estuarine waters. Using natural estuarine waters and sediments, Hood and Ness (1982) have demonstrated that V. cholerae remains viable for long periods of time. Singleton et al. (1982) have shown the relationship between the survival and growth of V. cholerae and the parameters of salinity, temperature, and nutrient levels. Their results clearly illustrate that V. cholerae survives and grows under conditions typical of the estuarine environment.

Not only does V. cholerae survive well in estuarine waters, but it appears that the organism inhabits a variety of niches within the estuary. The fact that V. cholerae readily attaches to a number of substrates including chitin (both natural crab and shrimp exoskeleton and commercial chitins), cellulose, glass, and $CaCO_3$ (Belas and Colwell, 1982; Hood, unpublished data) and has been found attached to shellfish, plankton (Huq, this volume), and aquatic plants (Lee and West, this volume) suggests that it lives in an epibiotic stage.

The organisms also appears to survive unattached in the water column as a free-living form. The isolation of V. cholerae from estuarine waters filtered through a $0.4-\mu$ membrane filter (MacDonell and Hood 1982), as well as the abundance of Vibrio spp. in marine waters which pass through $0.45-\mu$ membrane filters (Tabor et al. 1981), suggests that the organism exists as a planktonic bacterium. However, recent experiments in our laboratory (unpublished data) reveal that the viability of V. cholerae is reduced in seawater in the absence of particulates. When V. cholerae was added to filtered and centrifuged seawater, viable numbers of cells (but not direct counts) decreased in proportion to the size of the filter and the speed and force of centrifugation. Since filtering and centrifugation reduces the particulate load, the viability of V. cholerae may be related to the presence of particulates. This would suggest that the organism's preferred habit is probably an epibiotic one. However, the fact that the organism can be isolated from filtered estuarine or seawater and is recoverable from particulate-free water suggests that it can survive for a certain period of time as a planktonic form.

Free-living or planktonic cells appear to give rise to forms which we have called microvibrios. It was observed (unpublished data) that when freshly cultured V. cholerae cells were inoculated into estuarine waters, a number of morphological changes in the cells took place. Cells were observed to round up, while others became very small, retaining their vibrio shape. After several months in the systems, some of the cells were filterable through a 0.2-μ membrane filter and, upon reculturing, developed into normal size cells again. The fact that these forms may represent spheroplasts was one possibility that was considered since the salinity would certainly preserve the integrity of the cell wall osmotically. However, electron microscopy of the cells revealed that the cells had intact cell walls, although some cells exhibited a phenomenon in which the cell wall appeared to consist of small extrusions. A number of other morphological changes were observed in these cells and will be described elsewhere (Baker et al., in preparation). Further evidence of the occurrence of cell wall transformation was observed when it was discovered that the serotype of these cells changed (Hood, unpublished data). The nature of these morphological changes and the associated cell wall alterations is unclear, but the formation of these microcells are continuing to be investigated in our laboratory.

Other studies which may be relevant to the understanding of the nature of these microvibrios include the isolation and characterization of a group of organisms called the ultramicrobacteria (Torrella and Morita 1981) or mini-bacteria (Watson et al. 1977) which have been observed in the water column of numerous aquatic environments. In estuarine waters, MacDonell and Hood (1982) were able to isolate bacteria which passed through 0.4- and 0.2-μ membrane filters, and those which were 0.2-μ filterable cells, upon initial isolation, required low nutrients. Characterization of these isolates suggested that they represented strains which had adapted to low nutrients. The majority of the isolates were Vibrio spp. and several were phenotypic strains of V. cholerae.

There is a likely relationship between the ultramicrobacteria which can be isolated from environmental waters and the microvibrios which can be induced in laboratory systems. The small, morphologically altered cells formed in laboratory systems represent cells which have developed in response to a nutrient-depleted, particulate-free environment. It may be that the ultramicrobacteria are cells which form in the same manner. Studies are on going to demonstrate this relationship.

The mechanism by which V. cholerae survives in the aquatic environment is unclear but it may be that the formation of cells such as the microvibrios may serve a survival function. However, regardless of the mechanism by which these cells develop or their function, V. cholerae can survive for long periods of time in estuarine waters. Viable cells have been recovered from estuarine waters and seawaters (Hood and MacDonell, unpublished data) inoculated for over a year. Pollitzer (1959), in his review of the early literature, studies has also presented data which show that V. cholerae survives in marine and estuarine waters for very long periods of time.

Figure 2 presents a proposed model of how V. cholerae may survive in the estuary. In all likelihood, its preferred

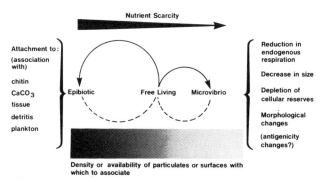

Figure 2. A model of the survival of Vibrio cholerae in Gulf Coast estuaries.

habitat is the epibiotic one in which it lives attached to a substrate. It also survives in a free-living state and under certain conditions such as nutrient depletion, develops into the small, cellular reduced forms called the microvibrios.

Outside the estuary, V. cholerae may inhabit the human; this is most dramatically demonstrated when outbreaks of cholera occur. Isolation of V. cholerae from gulls and other birds (Lee and West, this volume) and the possibility that other near-shore wildlife may harbor the organism (Depaola 1981) suggest that the organism occupies an even wider variety of niches. Thus, from an ecological view, it appears that V. cholerae has evolved a successful survival strategy based on habitat flexibility and its ability to adapt to environmental stresses encountered in the estuary.

SUMMARY AND CONCLUSIONS

From the studies of V. cholerae in the Florida estuaries as well as other distribution studies, it appears that the findings and conclusions first reported by Kaper et al. (1979) were accurate and that the organism is indeed an autochthonous species in U.S. estuaries. Although V. cholerae serotype non-O1 isolates were abundant in oysters, sediments, waters, and blue crabs collected from the Florida estuaries, serotype O1 strains were isolated from only one sample of oysters and comprised only 1% of the total V. cholerae strains isolated. Strong linear correlations between V. cholerae levels and salinity, temperature, other physical/chemical parameters, and fecal coliforms were not observed. However, a range of salinities and temperatures appeared relevant to the distribution of the organism. Highest concentrations of V. cholerae were observed when salinities were 12 to 25 ppt and temperatures were 20°C to 35°C. Seasonally, the organism was most abundant in late summer and fall.

The salinity, temperature, and nutrient levels typical of the Florida estuaries appear to provide a very suitable environment for V. cholerae. The fact that these estuaries are ideal environments for V. cholerae is reflected in both the abundance of the organism and the frequency of isolation. In the shellfish examined, V. cholerae was isolated from every monthly sample with two exceptions, suggesting that low levels of the organism persist throughout the year. Clearly, the warm, nutrient-rich estuaries of Florida and the Gulf Coast are excellent habitats for V. cholerae.

ACKNOWLEDGMENTS

We gratefully thank the following investigators for helpful discussions and advice: Dr. R.R. Colwell, Dr. R.J. Siebeling, Dr. R.J. Seidler, and Nell Roberts. We acknowledge John Cheney and Kathy Williams for their excellent technical support, Florida State Department of Natural Resources for their logistical support, and Dr. Mike Bundrick and the University of West Florida Institute of Statistical and Mathematical Modeling for statistical assistance. The work is a result of research sponsored by Florida Sea Grant, National Oceanic and Atmospheric Administration, Office of Sea Grant, Department of Commerce, under Grant NA 80AA-D-00038. The U.S. Government is authorized to produce and distribute any copyright portion that may appear herein.

REFERENCES

Belas, M.R., and R.R. Colwell. 1982. Adsorption kinetics of laterally and polarly flagellated Vibrio. J. Bacteriol. 151:1568-1580.

Colwell, R.R., R.J. Seidler, J. Kaper, S.W. Joseph, S. Garges, H. Lockman, D. Maneval, H. Bradford, N. Roberts, E. Remmers, I. Huq, and A. Huq. 1981. Occurrence of Vibrio cholerae serotype O1 in Maryland and Louisiana estuaries. Appl. Environ. Microb. 41:555-558.

Depaola, A. 1981. Vibrio cholerae in marine foods and environmental waters: A literature review. J. Food Sci. 46:66-70.

Hood, M.A., G.E. Ness, and G.E. Rodrick. 1981. Isolation of Vibrio cholerae serotype O1 from the eastern oyster, Crassostrea virginica. Appl. Environ. Microbiol. 41:559-560.

Hood, M.A., and G.E. Ness. 1982. Survival of Vibrio cholerae and Escherichia coli in estuarine waters and sediments. Appl. Environ. Microbiol. 43:578-584.

Kaper, J., H. Lockman, R.R. Colwell, and S.W. Joseph. 1979. Ecology, serology, and enterotoxin production of Vibrio cholerae in Chesapeake Bay. Appl. Environ. Microbiol. 37:91-103.

MacDonell, M.T., and M.A. Hood. 1982. Isolation and characterization of ultramicrobacteria from a Gulf Coast estuary. Appl. Environ. Microbiol. 43:566-571.

Pollitzer, R. 1959. Cholera. WHO Monogr. Series No. 43. World Health Organization, Geneva.

Singleton, F.J., R.W. Attwell, M.S. Jangi, and R.R. Colwell. 1982. Influence of salinity and organic nutrient concentration on survival and growth of Vibrio cholerae in aquatic microcosms. Appl. Environ. Microbiol. 43:1080-1085.

Tabor, P.S., K. Ohwada, and R.R. Colwell. 1981. Filterable marine bacteria found in the deep sea: distribution, taxonomy, and response to starvation. Microb. Ecol. 7:67-83.

Torrella, F., and R.Y. Morita. 1981. Microcultural study of bacteria size changes and microcolony and ultramicrocolony formation by heterotrophic bacteria in sea water. Appl. Environ. Microbiol. 41:518-527.

Twedt, R.M., J.M. Madden, J.M. Hunt, D.W. Francis, J.T. Peller, A.P. Duran, W.O. Hebert, S.G. McCay, C.N. Roderick, G.T. Spite, and T.J. Wazenski. 1981. Characterization of Vibrio cholerae isolated from oysters. Appl. Environ. Microbiol. 41:1475-1478.

Watson, S.W., T.J. Novitsky, H.L. Quinby, and F.W. Valois. 1977. Determination of bacterial number and biomass in the marine environment. Appl. Environ. Microbiol. 33:940-946.

Chapter 24

COMPUTER-ASSISTED ANALYSIS OF VIBRIO FIELD DATA: FOUR COASTAL AREAS

Ramon J. Seidler and Thomas M. Evans

Vibrio cholerae, especially the non-O1 serovar, has been widely isolated from marine environments, especially bays, estuaries, and other brackish waters around the world (Kaper et al. 1979; Bashford et al. 1979; Desmarchelier and Reichelt 1981; Centers for Disease Control 1981). Interest in the ecology of V. cholerae in the United States has risen sharply since it was isolated from Chesapeake Bay and was involved in food-borne cholera outbreaks in Louisiana, Texas, and Florida (Blake et al. 1980; DePaola 1981; Wilson et al. 1981). At least some non-O1 serovars of environmental origins produce one or more virulence factors including enterotoxin (Kaper et al. 1979; Craig et al. 1981). Cholera organisms are apparently present in most brackish waters or bays, but numbers vary over several orders of magnitude (Kaper et al. 1979; Bashford et al. 1979). Isolations of V. cholerae are more common in the summer months (Bashford et al. 1979), indicating that temperature may influence cell densities.

Studies have been underway to evaluate environmental factors which might correlate with changing numbers of cholera organisms in three major coastal regions of the United States. These studies are being conducted on samples collected along the Florida and Louisiana Gulf waters, the Chesapeake Bay, and on the Oregon Coast by four research teams. The purpose of this report is to summarize these studies of V. cholerae in the U.S. coastal waters which made possible the collation of extensive field data from three different geographic and climatic areas. The data in four areas were collected and analyzed by the same methods and procedures. A major effort was devoted to bringing order to the apparent diversity of field data, geographic, climatic, and water quality conditions existing in the various regions. The basic methodologies used in collecting samples and the microbiological analyses have previously been presented in these proceedings (Roberts and Seidler, this volume). V. cholerae were enumerated by 9-tube MPN involving alkaline peptone broth and 18-24 hours incubation at 35°C. A loopful of broth was then streaked onto thiosulfate citrate bile salts sucrose agar (TCBS). Fecal coliforms were enumerated by a 9-tube MPN using the A-1 medium (Hunt and Springer 1978). In all water samples the following parameters were measured using appropriate electronic sensing probes: dissolved oxygen (D.O.), pH, salinity, and temperature. The data presented cover the sampling period of January 1980 through June 1981.

Table 1 summarizes results of some of the measured parameters for the different regions. Substantial differences in mean parameter values are noted especially for temperature, salinity, and microbiological densities. Oregon and Maryland mean water temperature values were the lowest and mean D.O. values were the highest. Mean salinities in the Louisiana region were substantially less than Oregon and Florida. The differences reflect the intrusion of fresh water into the shallow sampling stations in Louisiana. Mean microbiological densities in Louisiana were two orders of magnitude greater than any of the other regions.

Figure 1 presents a scatter diagram of pH versus V. cholerae counts as observed in all regions. A few of the highest counts are excluded from the display since they exceed the top value selected for this scatter diagram. Overall hydrogen ion concentration fluctuated nearly 1000-fold during the sampling period. Figure 1 illustrates that

Table 1. Tabulation of Mean Sample Parameters on a Regional Basis

Region	No. Dates Sampled	Temp[a]	D.O.[b]	pH	Sal[c]	W-VC[d]	W-FC[e]	S-VC[f]	S-FC[g]
						Mean Parameter Values			
OR	34 (16%)	13.3	10.3	7.08	14.8	20	29	100	2,232
LA	110 (51%)	19.3	7.7	7.61	7.0	1913	9403	10,000	1,711
FL	32 (15%)	22.4	6.4	--	19.8	0.3	80	200	--
MD	41 (19%)	16.4	9.9	7.69	10.9	4	53	50	2,400

[a]Water temperature (°C).
[b]Dissolved oxygen.
[c]Water salinity (ppt.).
[d]Water V. cholerae counts/liter.
[e]Water fecal coliform counts/100 ml.
[f]Sediment V. cholerae counts/1000 g.
[g]Sediment fecal coliform counts/100 g.

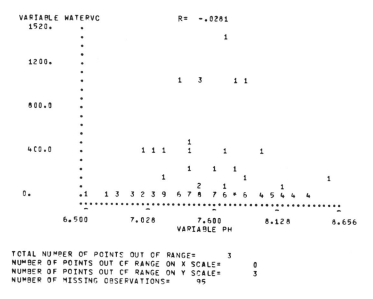

```
VARIABLE WATERVC                    R=  -.0281
1520.        .
             .                              1
             .
1200.        .
             .              1   3       1 1
             .
800.0        .
             .
             .
             .                  1
400.0        .       1 1 1      1       1       1
             .                  1   1   1
             .           1              1               1
             .              2   1           1
0.           .1   1 3  3 2 3 9  6 7 8   7 6 *  6   4 5 4 4   4
              ...........................................
                ‾           ‾            ‾
            6.500        7.028        7.600       8.128       8.656
                                    VARIABLE PH
```

TOTAL NUMBER OF POINTS OUT OF RANGE=   3
NUMBER OF POINTS OUT OF RANGE ON X SCALE=   0
NUMBER OF POINTS OUT OF RANGE ON Y SCALE=   3
NUMBER OF MISSING OBSERVATIONS=   95

Figure 1. Direct computer display tabulating water V. cholerae counts per liter with water pH for all regions. Scales of the ordinate and abscissa were arbitrarily selected so as to illustrate distribution of data points. Values of V. cholerae greater than 1520/liter were not printed. Numerals within the display indicate number of samples with identical coordinates.

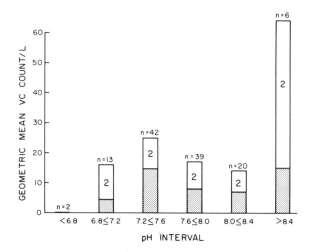

Figure 2. Geometric mean V. cholerae counts as a function of water pH interval. The numeral "2" within the bar graph represents geometric mean counts for Louisiana samples.

414

nearly all of the cholera isolations were recorded in the pH range of 7 to 8.

Geometric mean V. cholerae counts as a function of pH are summarized in Figure 2. The numeral "2" refers to counts for Region 2 (Louisiana). The elevated geometric mean counts for Louisiana at pH values over 8.4 is due to one sample containing very high V. cholerae numbers. Overall, there are no great fluctuations in geometric mean counts at different pH levels although the highest counts for all regions were in the range of pH 7.2-7.6.

Occurrences of V. cholerae in the water column were strikingly correlated with water temperature (Figure 3). Isolations were made from waters ranging from 8°C to 36°C. Counts of about 250/liter were made at temperatures ranging from 16°C to 29°C.

The highest geometric mean counts were recorded at temperatures of 21°C-28°C (Figure 4). Few V. cholerae were detected in water with temperatures less than 14°C or over 35°C. The temperature interval corresponding to the

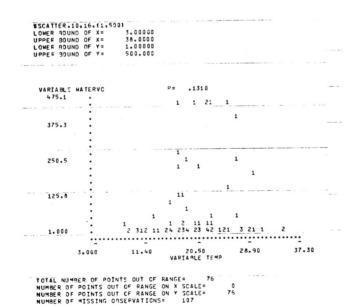

Figure 3. Direct computer display tabulating water V. cholerae/liter with water temperature.

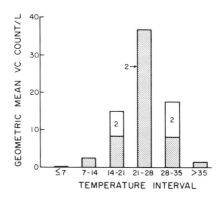

Figure 4. Geometric mean V. cholerae counts expressed as a function of water temperature interval. The numeral "2" represents geometric mean counts for Louisiana samples.

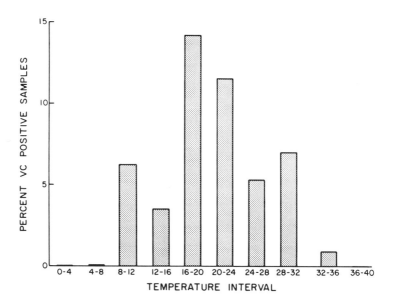

Figure 5. Percent of the V. cholerae positive samples expressed as a function of temperature interval.

```
$SCATTER,14,(0,30),16,(1,500)
LOWER  ROUND OF X=    0.
UPPER  ROUND OF X=      30.0000
LOWER  BOUND OF Y=     1.00300
UPPER  BOUND OF Y=     500.000
```

```
     VARIABLE WATERVC            R= -.2359
       475.1     .
                 .6      1
                 .
                 .1
       375.3     .
                 .
                 .
                 .1     1
       250.5     .1      1
                 .         1            1
                 .  1
                 .        1     1
       125.4     .1             1
                 .1     1
                 .        1
                 .2        1                  1
                 .1     1  1 1  1       1
       1.000     .*2 22  45 1 1211  1 2 1  32 1    1     2
                  .........................................
                0.      7.200     15.00    22.20   29.40
                          VARIABLE SALINITY
```

```
TOTAL NUMBER OF POINTS OUT OF RANGE=     78
NUMBER OF POINTS OUT OF RANGE ON X SCALE=       0
NUMBER OF POINTS OUT OF RANGE ON Y SCALE=      78
NUMBER OF MISSING OBSERVATIONS=     101
```

Figure 6. Direct computer display tabulating water V. cholerae with water salinity. Scales of the ordinate and abscissa were chosen so as to illustrate scatter of the data points. The number of missing observations result from water samples containing less than 1 V. cholerae/ liter or greater than 475/liter (limits of Y-axis plot). Numbers within the display indicate number of samples with identical coordinates. The counts decline asymptotically with increasing water salinity.

highest counts was the same for the combined regions as it was for Region 2.

Nearly 50% of all water samples analyzed from all regions were positive for V. cholerae (Figure 5). About one-half of all cholera cultures were isolated from samples with water temperatures in the range of 16°C-24°C. A relatively constant incidence (4-7%) of positive samples occurred in water temperatures of 8°C-16°C and 24°C-32°C.

Water salinity also influenced, or was associated with, major variations in numbers of V. cholerae (Figures 6, 7 and 8). V. cholerae were isolated over the entire salinity range monitored (< 1 to 30 ppt), but with a single exception, counts greater than 125/liter were not found at salinities over 14 ppt. The scatter diagram also illustrates a decay of occurrences and decreasing counts at higher salinities (Figure 6).

The highest geometric mean counts occurred in water specimens with less than 5 ppt salinity (Figure 7). The elevated counts at lower salinities also correlated with the highest incidence of cholera isolations (Figure 8). One-half of all positive samples came from waters with salinities less than 3 ppt.

To aid in understanding the interaction among the measured variables, data was coded and recorded in the CYBER computer and analyzed by a statistical interactive program system (SIPS) developed at Oregon State University. The goal of such analyses was to develop an equation which could be used to estimate numbers of cholera in the water column once specific physical, chemical, and/or biological data were specified. Parameters which were tested for relationships with V. cholerae numbers included fecal coliform counts, dissolved oxygen concentration, pH, temperature, salinity, turbidity, sampling region, and Julian date. It soon became obvious that V. cholerae numbers could not be correlated with any single measured parameter in a statistically significant fashion.

Analyses of sample correlation coefficients (R) were considered for arithmetic, logarithmic, and inverse counts of V. cholerae using various combinations of the measured parameters. Correlations between untransformed independent variables and numbers of V. cholerae in water were rejected since such relationships exhibited the lowest statistical significance (Table 2). Log and inverse transformations exhibited low correlation coefficients as well, but values were higher than any involving direct relationships with V. cholerae water counts. It therefore became necessary to build models based on complex combinations of several variables. Polynomial equations of the first, second, and third order were established and ● statistically tested for significance in predicting cholera counts. In all, several hundred equations were tested. Some 20 equations were found which generated predictable counts and the terms were statistically sound. One equation relating cholera counts to temperature and salinity cholerae counts from water specimens collected in Maryland, Louisiana, and Oregon. The straight line represents the points of equality between two relationships. Positive

Table 2. Some Sample Correlation Coefficients (R) Between V. cholerae Numbers in Water and Environmental Factors

	Log Temp.	Salinity	Inverse Salinity	Salinity Squared	ph x Salinity	ph Squared x Salinity	Temp.	Inverse Temp.	Log Salinity
Log V. cholerae Count (LNVC)	.38	.45	.38	.36	.46	.45	.34	-.36	-.46
Arithmetic V. cholerae Count	.10	-.13	.07	.10	-.11	-.05	.12	-.08	-.13
Inverse V. cholerae Count	-.40	.48	-.39	.40	.53	.47	-.33	.40	.36

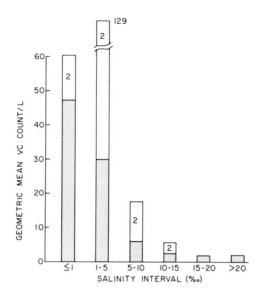

Figure 7. Geometric mean V. cholerae counts expressed as a function of water salinity.

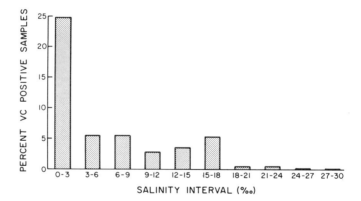

Figure 8. Percent of the V. cholerae positive samples expressed as a function of water salinity. One-half of all the cholera-positive samples came from waters with less than 3% ppt. salinity; none of the samples were actually zero salinity.

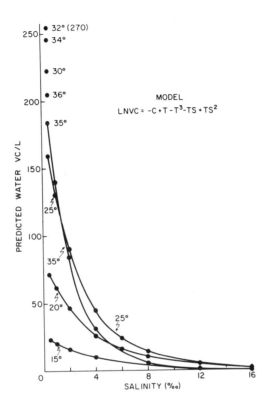

Figure 9. Family of curves generated from derived equation to predict numbers of V. cholerae as a function of water temperature and salinity.

specimens with counts in the range of 5-150 per liter are plotted against predicted counts using the equation in Table 3. All values except three are within the 95% confidence interval of the 9-tube MPN measurement used to recover and enumerate the cholera organism. Observed counts of V. cholerae in excess of 150 were generally underestimated by the equation.

is presented in Table 3 along with the statistical test results illustrating the significance of the terms in the equation.

A family of curves was generated from the equation which reveals the relationships between temperature, salinity, and V. cholerae counts (Figure 9). The maximum number of counts are predicted to occur at moderate temperatures and low salinities; this corroborates actual field data from all regions. The maximum counts are predicted at 32°C and numbers should decline in warmer waters. The influence of temperature on V. cholerae numbers is most pronounced at salinities less than 4 ppt. Numbers of V. cholerae increase abruptly with water temperatures above 15°C. It is tempting to speculate that warm waters promote the multiplication of V. cholerae, thus supporting the concept of its autochthonous nature in the estuary environment (Colwell et al. 1980). The equation continues to predict low level V. cholerae occurrences at salinity levels of 12-16 ppt and higher.

The value of the computer-derived equation lies in its ability to correctly estimate levels of the cholera organism. Figure 10 is a comparison of predicted and observed V.

Table 3. Evaluation of the Terms in an Equation to Predict Numbers of V. cholerae in Estuary Water[a]

Log V. cholerae count =	S.E. Regr. Coef.	T-Value	P-Value
$-C^a$	.670	-2.196	0.1
T	.053	6.424	0.005
$-T^3$	.00004	-2.825	0.05
-TS	.003	-4.970	0.01
TS^2	.0001	2.881	0.05

[a]Equation depicted in Figure 9 where C = constant, T = temperature and S = salinity.

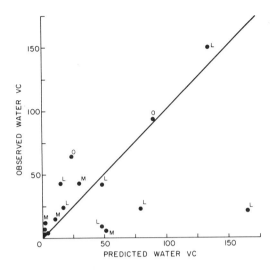

Figure 10. Representation of observed and predicted V. cholerae waters counts in samples collected from Louisiana, Maryland, and Oregon waters. The line represents points of equality between the two relationships.

CONCLUSION

A national coordinated field analysis for enumeration of V. cholerae was carried out over an 18-month period with sampling stations located along the three major U.S. coastal zones. Mean values for physical, chemical, and micro-biological water quality parameters were found to be significantly different in the various study areas. Nevertheless, many similarities were revealed in the computer-displayed profiles as seen in the Figures. The most significant similarities were the general agreements in all regions in peak geometric mean V. cholerae counts in waters of 21°C-28°C and salinities of less than 5 ppt. Individual occurrences of similar V. cholerae counts at different salinities or temperatures make it impossible for a single mathematical equation to predict all observed counts. However, an equation was derived which provides excellent predictive values of cholera in the range of 150 or less per liter of estuary water. Discrepancies between observed and predicted counts at higher cholera levels could reflect large variations expected from the 95% confidence limites of the MPN technique used to enumerate V. cholerae. In addition, field measurements may be spurious due to natural causes. This includes regrowth, sudden dilution, or microbial die-off due to changing natural elements. The development of mathematical models to predict elevated pathogen occurrences in aquatic environments is worthwhile and should be considered in investigations where sufficient field data warrant such efforts.

ACKNOWLEDGMENT

This study was supported by the Oregon State University Sea Grant College Program, National Oceanic and Atmospheric Administration Office of Sea Grant, Department of Commerce, under Grant NA79AA-D-00106, project R/FSD8. Oregon State University Agricultural Experiment Station Technical Paper No. 6622.

REFERENCES

Bashford, D.J., T.J. Donovan, A.L. Furniss, and J.V. Lee. 1979. Vibrio cholerae in Kent. Lancet 1:436-437.

Blake, P.A., D.T. Allegra, J.D. Snyder, T.J. Barrett, L. McFarland, C.T. Caraway, J.C. Feeley, J.P. Craig, J.V. Lee, N.D. Puhr, and R.A. Feldman. 1980. Cholera--a possible endemic focus in the United States. N. Engl. J. Med. 302:305-309.

Center for Disease Control. 1981. Cholera on a Gulf coast oil rig--Texas. Morbid. Mortal. Wkly. Rep. 30:589-590.

Colwell, R.R., R.J. Seidler, J. Kaper, S.W. Joseph, S. Garges, H. Lockman, D. Maneval, H. Bradford, N. Roberts, E. Remmers, I. Huq, and A. Huq. 1981. Occurrence of Vibrio cholerae O-group 1 from Maryland

and Louisiana estuaries. Appl. Environ. Microbiol. 41:555-558.

Craig, J.P., K. Yamamoto, Y. Takeda, and T. Miwatani. 1981. Production of cholera-like enterotoxin by a Vibrio cholerae non-O1 strain isolated from the environment. Infect. Immun. 34:90-97.

DePaola, A. 1981. Vibrio cholerae in marine foods and environmental waters: a literature review. J. Food. Sci. 46:66-70.

Desmarchelier, P.M., and J.L. Reichelt. 1981. Phenotypic characterization of clinical and environmental isolates of Vibrio cholerae from Australia. Curr. Microbiol. 5:123-127.

Hunt, D.A., and J. Springer. 1978. Comparison of two rapid test procedures with the standard EC test for recovery of fecal coliform bacteria from shellfish-growing waters. J. Assoc. Off. Anal. Chem. 61:1317-1323.

Kaper, J., H. Lockman, R.R. Colwell, and S.W. Joseph. 1979. Ecology, serology and enterotoxin production of V. cholerae in Chesapeake Bay. Appl. Environ. Microbiol. 37:91-103.

Wilson, R., S. Lieb, A. Roberts, S. Stryker, H. Janowski, R. Gunn, B. Davis, C.F. Riddle, T. Barrett, J.G. Morris, Jr., and P.A. Blake. 1981. Non-O-group 1 Vibrio cholerae gastroenteritis associated with eating raw oysters. Am. J. Epidemiol. 114:293-298.

Chapter 25

THE INCIDENCE AND DISTRIBUTION OF
V. CHOLERAE IN ENGLAND

J.V. Lee, D.J. Bashford, T.J. Donovan,
A.L. Furniss, and P.A. West

Between 1976 and 1979, several surveys were carried out in
Kent, England to establish the incidence of Vibrio cholerae
in the aquatic environment. V. cholerae occurred sporadically in all types of water during the summer but only in
very low numbers in water containing < 5 mmol Na^+/l.
Highest numbers of up to 700 cfu/ml appeared regularly in
static brackish water containing 25-200 mmol Na^+/l. They
were not introduced by sewage contamination of the water
and there was no correlation between the counts of Escherichia coli and V. cholerae. A wide range of serovars
including O1 was isolated. V. cholerae was not isolated
from sheep feces but was detected in 6% of cloacal swabs
taken from gulls caught at times when V. cholerae could not
be isolated from water. It was concluded that the presence
of these organisms in the environment in Kent does not
present any significant risk to health; aquatic birds may be
vectors of V. cholerae; V. cholerae occurs naturally in
static brackish water.

Vibrio cholerae has generally been accepted to be a
native of areas with warm climates and to occur only rarely
or spasmodically in temperate zones as a result of importa-
tion from hotter climates. In 1965 an outbreak of enteritis
occurred in Czechoslovakia due to non-O1 V. cholerae that

appeared to be indigenous (Aldova et al. 1968). Four cases of indigenous infections with non-O1 V. cholerae were reported in Sweden (Back et al. 1974) and "NAG-vibrios" that were probably non-O1 V. cholerae were detected in surface waters in West Germany (Ko et al. 1973). These three reports suggested that non-O1 V. cholerae at least may have been more common in temperate areas than previously thought and prompted us to look for them in the environment in Kent.

The aims of the surveys described here were to establish whether V. cholerae occurred in natural waters in Kent and, if so, to see if its incidence could be related to any other factors such as the input of sewage effluent into the environment. V. cholerae, although capable of growth in media containing no added NaCl, like all other species of Vibrio requires NaCl for optimum growth. V. cholerae might therefore be expected to survive better and occur more frequently in brackish water containing NaCl. We therefore intended to sample waters of a wide range of salinities.

The few surveys of the incidence of V. cholerae in natural waters that had been published at the time we began this work had not attempted to enumerate the V. cholerae occurring in water. We thought enumeration would give important clues as to the natural aquatic habitat of V. cholerae if one existed; therefore, we estimated the numbers of V. cholerae present in water samples examined throughout the surveys described here.

MATERIALS AND METHODS

The sites where water samples were collected are shown in Figure 1. Birds were caught by canon netting either at Richborough Refuse Tip or Margate Beach (Figure 1; sites 28 and 29, respectively), and cloacal swabs were taken after the birds had been ringed. The methods used to enumerate V. cholerae, Escherichia coli, and viable aerobic heterotrophic bacteria in water samples have been fully described elsewhere as have the methods used to isolate V. cholerae from cloacal swabs and animal feces, to determine

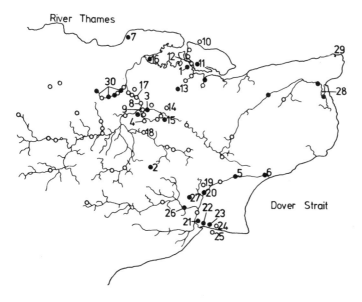

Figure 1. The locations of sites where samples were obtained in the surveys for V. cholerae between 1976 and 1981. ● V. cholerae detected in water; O V. cholerae not detected in water.

the physical and chemical parameters of water samples, to identify and serotype V. cholerae, and to determine the ability of V. cholerae to produce cholera toxin (Lee et al. 1982).

RESULTS

Preliminary Survey of 1976

During 1976, 45 samples of water that had been collected from 27 sites were examined. Eleven of the samples from seven sites were found to contain non-O1 V. cholerae and the results for these sites are summarized in Table 1. With the exception of the River Len (Site 3), the sites from

Table 1. Some Characteristics of Water from Sites where V. cholerae Was Detected during May–September 1976

Site[a]	Na+ mmol/1	E. coli MPN[b]/100 ml	V. cholerae Samples Positive	V. cholerae MPN or cfu[c]/100 ml
1 Chetney Marsh ditch	46	90[d]	3/3	400–70,000
2 Knoxbridge pond	<2	$\geq$ 180[d]	1/2	5
3 River Len	<2	$\geq$ 180	2/4	6,81
4 Bockingford pond	<2	$\geq$ 180	1/2[e]	5
5 Royal Military Canal	5	ND[f]	1/1	ND
6 Royal Military Canal	12	ND	1/1	ND
7 Cliffe Lake	111	$\geq$ 180	2/3[e]	5

[a]Sites are numbered as in Figure 1.
[b]Most probable number.
[c]Colony-forming units.
[d]Only estimated on one sample.
[e]Another sample was taken in October but did not contain V. cholerae.
[f]Not determined because of delay in samples reaching the laboratory.

which V. cholerae was isolated were all static water systems with concentrations of Na$^+$ in the range of < 2-111 mmol/l.

The water from Site 1 contained particularly high numbers of V. cholerae--up to 700/ml. This site is a drainage system containing static brackish water (46 mmol Na$^+$/l) and is situated on agricultural land reclaimed about 100 years ago from Chetney Marshes in the North of Kent (see Figure 1). The main ditches are 5-10 m wide and the water, depending on the time of year, is 1-2 m deep at its deepest point. These ditches are similar to the small bayous found in Louisiana. The ditch from which samples were taken in 1976 was a tributary of one of the main ditches and was only 2-3 m wide and up to 0.5 m deep. In subsequent years one of the main ditches was sampled. The nearest human habitation is at least half a mile away and the ditches are very unlikely to be contaminated by human sewage. Although low lying, the area is well protected by embankments and not susceptible to flooding from the adjacent area.

The 20 sites where V. cholerae was not detected varied in their characteristics. Some were static and other flowing water courses of different sizes. The water from 17 of the sites contained $\leq$ 5 mmol Na$^+$/l while the remaining 3 were estuarine sites where the water contained 406-434 mmol Na$^+$/l, which is only slightly less than in seawater.

The MPN method used for counting the E. coli was not sensitive enough to detect differences between most of the sites. At least 180/100 ml were present in water from 23 of the sites while 3 sites, including Site 1, had 90/100 ml and the remaining site had 5/100 ml.

1977 Survey

The sites examined during 1977 were numbers 1-4 which had contained V. cholerae during 1976 and Sites 8-9 which had not. Samples were collected at regular intervals between April and December with the intention of detecting any seasonal incidence of V. cholerae. The E. coli counts were determined more accurately than before to enable any correlation between the presence of E. coli and V. cholerae to be assessed. The results are summarized in Table 2.

Again the brackish water drainage ditch at Site 1 contained the highest numbers of V. cholerae. Although far fewer V. cholerae were present than in the exceptionally hot summer of 1976, this year 4 strains of V. cholerae O1 were isolated from 3 samples taken over a period of five weeks during August and September. Unfortunately we are not able to estimate how many were present in the water because the serotyping of all of our isolates was done several months later on a small sample of strains that had been retained from our original isolates.

The 4 strains were serologically typical V. cholerae O1 subtype Ogawa and none produced cholera toxin. Furthermore they lack the structural genes for cholera toxin (Kaper et al. 1981; Kaper and Lee, unpublished results). Their typing characteristics differ from those of epidemic strains. They are strongly hemolytic for sheep erythrocytes, positive in the Voges-Proskauer test, resistant to Polymyxin B (50 IU disc), and they agglutinate chicken erythrocytes--all characteristics of biovar El Tor strains except that most recently isolated epidemic strains are only poorly hemolytic. The strains were only sensitive to phages I, IV, e4, and 57--a pattern more like that of strains of the now rarely isolated classical biovar.

The only other site where V. cholerae was detected was Site 3 (the River Len), and there only low numbers (1-3/100 ml) were detected, although this was also the site with the highest E. coli counts. There did not appear to be any direct link between high counts of E. coli and the presence of V. cholerae. The site with the greatest population of V. cholerae had a relatively low population of E. coli. The results indicate a seasonal incidence of V. cholerae since they were only detected between August and November with the highest numbers in late August and early September.

Table 2. Results of the Survey for V. cholerae in Waters, April-December 1977

Site[a]	Na$^+$ mmol/l	E. coli cfu[b]/ 100 ml	V. cholerae Samples Positive	V. cholerae MPN[c] or cfu/100 ml
1 Chetney Marsh ditch	20-60	0-500	8/18[d]	2-160
2 Knoxbridge pond	<2	10-100	0/9	0
3 River Len	<2	1000-90000	3/21	1-3
4 Bockingford pond	<2	600-20000	0/9	0
8 River Medway	<2	<100-1500	0/8	0
9 Mote Park Lake	<2	400-70000	0/8	0

[a]Sites are numbered as in Figure 1.
[b]Colony-forming units.
[c]Most probable number.
[d]V. cholerae serovar O1 Ogawa was isolated in August.

1978 Survey

A total of 160 samples from 50 sites were examined between January and December 1978. Although each site was sampled an average of three times throughout the year, some sites were sampled more often than others, such as those along the Leybourne stream (Site 30, Figure 1). Seven pairs of the sites were chosen to be above and below the outfalls from sewage works with the intention of determining if the input of sewage effluent influenced the presence of V. cholerae in rivers.

Non-O1 V. cholerae was detected in water from 12 sites, including Site 1, but the O1 serovar was not detected in 1978. As can be seen from Table 3, the 2 sites with water containing 40-65 mmol Na^+/1 contained the highest number of V. cholerae. One of these sites was Site 1 and the other was a similar drainage ditch further east. Only low numbers of V. cholerae were detected at the other sites. Apart from the site with 390 mmol Na^+/1 the sites where V. cholerae was not detected had water with $\leq$ 4 mmol Na^+/1. With two exceptions, V. cholerae was only detected during the summer. Sewage did not appear to be an important source of these organisms in the waters examined since V. cholerae was detected in only 2 of the sites downstream of sewage outfalls and in both cases the upstream samples were positive as well.

1979 Survey

The previous surveys had indicated a relationship between the Na^+ content of a water sample and the presence of V. cholerae. However, only 2 sites with relatively large numbers of V. cholerae had been found and there were often considerable temporal differences between the samples from different sites. Because of limited manpower, in general no more than 3 or 4 sites had been sampled in one day, and rarely more than 12 in one week. In July 1979, we were able for the first time to sample a large number of sites in one day, thus eliminating major temporal differences between the samples from different sites. Studies of the

Table 3. Summary of the Results of the Survey for V. cholerae in 1978

	No. of Sites		V. cholerae
Na$^+$ mmol/l	Examined	Containing V. cholerae	MPN[a] or cfu[b]/100 ml.
≤ 10	43	8	1-3
11-15	1	1	1-5
40-65	2	2	100-10000
140	1	1	2
390	1	0	0
ND[c]	2	0	0

[a]Most probable number.
[b]Colony-forming units.
[c]Not determined.

annual incidence of V. cholerae in water at Site 1 during 1978 had indicated that the population of V. cholerae could be expected to near its maximum at the end of July (West et al. 1980; West and Lee 1982). The 20 sites listed in Table 4 and indicated in Figure 1 are situated approximately on a transect running across Kent from the north to south and were chosen to cover a complete range of salinities. Only non-O1 V. cholerae was detected and the results are summarized in Table 4.

On July 2, V. cholerae was detected in the water from 5 sites: 1 and 11 in the north and 21, 22, and 23 in the south. All of them contained static or, in the case of Site 21 nearly static brackish water with concentrations of Na$^+$ in the range of 31-181 mmol/l. The sites where V. cholerae was not detected contained water with Na$^+$ concentrations outside this range.

Table 4. Results of the Surveys for V. cholerae in water on 2 and 23 July, 1979[a]

Site[f]	Temp. (°C)	DO[d] mg/1	pH	Na+ mmol/1	AH[e] x10^4	MPN[b] or cfu[c]100/ml V. cholerae
1 Chetney Marsh ditch	16.0	3.6	7.64	33	3700	1600
	14.5	1.7	7.52	36	2600	800
2 Knoxbridge Pond	15.5	2.2	7.21	<1	2500	0
	16.0	3.2	6.93	<1	620	0
10 Seawater	16.5	5.1	8.08	466	48	0
	15.0	3.8	7.90	470	20	0
11 Minster Marshes ditch	17.0	3.9	8.16	144	21000	32000
	15.5	3.7	8.15	184	4700	2000
12 Tidal estuary	17.0	7.9	8.10	417	3300	0
	17.5	6.3	7.80	410	1200	0

No.	Type	Temp	O₂	pH		Cond.	
13	Village pond	16.5	3.7	7.63	11	30	0
		16.0	2.2	7.47	11	840	>18⁹
14	Village pond	11.0	7.1	6.97	<1	110	0
		12.0	4.5	7.04	<1	210	0
15	Bird-breeding pond	14.0	7.9	7.81	<1	160	0
		15.5	6.1	7.83	<1	500	16
16	Tidal estuary	17.5	5.0	7.42	256	90	0
		18.0	4.5	7.54	260	350	1
17	River, non-tidal	11.5	7.3	7.48	2	410	0
		17.5	6.7	7.28	2	45	0
18	River, non-tidal	16.5	6.1	7.42	2	250	0
		17.0	4.3	7.08	3	900	0
19	Ditch	16.5	13.1	8.88	3	310	0
		16.0	2.3	7.63	3	340	0

Table 4. Continued

Site[f]	Temp. (°C)	DO[d] mg/l	pH	Na+ mmol/l	AH[e] x10^4	MPN[b] or cfu[c]100/ml V. cholerae
20 Canal	16.5	4.8	7.49	5	1700	0
	16.0	2.5	7.37	5	7000	$\geq$18
21 Dammed creek, semi-tidal	17.0	11.9	8.37	181	11000	160
	18.0	10.8	8.22	129	12000	180-2000
22 Gravel pit	18.0	9.5	8.42	103	22	5
	18.0	8.0	8.38	104	150	30
23 Ditch	16.5	6.5	7.78	31	9000	200
	16.0	3.7	7.66	30	11000	1000
24 Ditch	18.0	10.4	8.60	289	6000	0
	17.5	9.6	8.60	295	2200	0
25 Seawater	17.0	7.6	8.13	529	25	0
	17.0	7.9	8.03	495	29	0

26	Tidal river	18.5	11.1	8.97	17	170	0
		19.0	9.5	8.67	54	1000	8
27	Ditch	18.0	9.8	8.22	5	230	0
		18.0	9.6	8.40	4	11000	8

[a] The first line of data for each site corresponds to 2 July and the second to 23 July.
[b] Most probable number.
[c] Colony-forming units.
[d] Dissolved oxygen.
[e] Aerobic heterotrophic bacteria.
[f] Sites are numbered as in Figure 1.
[g] This value was 90 on 30 July 1979.

On July 23, V. cholerae was detected at all of the sites (10 in all) with water containing 4–270 mmol Na^+/l and site 15, a pond used for the breeding of waterfowl, which contained < 1 mmol Na^+/l. The 5 sites where V. cholerae had been detected on July 2 still had the highest populations of V. cholerae. On both occasions there was no strong correlation between any factor except Na^+ concentration and the presence of V. cholerae.

Isolation of V. cholerae
from Animal Feces

During the surveys described here and intensive studies of the seasonal incidence of V. cholerae in Chetney Marsh ditches (Site 1) it became obvious that V. cholerae usually became undetectable in water and sediment during the winter months (West et al. 1980; West and Lee 1982). We wished to investigate the ways in which V. cholerae could survive the winter period and one such mechanism could be survival in an animal vector. The land at Site 1 is grazed by sheep that frequently drink the water from the ditches and, of course, the ditches are visited by aquatic birds.

V. cholerae was not detected in 177 samples of fresh droppings from sheep grazing on the land at Site 1 although they were sampled at a time when V. cholerae was present in the ditch water. In contrast, non-O1 V. cholerae was isolated from the freshly voided droppings of two mute swans (Cygnus olor) nesting at Site 1 in May 1979 on the same day that non-O1 V. cholerae first became detectable in the water column. The strains from the water and swan feces all belonged to serovar O2.

Birds were caught by cannon netting in March 1979, March 1980, and February 1981 at Richborough refuse disposal tip and in November 1980 at Sandwich beach. These are months of the year when V. cholerae is usually undetectable in the aquatic environment. Water samples taken from drainage ditches on Richborough refuse tip at the time the birds were caught did not contain V. cholerae except in 1980 when March, like the rest of the winter, was very mild. The numbers and species of birds caught and the numbers from which V. cholerae was isolated are shown in Table 5. Approximately 6% of all the gulls sampled were carrying V. cholerae. One of the herring gulls caught in March 1980 had previously been caught in East Germany and of the black-headed gulls caught in February 1981, one had previously been caught in Belgium and another in Sweden.

Serotyping of Isolates

When typed according to the schemes of Sakazaki et al. (1970) and Shimada and Sakazaki (1977), the strains collected in all these surveys belonged to a wide range of O serovars including 1, 2, 3, 4, 6, 8, 12, 14, 15, 19, 20, 25, 26, 27, 32, 34, 36, 38, 39, 40, 41, 45, 48, 51, 52, 64, 65, 67, and 73.

DISCUSSION

The evidence presented here clearly demonstrates that V. cholerae occurs sporadically in all types of water in Kent during the summer months but only in very low numbers in water containing < 5 mmol Na^+/l. The largest populations, which may approach 10^3 cfu/ml, occur regularly in static brackish water with concentrations of Na^+ in the range 25-300 mmol/l. Thus the incidence of V. cholerae in water is clearly related to the ionic content of the water. Sodium may not be the only important ion. We have also measured the concentrations of K^+, Mg^{++}, Ca^+, and Cl^- but in our samples relative to Na^+ these ions are always present in the same proportions found in seawater and therefore we have only reported Na^+ concentrations. There did not appear to be any significant introduction of V. cholerae into rivers from sewage effluent and there was no correlation between the E. coli count and the presence of V. cholerae. In these respects our results closely parallel those of Kaper et al. (1979), who found that V. cholerae occurred in Chesapeake Bay in waters of salinities

Table 5. Isolations of $\underline{V}$. cholerae from Birds Caught by Cannon Netting

Species	No. Containing $\underline{V}$. cholerae/No. Sampled				
	March 1979	March 1980	Nov. 1980	Feb. 1981	Totals
Blackheaded gull (Larus ridibundus)	1/6	5/98	0/12	1/26	7/142
Greater blackbacked gull (Larus marinus)	0/1	NT[a]	NT	3/14	3/15
Herring gull (Larus argentatus)	3/31	0/3	0/1	2/53	5/88
Jackdaw (Corvus monedula)	NT	NT	NT	0/2	0/2
Rook (Corvus frugilegus)	NT	NT	NT	1/28	1/28
Sanderling (Calidris alba)	NT	NT	0/105	NT	0/105
Turnstone (Arenaria interpres)	NT	NT	0/15	NT	0/15

[a]Not tested.

in the range of 4-17% (approximately 7-290 mmol Na^+/l) and that there was no correlation between the fecal coliform count and the presence of V. cholerae. There was no correlation between the other parameters that we measured (pH, dissolved oxygen, total heterotrophic count) and the presence of V. cholerae.

There have been few extensive studies of the occurrence of V. cholerae in waters in temperate areas. The most comprehensive studies published so far are those of Kaper et al. (1979) and Colwell et al. (1981). There have also been several reports of the isolation of "NAG" or "non-cholera" vibrios from surface waters and sewage in West and East Germany (Ko et al. 1973; Muller 1978; Juras et al. 1979). Unfortunately it is not possible to be absolutely certain that these "NAG" or "non-cholera" vibrios were all non-O1 V. cholerae because the tests used were not adequate to distinguish V. cholerae from V. alginolyticus and similar vibrios. In particular, the strains were not examined for their ability to grow in the absence of Na^+. All of our strains conformed to the species V. cholerae as defined by Furniss et al. (1978), and the identification of 55 of our isolates, mostly from Site 1, was confirmed in a numerical taxonomic study (West 1980). The populations of V. cholerae (1-10 cells/l) detected by Kaper et al. (1979) were much lower than some of the populations detected in Kent. In the only other quantitative study that we know of, Barbay et al. (1981) found V. cholerae populations comparable to ours--up to 110/ml in water in Louisiana.

Our surveys suggested that there was a distinct seasonal incidence of V. cholerae with the highest frequency of isolation and counts occurring during the summer months. Seasonality was also suggested by the data of Muller (1977), Muller (1978), and Juras et al. (1979), but Kaper et al. (1979) were unable to study seasonality because of the very low numbers of V. cholerae present in their samples. The high numbers of V. cholerae found in the brackish-water drainage ditches on Chetney Marsh (Site 1) have enabled us to confirm that there is a marked seasonal incidence of V. cholerae in these ditches (West et al. 1980; West and Lee 1982). The organism was present in the water column from May to November, with the highest numbers of up to 400 cfu/ml occurring in late August, but not during the rest of 1978 and 1979. V. cholerae was also not detected from the sediment and vegetation during the winter months (West and Lee 1982).

Inevitably it will be asked if the presence of these organisms presents any health hazard to the public. In addition to the serovar O1 strains discussed above, over 300 V. cholerae strains isolated from water and bird samples in Kent have been examined using the E. coli LT gene probe and none of them possess the gene for cholera toxin (Kaper and Lee, unpublished results). On initial examination, one strain--VL 3944, isolated from Site 1--appeared to produce cholera toxin (Bashford et al. 1979) but the strain does not possess the gene coding for cholera toxin (Kaper et al. 1981). Thus, none of the isolates examined so far, including these of the O1 serovar, produce cholera toxin. We cannot be certain that there are no cholera toxin producers in these environments for if such strains represented only a small proportion of the population--for example less than 1%--then they would be extremely difficult to detect. We do not believe that the presence of these strains of V. cholerae in the aquatic environment in Kent presents a significant health risk.

If cholera toxin-producing strains are present, they must be in such low numbers that an individual would have to ingest a large volume of the water to become infected. Deliberate ingestion of these waters is also extremely unlikely, particularly as many are brackish. The standards of sanitation and hygiene in the area are high and it is therefore highly improbable for these vibrios to get into the drinking water supply. Of course it is possible that shellfish in the estuaries may become contaminated with V. cholerae but, provided they were adequately cooked and processed, this would not present a risk of infection. In the whole of Kent during 1977-1980, there were only four cases of diarrhea from which V. cholerae was isolated and the patients had all been infected abroad (Public Health Laboratory Service, unpublished results). The serovars of the strains were O1 subtype Ogawa, O58 and O76, and one strain was not typeable. One of the non-O1 strains was isolated at Maidstone where all stool specimens are examined for the presence of vibrios. If indigenous infections do occur they are obviously very rare, and for these various reasons we can only conclude that the presence of the V. cholerae strains in waters in Kent presents no significant health risk.

One source of V. cholerae in these water samples could be fecal contamination from humans or other animals that are harboring the organisms. The lack of correlation between the presence of V. cholerae and the input of sewage on the E. coli count suggests that fecal contamination was not a source of V. cholerae. However, similar results could perhaps be explained by the better survival of V. cholerae in the brackish water environments although they are of fecal origin. Humans, we have already seen, are an unlikely source since vibrio infections are extremely rare in this area and those detected have all been at least 10 miles from those sites where V. cholerae occurs in high numbers. Farm animals are also an unlikely source since we failed to isolate V. cholerae from the feces of sheep that actually drink water containing high numbers of the organism. In addition, at the Veterinary Investigation Centre in Wye, Kent, V. cholerae could not be isolated from fecal specimens from 225 cattle, 110 sheep, 138 pigs, 43 birds (mostly poultry), and 69 other animals (Ministry of Agriculture, Fisheries and Food, unpublished results). Most of these animals had some enteric disorder.

V. cholerae was isolated from 6% of the gulls sampled, which all appeared to be healthy, at times when V. cholerae was not normally detectable in water samples. Non-O1 V. cholerae has also been isolated in Denmark from farmed ducks which became colonized very rapidly after release onto open farmland (Bisgaard and Kristensen 1975; Bisgaard et al. 1978). These birds may have been transient hosts to V. cholerae as a result of having eaten other animals such as molluscs or crustaceans that were harboring the vibrios. Alternatively they may be longer-term hosts; the possibility that V. cholerae could survive the winter in the guts of aquatic birds cannot be excluded. If V. cholerae can survive for only a few days in the gut of these birds it may be long enough for the vibrios to be carried considerable distances. Three of the birds we caught had travelled several hundred miles. Thus, the possibility that aquatic birds may be vectors of V. cholerae including epidemic strains warrants further investigation.

Although birds may be vectors of V. cholerae, the numbers that they carry must be quite low because on the one occasion when we attempted isolation by direct plating (March 1979), we only detected the vibrios after enrichment. Thus, we do not believe that the numbers of V. cholerae found regularly in brackish waters could be the result of fecal contamination by birds. Even if the V. cholerae are introduced by birds, they must be capable of multiplication in the water column or elsewhere in the aquatic environment to achieve the populations detected regularly at some of our sites. It is most likely that the strains of V. cholerae we have detected are indigenous to the aquatic environment. This theory was favored by Colwell et al. (1981) and Kaper et al. (1979). Experiments with membrane-diffusion chambers to demonstrate that these V. cholerae strains are able to grow in the water at Site 1 are reported elsewhere (West and Lee 1982). We conclude that non-toxin-producing strains of V. cholerae have a natural ecological niche in the aquatic environment and that this will be found in static or near-static brackish water environments with water containing Na^+ at concentrations of 25-200 mmol/l.

The possible survival of toxigenic virulent V. cholerae O1 in the environment along the Gulf Coast of the United States from 1973 until 1981 (Blake et al. 1980) and the persistence of toxigenic V. cholerae O1 in rivers in Australia for over 22 months in the absence of clinical cases (Rogers et al. 1980) are leading microbiologists to consider seriously the possibility that toxigenic V. cholerae has a natural ecological niche in the aquatic environment. Such a niche could explain its survival in interepidemic periods. Considering the extremely close similarity of the pathogenic to the nonpathogenic strains of V. cholerae it seems likely that any such niche, if it exists, will be found in static or near-static brackish water environments.

CONCLUSIONS

1. V. cholerae occurs spasmodically in all types of water in the summer months but only in very low numbers in water containing < 5 mmol Na^+/l or > 200 mmol Na^+/l.

2. High numbers (up to nearly 10^3/ml occur regularly in the summer in static or near-static brackish water containing 25-200 mmol Na^+/l.

3. V. cholerae are not introduced significantly by sewage contamination of the water.

4. There is no correlation between the E. coli count and the presence of V. cholerae in water.

5. Estuarine birds, in particular gulls, even if they do not represent a significant reservoir of V. cholerae, may be important vectors.

6. V. cholerae, including the O1 serovar, occurs naturally in Kent and is indigenous to brackish water environments.

ACKNOWLEDGMENTS

The figure, tables, and much of this paper have previously been published in the Journal of Applied Bacteriology (Lee et al. 1982); we are extremely grateful to that Journal for permission to reproduce the material here. P.A. West thanks the Science Research Council for a CASE Research Studentship.

REFERENCES

Aldova E., K. Laznickova, E. Stepankova, and J. Lietava. 1968. Isolation of non-agglutinable vibrios from an enteritis outbreak in Czechoslovakia. J. Infect. Dis. 118:25-31.

Back, E., A. Ljunggren, and H. Smith. 1974. Non-cholera vibrios in Sweden. Lancet 1:723-724.

Barbay, J.R., H.B. Bradford, N.C. Roberts, and R.J. Siebeling. 1981. Vibrios in Louisiana coastal regions. Page 215 in Abst. Ann. Mtg. Am. Soc. Microbiol.

Bashford, D.J., T.J. Donovan, A.L. Furniss, and J.V. Lee. 1979. Vibrio cholerae in Kent. Lancet 1:436-437.

Bisgaard M., and K.K. Kristensen. 1975. Isolation, characterization and public health aspects of Vibrio cholerae NAG isolated from a Danish duck farm. Avian Pathol. 4:271-276.

Bisgaard M., R. Sakazaki, and T. Shimada. 1978. Prevalence of non-cholera vibrios in cavum nasi and pharynx of ducks. Acta. Pathol. Microbiol. Scand., Sect. B. 86:261-266.

Blake, P.A., D.T. Allegra, J.D Snyder, T.J. Barrett, L. McFarland, C.T. Caraway, J.C. Feeley, J.P. Craig, J.V. Lee, N.D. Puhr, and R.A. Feldman. 1980. Cholera--a possible endemic focus in the United States. N. Engl. J. Med. 302:305-309.

Colwell, R.R., R.J. Seidler, J. Kaper, S.W. Joseph, S. Garges, H. Lockman, D. Maneval, H. Bradford, N. Roberts, E. Remmers, I. Huq, and A. Huq. 1981. Occurrence of Vibrio cholerae serotype O1 in Maryland and Louisiana estuaries. Appl. Environ. Microbiol. 41:555-558.

Furniss, A.L., J.V. Lee, and T.J. Donovan. 1978. The vibrios. Public Health Laboratory Service Monograph Series No. 11 London: HMSO.

Juras, H., U. Futh, D. Winkler, J. Friedmann, and T. Hillig. 1979. Vorkommen von NAG-vibrionen in Berliner gewassern. Zeits. Allem. Mikrobiol. 19:403-409.

Kaper, J., H. Lockman, R.R. Colwell, and S.W. Joseph. 1979. Ecology, serology and enterotoxin production of Vibrio cholerae in Chesapeake Bay. Appl. Environ. Microbiol. 37:91-103.

Kaper, J.B., S.L. Moseley, and S. Falkow. 1981. Molecular characterization of environmental and non-toxigenic strains of Vibrio cholerae. Infect. Immun. 32:661-667.

Ko, H.L., R. Lutticken, and G. Pulverer. 1973. Vorkommen von NAG-vibrionen (nicht-cholera-vibrionen) in Westdeutschland. English summary. Deuts. Medizin. Wocken. 98:1494-1499.

Lee, J.V., D.J. Bashford, T.J. Donovan, A.L. Furniss, and P.A. West. 1982. The incidence of V. cholerae in water, animals and birds in Kent, England. J. Appl. Bacteriol. 52:281-291.

Muller, G. 1977. Non-agglutinable cholera vibrios (NAG) in sewage, riverwater, and seawater. Zentralbl. Bakteriol. Parasitenkd. Infektionskr. Hyg. Abt. 1 Orig. B. 165:487-497.

Muller, H.E. 1978. Occurrence and ecology of NAG vibrios in surface waters. Zentralbl. Bakteriol. Parasitenkd. Infektionskr. Hyg. Abt. 1 Orig. B. 167:272-284.

Rogers, R.C., R.G.C.J. Cuffe, Y.M. Cossins, D.M. Murphy, and A.T.C. Bourke. 1980. The Queensland cholera incident of 1977:2. The epidemiological investigation. Bull. W.H.O. 58:665-669.

Sakazaki, R., K. Tamura, C.Z. Gomez, and R. Sen. 1970. Serological studies on the cholera group of vibrios. Jpn. J. Med. Sci. Biol. 23:13-20.

Shimada T., and R. Sakazaki. 1977. Additional serovars and inter-O antigen relationships of V. cholerae. Jpn. J. Med. Sci. Biol. 30:275-277.

West, P.A. 1980. Ecology and taxonomy of the genus Vibrio. Ph.D. Thesis, University of Kent.

West, P.A., C.J. Knowles, and J.V. Lee. 1980. Ecology of Vibrio species, including Vibrio cholerae, in waters of Kent, United Kingdom. Soc. Gen. Microbiol. Quart. 7:80.

West, P.A., and J.V. Lee. 1982. Ecology of Vibrio species, including Vibrio cholerae, in natural waters of Kent, England. J. Appl. Bacteriol. 52:435-448.

Chapter 26

DISTRIBUTION AND GROWTH OF VIBRIO CHOLERAE IN A NATURAL BRACKISH WATER SYSTEM

Paul Andrew West and John Vincent Lee

Between 1978 and 1980, a pronounced seasonal incidence (highest number 400 cfu/ml) of non-O1 serovar Vibrio cholerae was observed in a natural ditch containing static, brackish water. Strains were isolated only from May to November each year. The presence of non-O1 V. cholerae was not dependent on the input of human sewage. All strains of non-O1 serovar V. cholerae, representing isolates collected throughout the sampling period, failed to produce cholera toxin when tested by an enzyme-linked immunosorbant assay (ELISA). The hypothesis that nontoxigenic V. cholerae can survive and multiply in a ditch was tested by the use of submersible chambers constructed of polycarbonate membranes and plexiglass. The seasonal incidence of non-O1 V. cholerae could be explained by the ability of the organism to multiply when the ditch water temperature exceeded 9°C. The implications for the epidemiology of cholera are discussed.

Many serovars, including O1, of V. cholerae have been isolated from the natural aquatic environment of Kent, England. Studies demonstrated that V. cholerae occurred regularly, and in high numbers, in brackish water (25-200 mmol Na^+/liter). The frequency of isolation was higher in the summer months. No correlation with input of human sewage was apparent and it was concluded that V. cholerae (nontoxigenic) was a naturally occurring member of brackish water environments where its seasonal incidence may be due to the organism multiplying in the warmer waters (Lee et al. 1982; this volume). Further studies to elucidate the seasonal distribution of V. cholerae and its ability to multiply in brackish water are described here.

MATERIALS AND METHODS

The temporal distribution of non-O1 V. cholerae in an agricultural drainage ditch containing static brackish water was studied between April 1978 and February 1980. The ditch is not polluted by human sewage. The location of Chetney Marsh ditch and collection of samples (water, sediment, plant material) have been described (Lee et al. 1982; West and Lee 1982).

Throughout the sampling period, the number of V. cholerae strains in the water varied from a few cells per liter up to several hundred per milliliter. Depending on the numbers likely to be encountered, the following isolation and enumeration methods were used: a) concentration by filtration through pulverized diatomaceous earth, b) a 5-tube, 3-dilution most probable number technique, c) direct plating onto thiosulphate citrate bile salts sucrose agar (West and Lee 1982). Other bacteriological examinations of water, sediment, and plant material, the identification tests for V. cholerae, and the ELISA assay for cholera toxin have been previously described (Lee et al. 1982; West and Lee 1982).

In situ survival growth experiments were performed using submersible chambers of polycarbonate membrane (0.4-μm pore size, Nucleopore Co.) and plexiglass constructed to the original design of McFeters and Stuart (1972). These semipermeable membrane chambers sequester the bacteria under study from the aquatic microbial community without sacrificing interaction of the test organisms with the abiotic environment. Sampling ports in the chambers allow the bacteria in the membrane-enclosed area of the chamber to be counted and their response rates assessed. For use, cells were grown to stationary phase in

T_1N_1 broth (1% w/v tryptone, 1% w/v NaCl, pH 7.2) and diluted in sterile ditch water so that chambers were inoculated with bacterial numbers similar to those found in the water column in the summer. Strains were tested in duplicate chambers. Chambers were incubated 30 cm below the water surface and samples taken daily for six or seven days. Counts were determined on heart-infusion agar (Difco). The strains and their serovars studied--V. cholerae O1 (Lee et al. 1982), V. cholerae O6 (ditch isolate), and V. cholerae O6 (gull isolate)--were randomly selected from representative cultures (West and Lee 1982). All of these strains have been shown to lack the structural gene coding for cholera toxin production (Kaper et al. 1981; J.B. Kaper, personal communication).

RESULTS

The temporal distribution of non-O1 V. cholerae in Chetney Marsh ditch water is presented in Figure 1. A distinct seasonal cycle was observed as strains were isolated from May to October (1978) and May to November (1979). Concentration techniques using up to 9 liters of water failed to isolate strains during the other months. Strains could not be isolated from six 100g sediment samples between December 1978 and March 1979 although non-O1 V. cholerae strains were isolated from one out of three 100g samples taken during January 1980. Strains appeared when the water temperature rose above 9°C. Maximum counts of non-O1 V. cholerae were 70 colony-forming units (cfu)/ml in September 1978 and 400 cfu/ml in August 1979. Strains of non-O1 V. cholerae were only isolated from plant material when strains were present in the water column as well. Counts of non-O1 V. cholerae were higher on plant material than in the water column. The ELISA assay for cholera toxin production was negative for 71 strains representing isolates throughout the sampling period.

The data in Figures 2A to 2J demonstrate the survival and growth curves of each test strain in Chetney Marsh ditch water between May 1979 and February 1980. The date on each figure represents the start of a chamber run. The

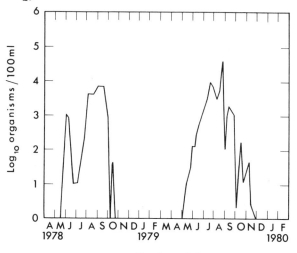

Figure 1. The incidence of non-O1 <u>Vibrio</u> <u>cholerae</u> in water of Chetney Marsh ditch. Counts (c) have been plotted after a $\log_{10}$ (c+1) transformation.

ability of <u>V</u>. <u>cholerae</u> O6 (ditch isolate) to grow and survive in the chambers followed closely the rise and fall of the population of non-O1 <u>V</u>. <u>cholerae</u> in the water column. During May to August, the population of non-O1 <u>V</u>. <u>cholerae</u> steadily increased and strains were able to multiply in the chambers. In August, there was a sharp fall in the water column population and simultaneously the test strains lost the ability to grow in the chambers (Figure 2F). The sudden decline was eventually attributed to a period of stagnation and production of toxic levels of hydrogen sulphide in the ditch. When the population of non-O1 <u>V</u>. <u>cholerae</u> gradually increased again in the water column in late August, the ditch test strain regained its ability to multiply in the chambers (Figure 2G). Counts of non-O1 <u>V</u>. <u>cholerae</u> in the water column then fell slowly to below detectable levels between September and November with a corresponding loss of the ability of the ditch and gull test strains to multiply in the chambers (Figure 2H and 2I). The ditch test strain failed to multiply in the chambers when tested in February 1980 (Figure 2J).

The gull isolate behaved similarly to the ditch isolate of <u>V</u>. <u>cholerae</u>. Interestingly, the gull isolate appeared more sensitive to apparently unfavorable growth conditions than the ditch isolate (Figure 2F, 2I, and 2J). A strain of $\underline{V.\ cholerae}$ O1 was tested only once and it multiplied in the chambers studied in July 1979.

DISCUSSION

Results for Chetney Marsh ditch are the first clear demonstration of the seasonal incidence of non-O1 $\underline{V.\ cholerae}$ in the aquatic environment of a temperate, cholera nonendemic area. No cholera toxin-producing strains were isolated from this site nor have any been isolated from other waters in Kent (Lee et al. 1982; unpublished observations).

Strains of nontoxigenic, non-O1 $\underline{V.\ cholerae}$ were not detected in the water column each year until the water temperature rose above 9°C. No correlation between non-O1 $\underline{V.\ cholerae}$ and $\underline{Escherichia\ coli}$ was observed. The count of non-O1 $\underline{V.\ cholerae}$ peaked in the months of August or September, then gradually declined as the water temperature dropped until the count became undetectable at the end of the year. In the winter months, strains could not be isolated from plant material and were only detected once in sediment. The low isolation rate suggests that non-O1 $\underline{V.\ cholerae}$ did not overwinter in sediment or on plant material between seasonal appearances. Evidence is accumulating that an animal reservoir may be significant in the transmission and maintenance of non-O1 $\underline{V.\ cholerae}$ in the local aquatic environment. Lee et al. (1982) demonstrated the isolation of non-O1 $\underline{V.\ cholerae}$ from estuarine birds during the winter months when numbers in the water were very low and occurred sporadically. The present study has shown that, under favorable conditions, a strain from a gull will survive and grow in brackish water.

It was concluded from the in situ survival studies that the seasonality of non-O1 $\underline{V.\ cholerae}$ in the ditch reflected the ability of strains to survive and grow when the water temperature exceeded 9°C. Submersible chambers employed as survival studies under laboratory culture provide only limited information on the responses of bacteria in their

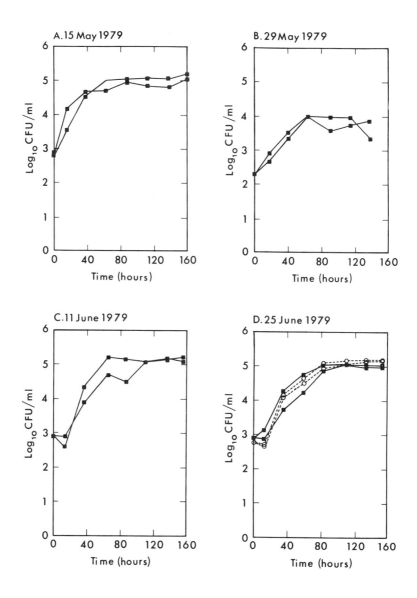

Figure 2A-2D. Growth and survival of <u>Vibrio</u> <u>cholerae</u> in submersible membrane diffusion chambers in Chetney Marsh ditch water. Counts (c) have been plotted after a $\log_{10}$ (c+1) transformation. Symbols: ■—— <u>V</u>. <u>cholerae</u> O6 (ditch isolate); O--O <u>V</u>. <u>cholerae</u> O6 (gull isolate).

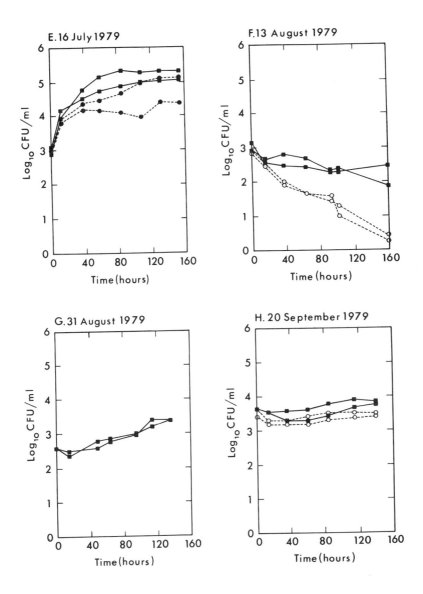

Figure 2E-2H. Growth and survival of <u>Vibrio cholerae</u> in submersible membrane diffusion chambers in Chetney Marsh ditch water. Counts (c) have been plotted after a log$_{10}$ (c+1) transformation. Symbols: ■—■ <u>V</u>. <u>cholerae</u> O6 (ditch isolate); O‑‑O <u>V</u>. <u>cholerae</u> O6 (gull isolate); ●‑‑● <u>V</u>. <u>cholerae</u> O1.

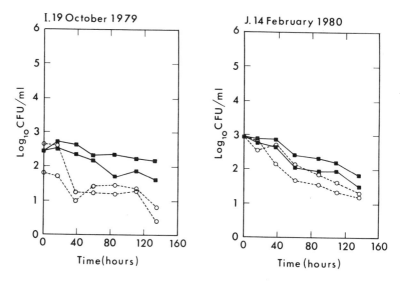

Figure 2I-2J. Survival of <u>Vibrio</u> <u>cholerae</u> in submersible membrane diffusion chambers in Chetney Marsh ditch water. Counts (c) have been plotted after a $\log_{10}$ (c+1) transformation. Symbols: ■——■ <u>V</u>. <u>cholerae</u> O6 (ditch isolate); O– –O <u>V</u>. <u>cholerae</u> O6 (gull isolate).

natural environments. Many historical studies on the survival of toxin-producing <u>V</u>. <u>cholerae</u> O1 strains have been conducted in vitro and have concluded that these strains do not multiply nor survive for long periods outside the human intestine in natural waters. However, the initial cell numbers were often unrealistically high in these studies when compared to the cell numbers reported in field data. Indeed, many of these survival experiments were stopped when the population had reached a level that would normally be detected in the environment and the decline to this level was interpreted as failure to survive outside the human intestine. Reviews of these types of survival studies have been published by Pollitzer (1959) and Felsenfeld (1974).

In our experiments, the behavior of nontoxigenic non-O1 <u>V</u>. <u>cholerae</u> in Chetney Marsh ditch water was investigated by the use of submersible chambers which were inoculated with a realistic population when compared to our field data. We have demonstrated that these strains can survive and multiply in the water under favorable conditions. It may be argued that chambers are not suitable for survival studies because they provide large surface areas for colonization which would not normally be present in the natural environment. Nonetheless, the responses of the test strains in the chambers were closely mirrored by the behavior of the population of non-O1 V. cholerae occurring naturally in the surrounding water column. Indeed, if an organism is unable to grow and survive in the aquatic environment inside these chambers, it is unlikely to do so in the water naturally as a free-living organism.

Previous studies have demonstrated the presence of nontoxigenic strains of V. cholerae in temperate, cholera nonendemic areas (Juras et al. 1979; Kaper et al. 1979; Lee et al. 1982). The present study is the first demonstration, using techniques which more closely approached field conditions, that nontoxigenic strains of O1 and non-O1 V. cholerae can grow in brackish water when the temperature is high enough. The theory that V. cholerae is a natural resident of aquatic microbial communities was originally proposed by Colwell et al. (1977). The evidence presented here strongly supports this hypothesis for strains unable to produce cholera toxin.

From the present study and others reported in this volume, water temperature is emerging as a major environmental parameter controlling the distribution and population of nontoxigenic V. cholerae in the aquatic environment. The possibility that toxigenic strains of V. cholerae O1 can also multiply and maintain themselves in natural waters would explain the reoccurrence and persistence of toxigenic strains in the warm Gulf Coast States waters between 1973 and 1978, a feature of the Louisiana cholera outbreak of 1978 (Blake et al. 1980).

Can the results and conclusions from the survival studies with nontoxigenic, non-O1 serovars be extrapolated to the toxigenic O1 and non-O1 serovars? The recurrent isolation of toxigenic V. cholerae O1 from cholera nonendemic areas such as the Gulf Coast States (Blake et al. 1980), Chesapeake Bay (Colwell et al. 1981), and rivers of Queensland, Australia (Rogers et al. 1980) strongly suggests that toxigenic V. cholerae O1 strains also have an ecological niche in brackish aquatic environments. The ecology and survival of cholera toxin-producing V. cholerae

O1 strains should now be studied, using techniques described in the present study and this volume, in cholera-endemic areas where these strains are naturally found. The influence of cholera toxin production, plasmid carriage, physiological and serological differences, and the attachment or otherwise to plankton on the survival of toxigenic V. cholerae strains in the aquatic environment, as well as subsequent transmission to the human population, are fundamental questions requiring urgent attention. Indeed, the epidemiology of cholera and non-O1 V. cholerae enteritis may need to be radically revised as the ecology of the causative bacteria becomes better understood.

ACKNOWLEDGMENTS

P.A.W. thanks the Science Research Council of Great Britain for a CASE research studentship. We are grateful to Blackwell Scientific Publications Limited, Oxford, England and the Journal of Applied Bacteriology for permission to reproduce figures and data.

REFERENCES

Blake, P.A., D.T. Allegra, J.D. Snyder, T.J. Barrett, L. McFarland, C.T. Caraway, J.C. Feeley, J.P. Craig, J.V. Lee, N.D. Puhr, and R.A. Feldman. 1980. Cholera--a possible endemic focus in the United States. N. Engl. J. Med. 302:305-309.

Colwell, R.R., J. Kaper, and S.W. Joseph. 1977. Vibrio cholerae, Vibrio parahaemolyticus, and other vibrios: occurrence and distribution in Chesapeake Bay. Science 198:394-396.

Colwell, R.R., R.J. Seidler, J. Kaper, S.W. Joseph, S. Garges, H. Lockman, D. Maneval, H. Bradford, N. Roberts, E. Remmers, I. Huq, and A. Huq. 1981. Occurrence of Vibrio cholerae serotype O1 in Maryland and Louisiana estuaries. Appl. Environ. Microbiol. 41:555-558.

Felsenfeld, O. 1974. The survival of cholera vibrios. Pages 359-366 in D. Barua and W. Burrows (Eds.), Cholera. W.B. Saunders, London.

Juras, H., U. Futh, D. Winkler, J. Friedmann, and T. Hillig. 1979. Vorkommen von NAG--vibrionen in Berliner gewassern. Zeitschrift fur Allemeine Mikrobiologie 19:403-409.

Kaper, J., H. Lockman, R.R. Colwell, and S.W. Joseph. 1979. Ecology, serology and enterotoxin production of Vibrio cholerae in Chesapeake Bay. Appl. Environ. Microbiol. 37:91-103.

Kaper, J.B., S.L. Moseley, and S. Falkow. 1981. Molecular characterization of environmental and nontoxigenic strains of Vibrio cholerae. Infect. Immun. 32:661-667.

Lee, J.V., D.J. Bashford, T.J. Donovan, A.L. Furniss, and P.A. West. 1982. The incidence of Vibrio cholerae in water, animals and birds in Kent, England. J. Appl. Bacteriol. 52:281-291.

McFeters, G.A., and D.G. Stuart. 1972. Survival of coliform bacteria in natural waters: field and laboratory studies with membrane filter chambers. Appl. Microbiol. 24:805-811.

Pollitzer, R. 1959. Cholera. World Health Organization monograph series no. 43. W.H.O., Geneva.

Rogers, R.C., R.G.C.J. Cuffe, Y.M. Cossins, D.M. Murphy, and A.T.C. Bourke. 1980. The Queensland cholera incident of 1977: 2. The epidemiological investigation. Bull. W.H.O. 58:665-669.

West, P.A., and J.V. Lee. 1982. Ecology of Vibrio species, including Vibrio cholerae, in natural waters of Kent, England. J. Appl. Bacteriol. 52:435-448.

Chapter 27

TOXIGENIC O1 AND NON-O1 V. CHOLERAE FROM PATIENTS AND THE ENVIRONMENT IN TEXAS

Michael T. Kelly, Johnny W. Peterson, Michael Romanko,
Harry E. Sarles, Jr., Deborah Martin,
and Barry Hafkin

Cholera has recently been recognized in the United States in low-lying coastal areas on the Gulf of Mexico. The first indication of cholera in this region came from a single case that occurred in Port Lavaca, Texas, in 1973 (Weissman et al. 1973). Subsequently, an outbreak of 11 cases of Vibrio cholerae O1 infection was detected in Louisiana in 1978 (Blake et al. 1980), and the occurrence of sporadic cases of non-O1 V. cholerae infection has recently been reported in the United States, although most of the latter cases were due to nontoxigenic strains (Morris et al. 1981). We report here 2 cases of cholera with classical clinical presentation. Toxigenic strains of V. cholerae were isolated from both patients. One isolate was the first O group 1 V. cholerae encountered in Texas since 1973, and the other isolate was the non-O group 1 V. cholerae. We also report the isolation of V. cholerae from the home environments of these patients.

Case 1

On May 7, 1981, a 42-year-old black male who lived in Jefferson County, Texas, and had a history of ethanol abuse collapsed upon arrival in the emergency room at the University of Texas Medical Branch. He was grossly dehydrated with decreased skin turgor, sunken eyes, and bony fingers. His blood pressure was 60 mm Hg by palpation, pulse 130 beats per minute, and respirations 24 per minute. His blood hemoglobin was 20.7g per 100 ml and the hematocrit was 62.7%. The serum sodium was 135mmol per liter, chloride 99mmol per liter, potassium 3.8mmol per liter, and carbon dioxide content 17mmol per liter. Intravenous fluids were administered, and the patient's condition stabilized. Shortly after admission to the hospital, the patient was noted to be producing large quantities of "rice-water" stools, and specimens were sent for culture. Massive fluid replacement (up to 1.5 liters per hour) was required for several days to maintain blood pressure and renal function. Oral tetracycline and aspirin were administered; the diarrhea was controlled after 5 days. The patient was discharged in good health after 12 days of hospitalization. Gastric contents were tested and found to have a pH of 4.8. Questioning as to possible sources of the infection revealed that the patient frequently went wading and fishing in bayous. In the week prior to his illness, he caught and ate a turtle from a ditch near his home and fish from a bayou that had been contaminated by untreated sewage 4 days prior to his fishing trip. He had no history of travel outside his immediate area of residence, and he had no guests in the month prior to his illness. Nor had he frequented any restaurants or taverns in the month prior to his illness. Family members were interviewed, but none gave a positive history of recent illness. Stool cultures were taken from each family member at the time of the patient's discharge from the hospital.

Case 2

On August 4, 1980, a previously healthy 14-year-old Latin American male presented to the emergency room at the University of Texas Medical Branch. The patient had a history of accidental consumption of ditch water 2 days before onset of symptoms, and the day before admission to the hospital the patient complained of increased thirst and malaise followed by repeated vomiting. Upon admission to the hospital, the patient was cachectic with sunken eyes, decreased skin turgor, and dry mucous membranes. He was unresponsive and had a blood pressure of 90/60 mm Hg supine. Intravenous fluids were administered, and after completion of a 1000-ml infusion the patient became more responsive. After resuscitation he spoke with a weak, high-pitched voice. His blood pressure was 90/60 mm Hg supine and 70/50 mm Hg sitting. His pulse was 110 beats per minute; respiration, 24 per minute; and temperature, 38°C. The blood hemoglobin was 18.3g per 100 ml, hematocrit 55.5%, and leukocyte count 24,900 per ml. On the day of admission and after rehydration, the patient passed 2000 ml of rice-water stool, and specimens were sent for culture and Gram stain. Over the following 4 days, the patient passed 2000, 2170, 2625, and 1150 ml of rice-water stool. Oral tetracycline therapy was initiated on day 2 and continued for 7 days. The patient was discharged in good health after 7 days of hospitalization. Questioning of the patient and family members revealed no history of recent travel outside the immediate area of residence. A grandfather living with the family had a history of a vomiting episode 2 days prior to the patient's illness, but no other family members complained of any recent illness. Stool cultures of all family members were taken at the time of the patient's discharge from the hospital.

METHODS

Stool specimens were cultured on blood agar, Hektoen enteric (HE) agar, thiosulfate citrate bile salts sucrose (TCBS) agar, peptone-water enrichment, and selenite broth. The peptone-water enrichment was subcultured to TCBS after 6 and 18 hours of incubation, and the selenite broth was subcultured to HE agar after 18 hours of incubation. All cultures were incubated at 37°C. Opaque, yellow colonies on TCBS agar were subcultured to blood agar and tested for indophenol oxidase by the Kovac method. Oxidase-positive organisms were identified by the Automicrobic System EBC card (Vitek, Hazelwood, MO), and identifications were confirmed by classical biochemical tests (Wachsmuth et al. 1980). Serological confirmation was done by slide agglutination using polyvalent O1 antiserum (Difco, Detroit, MI). Biochemical and serological identification was also confirmed by the Texas Department of Health (TDH) and the Centers for Disease Control (CDC).

For toxin testing, isolates were grown in Syncase broth (Finkelstein and LaSpalluto 1970) at 37°C for 18 hours. Cells were removed by centrifugation, and the supernatants were passed through 0.22-μm membrane filters (Millipore). The sterile filtrates were stored at 4°C prior to assay. Analyses for cholera toxin were performed using Chinese hamster ovary (CHO) cell assays in which cell elongation and the number of floating cells were monitored (Peterson et al. 1981; Houston et al. 1981). Antigenic identity of cholera toxin in the filtrates was confirmed by neutralization with serial dilutions of monospecific cholera antitoxin made in rabbits (Peterson et al. 1979). This antiserum contained 810 antitoxin units/ml (au/ml).

Environmental water and mud samples, were collected in sterile whirl-pak bags or plastic bottles. Surface and well water samples were also collected by immersing sterile gauze bundles (Moore swabs) in the water sources for 24 hours. The samples were transported immediately to the laboratory at ambient temperature. Water and mud samples were cultured directly by inoculation of 0.1 ml volumes to the surface of TCBS plates, and 10 ml-peptone-water enrichments were inoculated with 0.5 ml volumes of each sample. Water samples were also analyzed by filtration of 20 to 200 ml volumes (depending on particulate content) through sterile, 0.45-μm pore size membrane filters (Millipore, Bedford, MA). The filters were cultured on the surface of TCBS agar plates. Moore swabs were cultured in peptone-water enrichment which was subcultured onto TCBS agar. Organisms isolated from environmental samples were processed and identified as described above.

RESULTS

Stool samples from the patient described in Case 1 yielded a nearly pure culture of sucrose-positive, oxidase-positive, curved Gram-negative bacilli which had the biochemical reactions of V. cholerae (Table 1). This organism agglutinated in polyvalent O group 1 antiserum, and it was beta hemolytic on blood agar. The isolate was resistant to colistin but susceptible to ampicillin, carbenicillin, chloramphenicol, gentamicin, sulfamethoxyzole-trimethoprim, and tetracycline. These results were confirmed by the Texas Department of Health and by the Centers for Disease Control where the isolate was found to be V. cholerae O1 biotype El Tor and serotype Inaba. Culture filtrates of this isolate produced marked elongation of CHO cells (Figure 1) and positive floating cell responses, indicative of the presence of active cholera toxin. These culture filtrates contained approximately 7.5 ng/ml of cholera toxin, based on comparison of CHO cell responses to serial dilutions of the filtrate and purified cholera toxin standards. Both the elongation effect and the floating cell response were prevented by preincubation of the filtrates with monospecific cholera antitoxin. The toxin activity in the filtrates could be neutralized by an antiserum dilution containing 8.1 au/ml but not 0.81 au/ml. This organism was also positive for cholera toxin production as determined by an ELISA assay performed at the CDC (Don Brenner, personal communication). Follow-up stool cultures prior to the patient's discharge from the hospital and two weeks later failed to yield V. cholerae, and cultures of family members were negative for enteric pathogens.

Gram stain of the initial stool specimen from Case 2 showed abundant curved, gram-negative bacilli (Figure 2). Cultures of this specimen yielded abundant growth of an organism with the biochemical characteristics of V. cholerae (Table 1). However, this isolate failed to agglutinate in

Table 1. Biochemical Characteristics of V. cholerae Isolates

Test	Case #1	Case #2	% Positive Predicted[a]
Arginine dihydrolase	−	−	0
Citrate utilization	+	+	(74)[b]
Gelatin hydrolysis	+	+	97
Glucose fermentation	+	+	100
Indole	+	−	100
Lactose fermentation	−	−	(100)
Lysine decarboxylase	+	+	100
Motility	+	+	97
Ornithine decarboxylase	+	+	100
Oxidase	+	+	100
Phenylalanine deaminase	−	−	0
Salicin fermentation	−	−	0
Sucrose fermentation	+	+	96
Urease	−	−	0
Voges-Proskauer	+	−	47
Growth in nutrient broth plus:			
0% NaCl	+	+	100
3% NaCl	+	+	100
10% NaCl	−	−	0

[a]Percentage of positive reactions according to Wachsmuth et al. (1980).
[b]( ) Delayed or weak reactions.

polyvalent O group-1 antiserum and was identified by the CDC as V. cholerae, Smith type 59. This organism was resistant to colistin but susceptible to all other antimicrobial agents tested. Culture filtrates of this isolate also produced marked elongation of CHO cells (Figure 1) and positive floating cell responses that were neutralized by preincubation with monospecific cholera antitoxin. However,

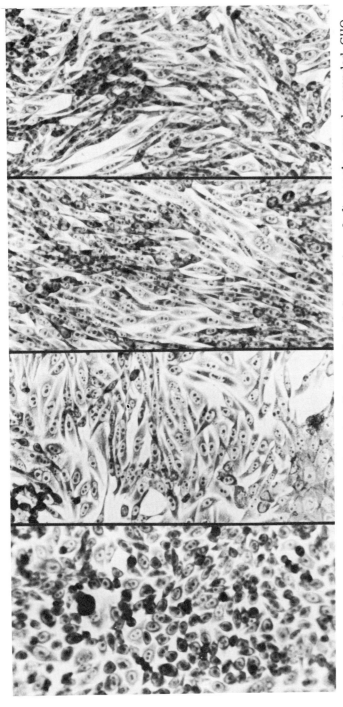

Figure 1. Chinese hamster ovary (CHO) cell assay for cholera toxin. Left panel: normal, rounded CHO cell morphology in the absence of cholera toxin. Left middle panel: elongated CHO cells exposed to 1 ng of purified cholera toxin. Right middle panel: CHO cells exposed to 50 μl of undiluted syncase culture filtrate of the V. cholerae isolate from Case 2. Right panel: CHO cells exposed to 50 μl of undiluted syncase culture filtrate of the V. cholerae isolate from Case 1.

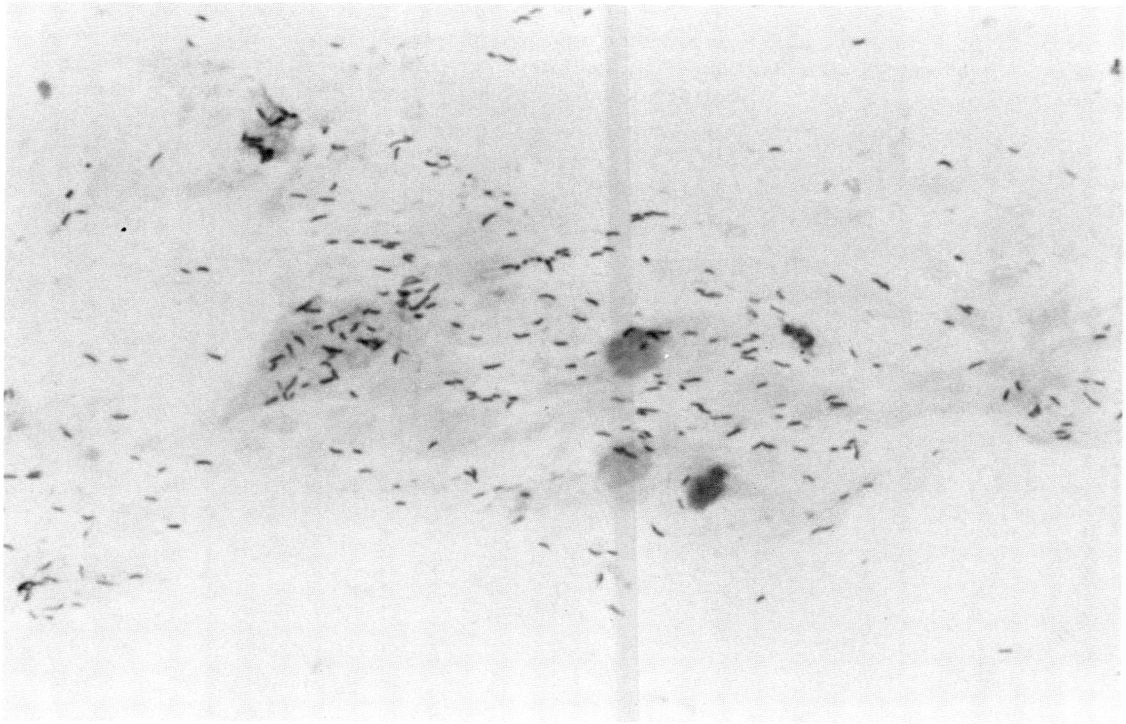

Figure 2. Gram stain of stool from Case 2. Abundant curved, gram-negative bacilli are observed with few normal flora organisms present.

Table 2. Isolation of Toxigenic V. cholerae O1 from Environmental Sources

Site	Sample[a]	Culture Result
Bayou near home	Water	--[b]
Ditch across road	Water	--
Ditch beside house	Water	--
Well water	Water & Moore Swab	--
Sewage upwelling	Water & Moore Swab	--
Standing water	Water	V. cholerae O1
Mud in yard	Mud	V. cholerae O1
Beaumont water	Moore Swab	--
Beaumont sewage	Moore Swab	--

[a]Processing of samples: Water--peptone-water enrichment and filtration, Moore Swab--enrichment, Mud--direct plating and enrichment.
[b]No V. cholerae or other enteric bacteria isolated.

culture filtrates of this organism contained only 1.5 ng/ml of toxin. This level of toxin production is at the lower limit of detection by the CHO cell assay, and the filtrates were positive at a 1:2 dilution but negative at 1:10. Toxin production by this organism was also confirmed by an ELISA assay performed at the CDC (Don Brenner, personal communication). Follow-up stool cultures prior to the patient's discharge from the hospital and two weeks later were negative for enteric pathogens, as were cultures from family members.

Environmental investigations were conducted in follow-up to both cases. Thirteen sites near the home of the first patient were sampled for V. cholerae 12 days after the illness was first recognized (Table 2). The homestead was in a low-lying rural area approximately 100 km from the Gulf of Mexico. Several bayous and drainage ditches were in the vicinity of the home. Well water, ditch water, and bayou water from near the house were collected by direct sampling and by immersion of Moore swabs. Water from an upwelling of sewage under the house was also sampled by both methods. In addition, Moore swabs were used to sample a bayou where the patient fished, a canal that supplies drinking water to the city of Beaumont, and un- treated sewage from the city of Beaumont. None of these samples yielded V. cholerae O1. However, cultures of shallow standing water in the yard near the house and cultures of mud from an adjacent site were positive for V. cholerae. These isolates were beta hemolytic V. cholerae O1, biotype El Tor and serotype Inaba (confirmed by the CDC). They were markedly positive for cholera toxin production in CHO cell assays, and they were otherwise indistinguishable from the patient isolate.

The second patient lived near Alvin, Texas in a rural environment. He had been swimming in a local drainage ditch two days before onset of illness and swallowed water inadvertently. Fourteen samples--including fish, crayfish, water and bottom samples from the drainage ditch, well water and mud samples from around the home--were cul- tured 8 days after the onset of the patient's illness (Table 3). Organisms biochemically identified as V. cholerae were isolated from 10 of the 15 samples. V. cholerae was recovered from mud samples collected at the patient's home and from ditch water, ditch bottom mud samples, fish and crayfish collected from the drainage ditch. The organism was not recovered from well water. Six of the environmental isolates were subjected to detailed analysis, but none of the six was identical to the clinical isolate. They failed to produce cholera toxin, and they were biochemically distinct. One isolate each of Smith types 17, 24, and 40 was detected, and three isolates were untypeable.

DISCUSSION

Case 1 represents the first V. cholerae O1 infection encountered in Texas since 1973 (Weissman et al. 1973), and it brings the total number of cholera cases reported

Table 3. Isolation of _V. cholerae_ non-O1 from Environmental Sources

Site	Sample[a]	Culture Result
Ditch bottom	Mud (4)[b]	_V. cholerae_, non-O1 (2/4)[c]
Ditch	Water (4)	_V. cholerae_, non-O1 (2/4)
Ditch	Fish	_V. cholerae_, non-O1
Ditch	Crayfish (3)	_V. cholerae_, non-O1 (3/3)
Well	Water	--[d]
Yard	Mud	_V. cholerae_, non-O1

[a] Processing of samples: Mud--enrichment and direct plating, Water--peptone-water enrichment, Animals--direct plating and enrichment.
[b] ( ) Number of samples tested.
[c] ( ) Samples positive/number tested.
[d] No _V. cholerae_ or other enteric bacteria isolated.

from the Texas-Louisiana Gulf Coast in modern times to 13. This case provides further evidence that an endemic focus of cholera exists in this area as suggested by Blake et al. (1980), and the results of our environmental studies represent the first instance of environmental isolation of _V. cholerae_ O1 in direct association with a cholera case in the United States. This case demonstrates the classical and life-threatening clinical presentation that may be encountered. Case 2 demonstrates that non-O1 _V. cholerae_ infections may also present with copious watery diarrhea and severe dehydration, clinically indistinguishable from disease caused by _V. cholera_ O1. The environmental studies done in association with Case 2 suggest that non-O1 _V. cholerae_ is commonly present in the Gulf Coast environment, possibly providing a source for these infections.

As summarized by Blake et al. (1980) cholera was not detected in the United States between 1911 and 1973, when a single case was reported from Port Lavaca, Texas (Weiss-man et al. 1973). Subsequently, 11 cases were reported from Louisiana (Blake et al. 1980); however, until the occurrence of the case reported here, no further cases were reported from Texas. These 13 cases were all caused by a hemolytic V. cholerae O1, serotype Inaba and biotype El Tor, suggesting an endemic focus of cholera in the Texas-Louisiana region of the Gulf Coast.

Gastroenteritis due to non-O1 V. cholerae has also been recently recognized. Of 14 cases recently described, all 9 acquired in the United States were associated with consumption of raw oysters, and only one isolate produced cholera toxin (Morris et al. 1981). The case described here was apparently acquired directly from the environment, and the patient had copious watery diarrhea associated with the isolation from stool cultures of a toxigenic V. cholerae. These findings demonstrate that infections due to non-O1 V. cholerae may closely mimic classical cholera.

Environmental contamination has been implicated as a probable source of V. cholerae on the Gulf Coast (Blake et al. 1980). V. cholerae O1 was isolated from the sewage systems of six communities in Louisiana, and two estuarine samples from areas receiving sewage also yielded the or-ganism. Inadequately cooked crabs, presumably from contaminated estuarine environments, were implicated as the vehicle for acquisition of cholera in the Louisiana cases. Other environmental sources of V. cholerae have not been found, and the source of the infections in the Texas patients is unknown. Our environmental studies in associ-ation with the V. cholerae O1 and non-O1 infections de-scribed here suggest that cholera organisms of both types may be found in the environment. V. cholerae O1 was isolated from samples taken at the home of the first patient. These environmental organisms could have been the source of the patient's infection, or they may have been present as a result of fecal contamination. However, there was no evidence of fecal contamination of the sites that yielded the V. cholerae O1 isolates. This finding of V. cholerae O1 in the environment may lend support to the hypothesis that pathogenic strains may be able to multiply and/or persist as a free-living form in the Gulf Coast environment, as suggested by Blake et al. (1980) and by Levine (1980). Sampling of the environment frequented by the second patient yielded many V. cholerae isolates. Although none of these were the same strain isolated from the patient, the results suggest that the environment was the source of his infection, and the failure to detect the patient strain may have been due to limitations in sampling. Mud and water samples taken at both sites were positive, suggesting that bottom samples as well as surface water may be worthy of evaluation in environmental investigations of cholera cases.

Our results together with previously reported findings (Blake et al. 1980; Morris et al. 1981) suggest that O1 and non-O1 V. cholerae are endemic in the Gulf Coast region. The results also suggest that cholera organisms exist in the environment, and human infections occur sporadically after exposure to environments harboring V. cholerae. The incidence of such infections is unknown, but it may be significant because, to date, only severe infections with massive diarrhea and dehydration have been diagnosed directly. Of the 13 V. cholerae O1 infections reported to date, 10 were detected by epidemiological investigations, suggesting that many V. cholerae infections may occur in the endemic area but remain undetected. The routine use of methods for the detection and identification of V. cholerae is needed in laboratories serving the endemic region in order to better define the incidence of these infections. The severity of the infections described here and the epidemic potential of V. cholerae O1 emphasize the need for physician awareness and accurate laboratory diagnosis of cholera-like illnesses to insure adequate therapy and epidemiological investigation.

CONCLUSIONS

1. Classical cholera may be produced by toxigenic strains of non-O1 as well as O1 V. cholerae.

2. V. cholerae O1 infections continue to be detected on the Texas-Louisiana Gulf Coast.

3. <u>V. cholerae</u> non-O1 may be commonly isolated from coastal environments in Texas.

4. Toxigenic <u>V. cholerae</u> O1 has been isolated from the environment in direct association with a case of cholera.

5. Toxigenic <u>V. cholerae</u> O1 is capable of persisting in the environment for at least two weeks, lending support to the hypothesis that this organism may be endemic in the Gulf Coast region.

REFERENCES

Blake, P.A., D.T. Allegra, J.D. Snyder, T.J. Barrett, L. McFarland, C.T. Caraway, J.C. Feeley, J.P. Craig, J.V. Lee, N.D. Puhr, and R.A. Feldman. 1980. Cholera--a possible endemic focus in the United States. N. Engl. J. Med. 302:306-309.

Finkelstein, R.A., and J.J. LaSpalluto. 1970. Production of highly purified choleragen and choleragenoid. J. Infect. Dis. 121:563-571.

Houston, C.W., F.C.W. Koo, and J.J. Peterson. 1981. Characterization of <u>Salmonella</u> toxin released by mitomycin C-treated cells. Infect. Immun. 32:916-926.

Levine, M.M. 1980. Cholera in Louisiana: old problem, new light. N. Engl. J. Med. 302:345-347.

Morris, J.G., R. Wilson, B.R. Davis, et al. 1981. Non-O Group 1 <u>Vibrio cholerae</u> gastroenteritis in the United States: clinical, epidemiologic, and laboratory characteristics of sporatic cases. Ann. Int. Med. 94:656-658.

Peterson, J.W., K.E. Hejtmancik, D.E. Mardel, et al. 1979. Antigenic specificity of neutralizing antibody to cholera toxin. Infect. Immun. 24:774-779.

Peterson, J.W., C.W. Houston, and F.C.W. Koo. 1981. Influence of cultural conditions on mitomycin C-mediated induction and release of Salmonella toxin. Infect. Immun. 32:232-242.

Wachsmuth, I.K., G.K. Morris, and J.C. Feeley. 1980. Vibrio. Pages 226-234 in E.H. Lennette, A. Balows, W.J. Hausler, J.P. Truant (Eds.), Manual of clinical microbiology. 3rd ed. American Society for Microbiology, Washington, D.C.

Weissman, J.B., W.E. DeWitt, J. Thompson, C. N. Muchnick, B. L. Portnoy, J. C. Feeley and E. J. Gangarosa. 1973. A case of cholera in Texas. Am. J. Epidemiol. 1973: 100:487-498.

Chapter 28

PERSISTENCE AND DISTRIBUTION OF
MARINE VIBRIOS IN THE HARDSHELL CLAM

E.P. Greenberg, Heidi B. Kaplan,
M. DuBoise and B. Palhof

The marine bacterium <u>Vibrio</u> <u>parahaemolyticus</u> has been implicated as a causative agent in food poisoning resulting from the consumption of raw or partially cooked seafood (Beuchat 1976; Fujino et al. 1974; Miwatani and Takeda 1976). This has led to a number of investigations concerning the survival of <u>V</u>. <u>parahaemolyticus</u> in seafood products (Beuchat 1975; Goatcher et al. 1974; Johnson and Liston 1973; Johnson et al. 1973; Matches et al. 1971; Oliver 1981; Vanderzant and Nickelson 1972), but there is little information available regarding the occurrence and persistence of this bacterial pathogen in active marine animals. Marine vibrios, including <u>V</u>. <u>parahaemolyticus</u>, are considered as enteric marine bacteria because of numerous similarities between their physiology and the physiology of enteric bacteria (Baumann and Baumann 1977). Furthermore, marine vibrios have been isolated not only from seawater but also from intestinal contents of a variety of marine animals (Baumann and Baumann 1977). As such, the ecology of these organisms within animal hosts is of interest.

Many areas along the Northeast Coast of the United States have been closed to commercial shellfishing due to pollution by enteric pathogens from terrestrial runoff.

Some of these areas have been reopened on a conditional basis. In such cases, clams must be treated at purification or depuration plants. The depuration process takes advantage of the fact that filter-feeding invertebrates will clear themselves of foreign particles as they feed, and a decrease in terrestrial bacteria such as Escherichia and Salmonella can be achieved in a relatively short time (Arcisz and Kelly 1955; Hartland 1978; Houser 1964). However, the persistence of marine vibrios in clams during depuration has not been determined, and since these bacteria are marine organisms, they may survive the process.

One purpose of these investigations was to compare the persistence of two marine Vibrio species (V. parahaemolyticus and the nonpathogenic Vibrio harveyi) to the persistence of Escherichia coli in the hardshell clam, Mercenaria mercenaria under conditions of depuration. Another aspect of these investigations was to compare the occurrence of marine vibrios in M. mercenaria and seawater from a polluted harbor closed to shellfishing and a harbor open to shellfishing. Such information should be of use in determining the potential health hazard of pathogenic vibrios in commercially depurated clams and should also be of value in developing an understanding of the relationships between marine enteric bacteria and M. mercenaria.

MATERIALS AND METHODS

Bacteria and media. For depuration experiments, the marine vibrios employed were V. parahaemolyticus strain 117, which was isolated in Japan from a case of food poisoning (Baumann et al. 1971), and V. harveyi strain 392, a luminous marine isolate (Reichelt and Baumann 1973). A strain of E. coli, S321, carrying a chloramphenicol resistance marker was provided by N. Kleckner for use in these studies.

Cultures of the marine vibrios were grown in Seawater-Complete (SWC) broth, a seawater-based medium containing peptone, yeast extract, and glycerol (Ruby et al. 1980). Cultures of E. coli were grown in Nutrient Broth (Difco). The medium used for plate counts of V. parahaemolyticus was thiosulfide citrate bile salts sucrose agar (TCBS; BBL). Plate counts for colony-forming units (cfu) of V. harveyi were performed using SWC agar (SWC broth plus 1.5% agar). Plate counts of E. coli were on EMB-agar (Difco) supplemented with chloramphenicol (25 µg/ml).

Culture conditions. Cells of V. parahaemolyticus and V. harveyi used to inoculate M. mercenaria for depuration experiments were grown overnight at 25°C with shaking (100 RPM) in 5 ml of SWC broth contained in 16 by 150 mm test tubes. Cells of E. coli used to inoculate M. mercenaria were grown overnight in 5 ml of Nutrient Broth contained in 16 by 150 mm test tubes. Incubation was at 30°C with shaking (100 RPM).

For each of the bacterial species, cfu values were determined by performing plate counts on dilutions of homogenized tissues from specimens of M. mercenaria (see below). Generally plate counts of V. parahaemolyticus were performed by passing 1-ml samples through 0.22-µm filters (Millipore Corp., Bedford, MA) and placing the filters on TCBS agar plates. In the case of the depuration experiments, green colonies arising after 24 hours at 35°C were scored as V. parahaemolyticus cfu. In the case of isolations from in situ samples, green colonies arising after 18-24 hours at 38-41°C were scored as presumptive V. parahaemolyticus cfu. Confirmation of these colonies as V. parahaemolyticus requires further characterization (Food and Drug Administration 1976). Several presumptive V. parahaemolyticus colonies from each sampling site and time were cloned and stored as described elsewhere (Ruby et al. 1980; Ruby and Nealson 1977) for further taxonomic characterization. For the depuration experiments, plate counts of V. harveyi were performed by placing filters that were prepared as described above on SWC agar plates. After 15-20 hours at 35°C, the SWC agar plates were taken into a darkroom and luminous colonies were scored as V. harveyi. In the case of the studies of natural abundances of luminous vibrios, incubation was at 25°C for 18-24 hours and luminous vibrios were enumerated and distinguished from the luminous genus, Photobacterium, by previously described techniques that involve characterization of the light-emitting enzyme, luciferase (Ruby et al. 1980; Ruby and Nealson 1977). Plate counts to determine $\underline{E}$. $\underline{coli}$ cfu were performed by placing filters on EMB agar supplemented with chloramphenicol. After incubation at 30°C for 48 hours the characteristic $\underline{E}$. $\underline{coli}$ colonies were counted. All plate counts were performed in duplicate and only dilutions which yielded between 10 and 100 colonies per filter were used.

Inoculation of M. mercenaria with Bacteria. Unless otherwise specified, suspensions of the bacterial species were prepared by diluting cultures into artificial seawater (Rila Products, Teaneck, NJ) to densities of approximately 10^3 cells/ml. Specimens of $\underline{M}$. $\underline{mercenaria}$ were incubated in the bacterial suspensions for 2 hours (up to 40 specimens/5 liters of cell suspension) and then transferred to the depuration chamber.

The Depuration Chamber. A 50-gallon aquarium tank through which filtered U.V.-sterilized artificial seawater was flowing at a rate of approximately 1 liter/min was employed as the depuration chamber. U.V.-sterilization was accomplished by means of an ultraviolet sterilizer (Greenberg et al., 1982).

The Depuration Experiments. Specimens of $\underline{M}$. $\underline{mercenaria}$ which had been inoculated with bacteria as well as marked "control" specimens that had not been inoculated with bacteria were placed in the depuration chamber. At time intervals as indicated, subgroups consisting of three specimens were removed, shelled, and the remaining tissues were weighed and suspended in 100 ml of artificial seawater. The suspensions were homogenized in a Waring blender and dilutions of homogenates were prepared in artificial seawater for subsequent plate counts. Each data point is the average of the results of plate-counts on homogenates of two subgroups which had been removed from the depuration chamber at the same time. The number of cfu of each bacterial species in the control specimens of $\underline{M}$. $\underline{mercenaria}$ never exceeded 10% of the number detected in the inoculated specimens for any given time point.

The occurrence of Marine Vibrios In Situ. Samples of M. mercenaria and seawater were collected at various times throughout the year during low tide periods from two sites in Vineyard Sound, Massachusetts: Eel Pond, a polluted harbor that is closed to shellfishing due to fecal contamination; and Great Pond, an area open to shellfishing. Samples were returned to the laboratory and processed immediately. Seawater samples were plated directly and enumerated as described above. Specimens of M. mercenaria were processed as described above except that each data point represents the number of cfu from one group of three specimens only.

RESULTS

The Depuration Experiments. The number of E. coli cfu in specimens of M. mercenaria incubated at 25°C in the depuration chamber declined with time. A 6-hour incubation affected a greater than tenfold decrease and at 36 hours, E. coli could no longer be detected (Figure 1). These results are consistent with previous studies (Arcisz and Kelly 1955; Hartland 1978). The number of V. parahaemolyticus cfu and the number of V. harveyi cfu did not follow a similar pattern (Figure 1). While there was a decrease in the cfu of the vibrios within the first 6 hours of incubation, the numbers actually increased between 6 and 24 hours and detectable levels of these two marine organisms existed in the tissues of M. mercenaria for the duration of the experiment.

There exists a considerable body of evidence to indicate that temperature of incubation is an important parameter which can govern the survival of marine vibrios (Beuchat 1975). However, it is not clear if this is the case when the Vibrio cells are present as a part of the microbiota of marine animals. Thus, the effects of water temperature in the depuration chamber on the number of cfu of each bacterial strain in M. mercenaria were studied (Figure 2). The data are from three different experiments, one at each of the three temperatures. In each experiment all three of the bacterial species were monitored. Very little difference

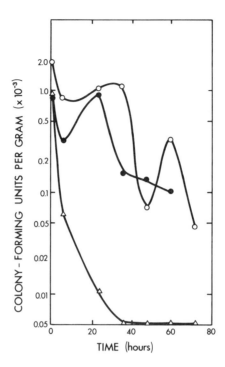

Figure 1. Persistence of V. parahaemolyticus (●), V. harveyi (○) and E. coli (△) in specimens of M. mercenaria incubated in the depuration chamber at 25°C.

in the persistence of a given bacterial species was observed over the range of temperatures employed. Both V. para-haemolyticus and V. harveyi persisted at considerable levels at all three temperatures while E. coli was rapidly elimi-nated.

Natural Populations of Presumptive V. parahaemolyticus and Luminous Vibrios in Seawater and in Specimens of M. mercenaria. A seasonal distribution of presumptive V. parahaemolyticus in specimens of M. mercenaria from the two sampling sites was observed (Figure 3A). This was consistent with a previous study concerning the distribution

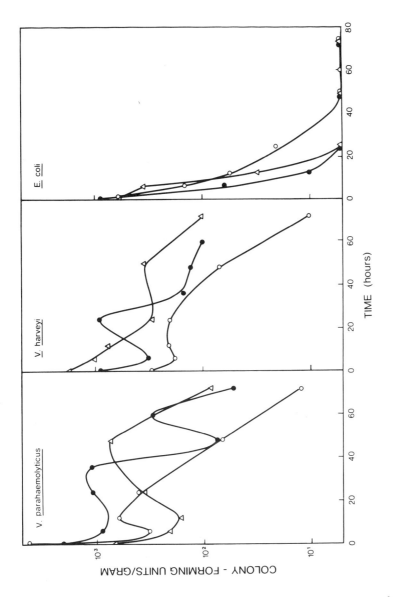

Figure 2. Relationship between incubation temperature and persistence of V. parahaemolyticus (A), V. harveyi (B) and E. coli (C) in M. mercenaria: 25°C (●), 15°C (○), and 8°C (△).

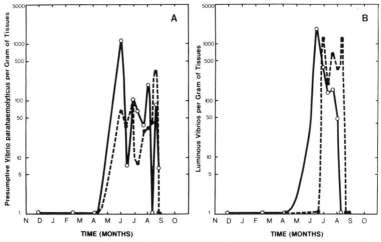

Figure 3. Seasonal distributions of (A) presumptive V. parahaemolyticus cfu and (B) cfu of luminous vibrios per gram of tissues in
specimens of M. mercenaria from Eel Pond (●---●) or Great Pond
(o—o).

of V. parahaemolyticus from various habitats in Chesapeake
Bay, Maryland (Kaneko and Colwell 1978). The organisms
were not detected until late spring, but they have been
found throughout the summer months, although there were
large fluctuations between results from one sampling point
to the next. Interestingly these data suggest that V.
parahaemolyticus does not necessarily occur at higher
population densities in M. mercenaria taken from the
polluted Eel Pond than from Great Pond. While this
suggests that the potential risk of parahaemolytic food
poisoning from clams obtained in polluted areas is no
greater than the risk from clams obtained from shellfishing
areas, the data are of a preliminary nature and a great
many questions remain unanswered. Most strains of V.
parahaemolyticus isolated from marine habitats are thought
to be nonpathogenic (Kudoh et al. 1974; Sakazaki et al.
1968) and the relationship between the occurrence of
pathogenic and nonpathogenic strains is not understood. It
may be that pathogenic strains are in greater abundance at
sewage-polluted sites than at other sites. We have not yet
addressed this question.

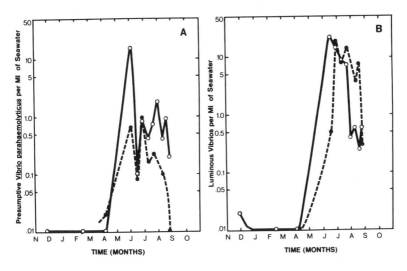

Figure 4. Seasonal distributions of (A) presumptive V. parahae-molyticus cfu and (B) cfu of luminous vibrios per ml of seawater from Eel Pond (●---●) or Great Pond (O—O).

A seasonal distribution of luminous vibrios in specimens of M. mercenaria similar to that of presumptive V. parahaemolyticus was observed (Figure 3B). Generally, the luminous vibrios detected were approximately tenfold more abundant than the presumptive V. parahaemolyticus detected although there were exceptions; for example, on June 13, luminous vibrios were not detected in tissues of M. mercenaria from Eel Pond (Figure 3).

Luminous vibrios and presumptive V. parahaemolyticus in seawater samples also showed a seasonal distribution (Figure 4) as has been reported elsewhere (Kaneko and Colwell 1978; Ruby et al. 1980; Ruby and Nealson 1977). The numbers detected of either taxon per ml of seawater were approximately 100-fold less than the numbers detected per gram of tissues from M. mercenaria and the day-to-day fluctuations were less erratic than the fluctuation in cfu from specimens of M. mercenaria.

Correlation Between Natural Abundances of Presumptive V. parahaemolyticus and Luminous Vibrios. The depuration experiments demonstrated that V. parahaemolyticus and

V. harveyi when fed to specimens of M. mercenaria, persisted to similar extents (Figures 1 and 2); that under the
conditions of the experiments there was a correlation
between the abundance of V. parahaemolyticus and of V.
harveyi. This was of interest since it suggested the
possibility that by monitoring the abundance of luminous
vibrios in natural samples, an indication of the presence or
abundance of V. parahaemolyticus could be obtained. This
would be of value since at present the identification of V.
parahaemolyticus from natural samples is costly and time
consuming (Food and Drug Administration 1976), while
identification of luminous vibrios is inexpensive and can be
accomplished in less than a day due to the rather unique
ability of these organisms to emit visible light (Ruby et al.
1980; Ruby and Nealson 1977). If natural populations of
these two groups of Vibrio showed a correlation it might be
possible to develop a test that could be used to provide
some indication of the levels of V. parahaemolyticus in the
environment.

At present, the data we have obtained regarding the
question of whether a correlation exists between abundances
of luminous vibrios and V. parahaemolyticus are of a preliminary nature. The fact that we have only presumptively
identified isolates as V. parahaemolyticus represents one
aspect of these preliminary data that needs to be addressed
by further investigation. Nevertheless, for each sample of
natural populations for each date, the log of the number of
luminous vibrio cfu was plotted against the log of the
number of presumptive V. parahaemolyticus cfu (Figure 5).
Clearly, the majority of points fall in clusters which
describe a straight line.

DISCUSSION

The results reported herein are consistent with the
conclusion that enteric bacteria such as E. coli are removed
from hardshell clams (M. mercenaria) under conditions of
artificial purification (Arcisz and Kelly 1955; Hartland 1978;
Houser 1964). However, we also present evidence that two
marine Vibrio species (V. harveyi, a luminous species; and

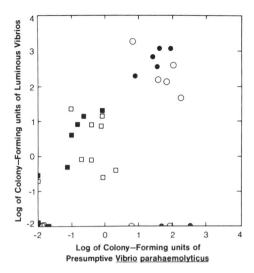

Figure 5. Relationship between cfu of presumptive V. parahaemoly-ticus and cfu of luminous vibrios. CFU per gram of tissues of M. mercenaria from Great Pond (O), per gram of tissues of M. mercenaria from Eel Pond (●), per ml of seawater from Great Pond (□), per ml of seawater from Eel Pond (■).

V. parahaemolyticus, a human pathogen) persist in speci-mens of M. mercenaria under a variety of conditions which result in elimination of E. coli (Figures 1 and 2). These data point to a possible health hazard associated with consumption of M. mercenaria fished legally from polluted areas and subjected to commercial purification procedures. This should not be taken to indicate that there is a greater risk of contracting a V. parahaemolyticus-associated disease from commercially depurated clams than from clams obtained in areas open to shellfishing. This would be true only if the occurrence of V. parahaemolyticus in clams from pol-luted areas open to shellfishing on a limited basis was greater than in clams from areas open to shellfishing. Preliminary investigations indicated that this is not neces-sarily the case (Figure 3).

At this time we have no evidence to indicate the loca-tion of the two Vibrio species within the host tissues.

Since these organisms are considered marine enteric bacteria (Baumann and Baumann 1977) it would seem possible that they were somehow associated with the digestive tract of M. mercenaria; however, elucidation of this point awaits experiments involving the dissection of specimens of M. mercenaria that have been inoculated with the Vibrio species. In performing the depuration experiments it was demonstrated that M. mercenaria will concentrate particles the size of bacteria and that once concentrated, the marine vibrios were capable of persisting within the host tissues for at least three days (Figures 1 and 2). We have also demonstrated that natural samples of M. mercenaria often contained levels of luminous vibrios and presumptive V. parahaemolyticus that were much higher than the levels found in the surrounding seawater (Figures 3 and 4). This could be due to the ability of M. mercenaria to concentrate these bacteria from seawater and for these bacteria to persist within the M. mercenaria or due to the ability of these bacteria to propagate within the invertebrate host or both.

Kaneko and Colwell (1978) found that there was a seasonal distribution of V. parahaemolyticus in Chesapeake Bay, Maryland. This bacterial species was found in greatest abundance during the summer months in seawater, on plankton, and in the sediment. In the winter, V. parahaemolyticus was only isolated from the sediments and relatively low numbers were detected. There was some information provided concerning the distribution of a subgroup of luminous vibrios. In most general terms this subgroup showed a similar distribution to V. parahaemolyticus but these luminous bacteria were detected in samples taken in the spring earlier than V. parahaemolyticus and they decreased in number earlier in the fall than V. parahaemolyticus. Ruby and Nealson (1977) observed a seasonal distribution of luminous vibrios in seawater samples from Mission Bay, California similar to the distribution of V. parahaemolyticus in Chesapeake Bay observed by Kaneko and Colwell (1978). We have initiated studies aimed at determining the relationship between natural populations of luminous vibrios and V. parahaemolyticus in seawater and in specimens of M. mercenaria (Figure 5). While these studies are incomplete they suggest a correlation between the abundance of these two bacterial taxa. If this is the case, enumeration of luminous vibrios could be used as an indication of contamination of seafoods with V. parahaemolyticus. However, it is clear that further investigations are required to establish the relationship between luminous vibrios and V. parahaemolyticus.

ACKNOWLEDGMENT

These investigations were supported by the New York State Sea Grant Institute.

REFERENCES

Arcisz, W., and C.B. Kelly. 1955. Self-purification of the soft clam Mya arenaria. Public Health Rep. 70:605-614.

Baumann, P., and L. Baumann. 1977. Biology of the marine enterobacteria: genera Beneckea and Photobacterium. Ann. Rev. Microbiol. 31:39-61.

Baumann, P., L. Baumann, and M. Mandel. 1971. Taxonomy of marine bacteria: the genus Beneckea. J. Bacteriol. 107:268-294.

Beuchat, L.R. 1975. Environmental factors affecting survival and growth of Vibrio parahaemolyticus. A review. J. Milk Food Technol. 38:476-480.

Beuchat, L.R. 1976. Parahaemolyticus food poisoning. Ga. Agric. Res. 18:17,18,22.

Food and Drug Administration. 1976. Bacteriological analytical manual for foods. Division of Microbiology, F.D.A. Washington, D.C.

Fujino, T., G. Sakaguchi, R. Sakazaki, and Y. Takada. (Eds.). 1974. International Symposium on Vibrio parahaemolyticus. Saikon Publishing Co., Tokyo.

Goatcher, L.J., S.E. Engler, D.C. Wagner, and D.C. Westhoff. 1974. Effect of storage at 5°C on survival of Vibrio parahaemolyticus in processed Maryland oysters (Crassostrea virginica). J. Milk Food Technol. 37:74-77.

Greenberg, E.P., M. DuBoise, and B. Palhof. 1982. The survival of marine vibrios in Mercenaria mercenaria, the hardshell clam. J. Food Safety. 4:113-123.

Hartland, B.J. 1978. Studies on antibacterial mechanisms in the American oyster, Crassostrea virginica, and the quahaug clam, Mercenaria mercenaria. M.S. Thesis, Cornell Univ., Ithaca, NY.

Houser, L.S. 1964. Depuration of shellfish. J. Environ. Health. 27:477-480.

Johnson, H.C., and J. Liston. 1973. Sensitivity of Vibrio parahaemolyticus to cold in oysters, fish fillets and crabmeat. J. Food Sci. 38:437-441.

Johnson, W.G., Jr., A.C. Salinger, and W.C. King. 1973. Survival of Vibrio parahaemolyticus in oyster shellstock at two different storage temperatures. Appl. Microbiol. 26:122-123.

Kaneko, T., and R.R. Colwell. 1978. The annual cycle of Vibrio parahaemolyticus in Chesapeake Bay. Microb. Ecol. 4:135-155.

Kudoh, Y., S. Sakai, H. Zen-Yoii, and R.A. LeClair. 1974. Epidemiology of food poisoning due to Vibrio parahaemolyticus in Tokyo during the last decade. Pages 9-14 in T. Fujino, G. Sataguchi, R. Sakazaki, and Y. Takeda (Eds.), International Symposium on Vibrio parahaemolyticus. Saikon Publishing Co. Tokyo.

Matches, J.R., J. Liston, and L.P. Daneault. 1971. Survival of Vibrio parahaemolyticus in fish homogenate during storage at low temperatures. Appl. Microbiol. 21:951-952.

Miwatani, T., and Y. Takeda. 1976. Vibrio parahaemolyticus, a causative bacterium in food poisoning. Saikon Publishing Co. Tokyo.

Oliver, J.D. 1981. Lethal cold stress of Vibrio vulnificus in oysters. Appl. Environ. Microbiol. 41:710-717.

Reichelt, J.L., and P. Baumann. 1973. Taxonomy of the marine luminous bacteria. Arch. Microbiol. 97:329-345.

Ruby, E.G., E.P. Greenberg, and J.W. Hastings. 1980. Planktonic luminous bacteria: species distribution in the water column. Appl. Environ. Microbiol. 39:302-305.

Ruby, E.G., and K.H. Nealson. 1977. Seasonal changes in the species composition of luminous bacteria in nearshore seawater. Limonol. Oceanogr. 23:530-533.

Sakazaki, R., K. Tamura, T. Kato, Y. Obara, S. Yamai, and K. Hobe. 1968. Studies on enteropathogenic, facultatively halophilic bacteria, Vibrio parahaemolyticus. III. Enteropathogenicity. Jpn. J. Med. Sci. Biol. 21:325-331.

Vanderzant, C., and R. Nickelson. 1972. Survival of Vibrio parahaemolyticus in shrimp tissue under various environmental conditions. Appl. Microbiol. 23:34-37.

Chapter 29

SURVEY OF VIBRIO ASSOCIATED WITH A NEW HAVEN HARBOR SHELLFISH BED, EMPHASIZING RECOVERY OF LARVAL OYSTER PATHOGENS

Stephen T. Tettelbach, Lisa M. Petti,
and Walter J. Blogoslawski

Advances in shellfish aquaculture techniques have led to the appearance of a greater number of hatcheries and an increased reliance upon the artificial propagation of shellfish "seed." An integral component in the development of such technology has been the increased awareness and routine monitoring of bacteria associated with hatchery operations. Certain species of Vibrio (V. anguillarum, V. alginolyticus) are known to be pathogenic to larval bivalve mollusks (Tubiash et al. 1965, 1970; Brown 1973; Tubiash 1975) and have been implicated in disease outbreaks at oyster hatcheries in different parts of the United States (Brown and Losee 1978; DiSalvo et al. 1978; Leibovitz 1979; Blogoslawski et al. 1981; Brown 1981; Elston et al. 1981).

While limited information exists on bacterial pathogens present in shellfish hatcheries (Murchelano et al. 1975; Leibovitz 1979), even less is known about the occurrence of these organisms in the natural environment. Colwell and Liston (1960; 1961) investigated the natural flora of the Pacific oyster, Crassostrea gigas, from the northwest United States. Lovelace et al. (1968) examined the bacteria present in water, mud, oyster (C. virginica) mantle fluid, and oyster gill tissue at two sites in Chesapeake Bay,

Maryland, and found a greater predominance of vibrios at the site where severe oyster mortalities were known to occur as compared to the more productive oyster ground. Murchelano and Brown (1970) enumerated the percentages of different genera and their relationship with season in a one-year study of the bacteria associated with a New Haven Harbor (Connecticut) oyster bed.

The purpose of this study was to obtain information about marine bacteria present at an oyster bed in New Haven Harbor over a two-year period (June 1979-June 1981). Major emphasis was placed on recovering larval oyster pathogens, in particular, those bacteria of the genus Vibrio.

MATERIALS AND METHODS

A natural oyster bed located approximately 185 meters NW (315° true) of the east end of the east breakwater in New Haven Harbor (41°14.4'N, 72°54.2'W) was chosen as the study site. Sampling of the surface and bottom waters and surficial sediments was conducted monthly during the period June 1979-June 1981, except during July and August when it was done semi-monthly. All sample and data collection was completed within one hour of the morning low tide (usually 0600-0900 hours) from the R/V Shang Wheeler.

In situ determination of the temperature and salinity of surface and bottom waters was conducted with a Yellow Springs Instrument Co. S-C-T meter. In situ dissolved oxygen measurements were taken with a YSI DO meter, while pH was determined on shipboard with an Orion portable pH meter or in the laboratory with a Beckman pH meter. Determination of in situ surface and bottom water parameters was conducted by suspending instrument probes at a point .25 m below the surface, and 1 m above the bottom, respectively.

Water and sediment samples for bacteriological analysis were collected as follows: Surface water was obtained by partially submerging a sterile bottle taped to a wooden stick; bottom water was obtained from a point 1 m above the bottom with a sterile Sieburth sampling bulb (Sieburth

1963) tripped by a messenger dropped along a steel cable. Surficial sediment was obtained via a modified gravity corer with an attached 50-ml sterile tube sealed with a sterile cork.

Three types of media were used to recover bacteria from the New Haven Harbor sampling site. Water and sediment were plated on Oppenheimer-ZoBell Reduced medium (OZR), which contained 0.1% yeast extract (Difco Labs., Detroit, MI), 0.1% Trypticase (BBL, Cockeysville, MD), and 1.0% agar (Difco) in 80% aged, 0.45-micron filtered seawater and 20% distilled water. OZR was employed to estimate the number of culturable heterotrophic marine bacteria. Thiosulfate citrate bile salts sucrose agar (TCBS; Difco) was prepared with distilled water according to the manufacturer's directions. Menhaden agar (Zapata Haynie Corp., Baltimore, MD), prepared from dried, 100% water-soluble Atlantic menhaden peptones, was dissolved in 80% aged, 0.45-micron filtered seawater and 20% distilled water. TCBS and menhaden agar were used to isolate potential shellfish pathogens.

Water and sediment samples were plated via the spread plate technique of Buck and Cleverdon (1960), using dilutions which varied in accordance with the type of medium used and the water temperature at the time of sample collection. Dilution ranges used for plating on the different media were as follows: OZR, 10^{-2}-10^{-6}; TCBS, 10^{-1}-10^{-2}; menhaden, 10^{-2}-10^{-3}. All samples were plated on board ship within 1 hour of collection. The plates were then returned to the laboratory, incubated at 15°C for one week, and the viable colonies counted.

Approximately 20-50 isolates were selected, depending on the color, morphology, and predominance of the bacterial colonies present, and the medium upon which colonies were found. Selection of isolates was predisposed toward those colonies which exhibited morphological characteristics similar to suspected or confirmed shellfish pathogens or toward those colonies which were unusual and/or which had not been selected previously.

Since TCBS is selective for vibrios and because these bacteria often produce yellow colonies on TCBS agar, this proved to be an ideal medium from which to isolate vibrios and, therefore, from which to recover potential shellfish pathogens.

Isolates selected from menhaden and OZR agar plates included those colonies which were brightly colored (e.g., yellow, orange, red, purple) and usually smooth, round, and convex; those which produced amorphous, spreading colonies, sometimes having a white to yellowish opalescent sheen; or those which were agarolytic. After isolates were selected and purified, they were either placed immediately into OZR broth cultures or on OZR slants and subsequently utilized in biochemical and/or larval oyster bioassay procedures. Six morphological and bacterial tests were conducted on each of the isolates: Gram stain, flagella stain, O/F, Tween 80, gelatin, and starch (Society of American Bacteriologists 1957; Leifson 1960; 1963), after which each of the isolates was identified to genus using the scheme presented by Murchelano and Brown (1970), which was adapted from Shewan et al. (1960).

The larval oyster bioassays were designed to test the pathogenicity of each of the isolates to freshly fertilized eggs of the American oyster, Crassostrea virginica. The initial step in the procedure was to inoculate OZR broth cultures and incubate them overnight (18-24 hours) at 26°C. Brood stock oysters, maintained at the Milford Laboratory, were induced to spawn by gradually raising the water temperature (Loosanoff and Davis 1963), and eggs were fertilized and counted. An inoculum of 15,000 freshly fertilized eggs was added to 1 liter of filtered, UV-treated seawater in glass beakers kept in a constant-temperature water table at 26°C as recommended by ASTM (1980). Subsequently, an appropriate inoculum of bacteria was added from the OZR broth cultures to attain an initial concentration of 10^2 to 10^4 cfu/ml in the challenge beakers. Cultures were maintained for 48 hours, which allowed ample time for normal development to the straight-hinge shelled veliger stage. Controls for the challenge beakers consisted of fertilized egg cultures to which 0.1 ml of sterile OZR broth was added, the inoculum volume being identical to that placed into the other beakers.

After 48 hours, samples were taken and the challenges terminated by sterilization. For the first five months, cultures were sampled by screening the entire culture through a 36-μm nylon mesh screen, resuspending the trapped larvae in 200 ml of filtered seawater, then collecting a 2-ml subsample, rinsing the pipet with 2 ml of seawater and preserving the sample with a few drops of 5% buffered formalin (Loosanoff and Davis 1963; Edwin Rhodes, personal communication, Milford Laboratory). For the following 19 months this procedure was replaced by that described by ASTM (1980), whereby a 10-ml sample was collected directly from each culture after thoroughly mixing with a perforated plunger; samples were preserved as described above and later examined with a compound microscope.

Larvae from challenge samples were counted and classified as normal or abnormal; normal larvae being those which were "D"-shaped, which is typical for straight-hinge, 48-hour oyster larvae; abnormal larvae being those which departed significantly from the "D" shape. Larvae were further classified as to whether they were alive or dead prior to fixing. Percent normal development in experimental cultures was computed relative to that in control cultures and those isolates which caused greater than 80% mortality were considered suspect and examined further.

RESULTS AND DISCUSSION

Salinity levels for the sampling period ranged from 16.7 to 28.5 parts per thousand (ppt) for surface water, and from 17.3 to 29.5 ppt for bottom water; pH values ranged from 7.3 to 8.4 for both surface and bottom waters. Temperature and dissolved oxygen (DO) levels for the two-year study ranged from -1.5° to 23.3°C, and 4.8 to 15.8 parts per million (ppm), respectively.

The plate counts for bacterial colonies present in bottom water and surficial sediment at the New Haven Harbor sampling site for June 1979-June 1981 are given in Figures 1 and 2, respectively. The total numbers of heterotrophic bacteria as given by the OZR plate counts ranged from 1.0×10^3 to 2.4×10^5 for bottom water and from 3.85×10^3 to 1.7×10^6 for sediment. The counts for the TCBS plates,

COMPARISON OF TOTAL PLATE COUNT

IN NEW HAVEN SEDIMENT.

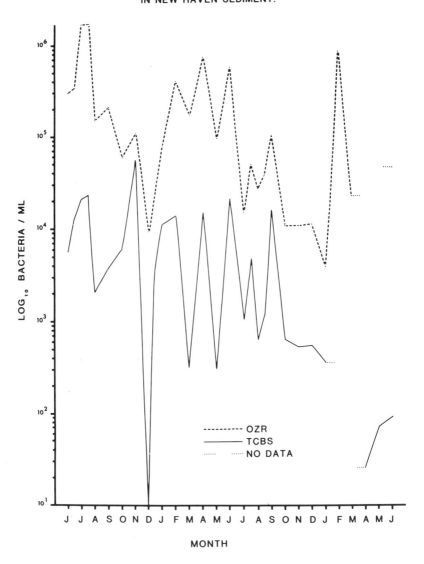

Figure 1. 24-month comparison of viable total-plate count using OZR versus TCBS media for New Haven Harbor surficial sediment.

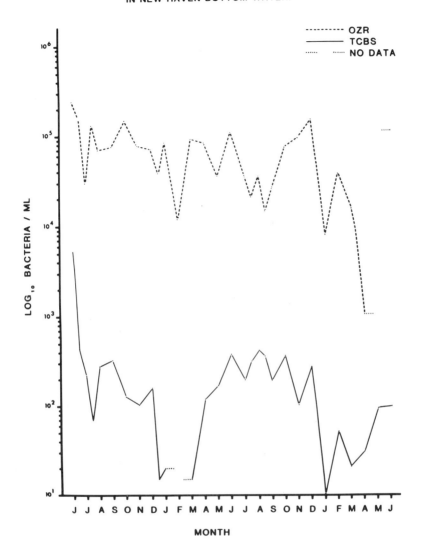

Figure 2. 24-month comparison of viable total-plate count using OZR versus TCBS media for New Haven Harbor bottom water.

which ranged from 1.0×10^1 to 5.3×10^5 for bottom water and from 1.0×10^1 to 5.5×10^4 for sediment, were lower than the OZR plate counts for each sample date, but roughly paralleled these counts. The menhaden plate counts (which are not graphed) ranged from 2.0×10^2 to 6.4×10^4 for bottom water and 1.25×10^2 to 4.25×10^5 for sediment over the period of February 20, 1980 to June 5, 1981 and exhibited no clearcut relationship to the OZR and TCBS data.

From a total of 35,172 bacterial colonies encountered during the two-year period, 366 isolates were selected for study. Of these isolates, 100 were Vibrio spp; other genera encountered included Flavobacterium, Pseudomonas, and Achromobacter. A breakdown of the numbers of isolates taken from different plates and the number of vibrios recovered is given in Table 1. As can be seen, the greatest percentage recovery of vibrios (numbers of vibrios isolated/numbers of isolates taken) based on our selection procedures was from TCBS plates. The next highest percentage recovery of vibrios was from menhaden plates, followed by OZR plates. The greatest percentage of vibrios isolated, regardless of the type of medium, was from sediment, followed by bottom water and surface water.

The morphological and color characteristics of the vibrios which were recovered generally agreed closely with those criteria used to select uncharacterized isolates. Several vibrios isolated from TCBS produced colonies which were not yellow, and ranged in color from cream to turquoise to dark green to brown. Overall, however, the percentage recovery of vibrios (100/366) or >27% seems to be fairly high, and this would tend to support the use of TCBS and the selection criteria which were employed. As a selective medium, TCBS agar has been used to isolate Vibrio parahaemolyticus from the marine environment (Baross and Liston 1970; Kaneko and Colwell 1973) and has also been employed to recover vibrios from water in a Long Island oyster hatchery while screening for larval pathogens (Leibovitz 1979). Menhaden agar was employed in this study because Vibrio anguillarum, which is reported to be responsible for mortalities of oyster larvae (Tubiash 1974; DiSalvo et al. 1978), is also known to be pathogenic to

Table 1. Isolates versus Media Used and Ratio of Vibrios Found versus Isolates Taken at a New Haven Station

| | OZR | | | Menhaden | | | TCBS | | | |
	Surface	Bottom	Sediment	Surface	Bottom	Sediment	Surface	Bottom	Sediment	Total
Number of isolates taken	68	48	93	9	6	14	9	60	59	366
Number of vibrios isolated	5	2	14	0	0	4	6	33	36	100
Percent recovery of vibrios	7.35	4.17	15.05	0	0	28.57	66.67	55.0	61.02	27.32

503

certain species of fish (Evelyn 1971; Egidius and Andersen 1977). On the basis of the number of vibrios recovered from this medium, menhaden agar does not appear to be selective for vibrios associated with shellfish beds.

Of the 100 vibrios isolated, only 1 was found to be pathogenic, causing approximately 82% mortality to oyster embryos at a concentration of 10^3 cells/ml when compared to controls. It is significant to note that 3 other non-Vibrio pathogens were isolated at New Haven, thus 4/366 or ~1% of the total number of isolates were pathogenic to oyster larvae.

While this study did not quantitatively assess seasonal changes in numbers of vibrios, the recovery of these bacteria did not appear to exhibit any apparent trend which might be related to the seasonal changes in temperature and dissolved oxygen. Other authors have demonstrated that greater numbers of vibrios are present in marine environments and shellfish when the water temperature is higher (Baross and Liston, 1970; Bartley and Slanetz 1971; Kaneko and Colwell 1973; Leibovitz 1979). It must be noted that some workers, however, have described a lack of seasonality to the distribution of vibrios in marine waters and shellfish (Sieburth 1967; Lovelace et al. 1968; Murchelano and Brown 1970).

Leibovitz (1979) demonstrated the importance of vibrios in causing disease of oyster larvae in hatcheries. He reported that the incidence of vibrios in influent waters was very high just prior to an epizootic within the facility; he therefore surmised that vibrios in the estuarine environment represent the greatest potential source of exposure to larval pathogens.

Lovelace et al. (1968), working in Chesapeake Bay, found that the level of vibrios present in an area of severe oyster mortalities was much higher than in a commercially productive oyster ground. This would seem to suggest the importance of vibrios in contributing to, or being involved in, mortalities of oysters in the natural environment.

Kaneko and Colwell (1973) found that while vibrios were not present in the water column of the Rhode River area of Chesapeake Bay during the winter, they were released from the sediment and attached to zooplankton in late spring and early summer, proliferating as the water temperature rose. They observed that the ecological role of Vibrio spp. was significant with respect to the population dynamics of zooplankton within Chesapeake Bay.

A very interesting study, which relates the ideas given by Lovelace et al. (1968), Kaneko and Colwell (1973), and Leibovitz (1979), is currently in progress (Petti, unpublished data). A natural oyster bed off Stratford, Connecticut, is being examined in an attempt to relate the high levels of vibrios and other bacterial pathogens found here to the historical lack of setting of oyster larvae in this area. Bacteriological analyses of oyster tissue and shell surfaces, as well as surface and bottom waters and surficial sediments, particularly at the time of natural oyster spawning, are being conducted toward this end.

Author's Note

Reference to trade names does not imply endorsement by the University of Connecticut or the National Marine Fisheries Service, NOAA.

ACKNOWLEDGMENTS

The authors are indebted to Elizabeth North Wikfors, Central Connecticut State College, New Britain, Connecticut, for the idea to initiate the study, and to Barry Nawoichik, Lynne Gilson, and Philip McDermott, Northeastern University, Boston, Massachusetts, for cruise assistance.

We appreciate the navigational skill and vessel operation of Captains Leroy Speer, Stephen Haynes, and Robert Alix, and are most grateful to Mr. John Baker, State of Connecticut Aquaculture Division, and Dr. James Hanks, Laboratory Director, Milford Laboratory, for providing vessel time.

Peter Pendoley, Schooner Inc., New Haven, Connecticut, collected additional site data from the sailing ketch, J.N. Carter. We thank Dr. Carolyn Brown for providing assistance in bacterial identification, Rita Riccio for editing and typing, and Dr. Rita Colwell, University of Maryland, College Park, Maryland, for providing technical review of the manuscript.

REFERENCES

American Society for Testing and Materials. 1980. Designation: E 724-80. Standard practice for conducting static acute toxicity tests with larvae of four species of bivalve molluscs. ASTM, Philadelphia, PA.

Baross, J., and J. Liston. 1970. Occurrence of Vibrio parahaemolyticus and related hemolytic vibrios in marine environments of Washington State. Appl. Microbiol. 20:179-186.

Bartley, C.H., and L.W. Slanetz. 1971. Occurrence of Vibrio parahaemolyticus in estuarine waters and oysters of New Hampshire. Appl. Microbiol. 21:965-966.

Blogoslawski, W.J., S.T. Tettelbach, L.M. Petti, and B.A. Nawoichik. 1981. Isolation, characterization, and control of a Vibrio sp. pathogenic to Crassostrea virginica and Ostrea edulis larvae. J. Shellfish Res. 1:109.

Brown, C. 1973. The effects of some selected bacteria on embryos and larvae of the American oyster, Crassostrea virginica. J. Invertebr. Pathol. 21:215-223.

Brown, C. 1981. A study of two shellfish-pathogenic Vibrio strains isolated from a Long Island hatchery during a recent outbreak of disease. J. Shellfish Res. 1:83-87.

Brown, C., and E. Losee. 1978. Observations on natural and induced epizootics of vibriosis in Crassostrea virginica larvae. J. Invertebr. Pathol. 31:41-47.

Buck, J.D., and R.C. Cleverdon. 1960. The spread plate as a method for the enumeration of marine bacteria. Limnol. Oceanogr. 5:78-80.

Colwell, R.R., and J. Liston. 1960. Bacteriological study of the natural flora of Pacific oysters (Crassostrea gigas). Appl. Microbiol. 8:104-109.

Colwell, R.R., and J. Liston. 1961. A bacteriological study of the natural flora of Pacific oysters (Crassostrea gigas) when transplanted to various areas in Washington. Proc. Nat. Shellfish. Assoc. 50:181-188.

DiSalvo, L.H., J. Blecka, and R. Zebal. 1978. Vibrio anguillarum and larval mortality in a California coastal shellfish hatchery. Appl. Environ. Microbiol. 35:219-221.

Egidius, E., and K. Andersen. 1977. Norwegian reference strains of Vibrio anguillarum. Aquaculture 10:215-219.

Elston, R., L. Leibovitz, D. Relyea, and J. Zatila. 1981. Diagnosis of vibriosis in a commercial oyster hatchery epizootic: diagnostic tools and management features. Aquaculture 24:53-62.

Evelyn, T.P.T. 1971. First records of vibriosis in Pacific salmon cultured in Canada, and taxonomic status of the responsible bacterium, Vibrio anguillarum. J. Fish. Res. Board Can. 28:517-525.

Kaneko, T., and R.R. Colwell. 1973. Ecology of Vibrio parahaemolyticus in Chesapeake Bay. J. Bacteriol. 113:24-32.

Leibovitz, L. 1979. A study of vibriosis at a Long Island shellfish hatchery. NYSG-RR-79-02, Sea Grant Reprint Series, Albany, New York.

Leifson, E. 1960. Atlas of bacterial flagellation. Academic Press, New York.

Leifson, E. 1963. Determination of carbohydrate metabolism of marine bacteria. J. Bacteriol. 85:1183-1184.

Loosanoff, V.L., and H.C. Davis. 1963. Rearing of bivalve mollusks. Pages 1-136 in F.S. Russell (Ed.), Advances in Marine Biology, Vol. 1. Academic Press, New York.

Lovelace, T.E., H. Tubiash, and R.R. Colwell. 1968. Quantitative and qualitative commensal bacterial flora of Crassostrea virginica in Chesapeake Bay. Proc. Nat. Shellfish Assoc. 58:82-87.

Murchelano, R.A., and C. Brown. 1970. Heterotrophic bacteria in Long Island Sound. Mar. Biol. 7:1-6.

Murchelano, R.A., C. Brown, and J. Bishop. 1975. Quantitative and qualitative studies of bacteria isolated from sea water used in the laboratory culture of the American oyster, Crassostrea virginica. J. Fish. Res. Board Can. 32:739-745.

Shewan, J.M., G. Hobbs, and W. Hodgkiss. 1960. A determinative scheme for the identification of certain genera of Gram-negative bacteria, with special reference to the Pseudomonadaceae. J. Appl. Bacteriol. 23:379-390.

Sieburth, J. McN. 1963. A simple form of the ZoBell bacteriological sampler for shallow water. Limnol. Oceanogr. 8:489-492.

Sieburth, J. McN. 1967. Seasonal selection of estuarine bacteria by water temperature. J. Exp. Mar. Biol. Ecol. 1:98-121.

Society of American Bacteriologists. 1957. Manual of Microbiological Methods. McGraw-Hill, New York.

Tubiash, H.S. 1974. Single and continuous exposure of the adult American oyster, Crassostrea virginica, to marine vibrios. Can. J. Microbiol. 20:513-517.

Tubiash, H.S. 1975. Bacterial pathogens associated with cultured bivalve mollusk larvae. Pages 61-71 in W.L. Smith and M.H. Chanley (Eds.), Culture of marine invertebrate animals. Plenum Press, New York.

Tubiash, H.S., P.E. Chanley, and E. Leifson. 1965. Bacillary necrosis, a disease of larval and juvenile bivalve mollusks. I. Etiology and epizootiology. J. Bacteriol. 90:1036-1044.

Tubiash, H.S., R.R. Colwell, and R. Sakazaki. 1970. Marine vibrios associated with bacillary necrosis, a disease of larval and juvenile bivalve mollusks. J. Bacteriol. 103:271-272.

Chapter 30

THE OCCURRENCE OF HALOPHILIC VIBRIOS
IN LOUISIANA COASTAL WATERS

Joan R. Barbay, Henry B. Bradford, Jr.,
and Nell C. Roberts

Louisiana coastal waters show a high incidence of Vibrio cholerae (Roberts et al., this volume). To determine distribution of the halophilic vibrios as well, most probable number (MPN) determinations were performed for Vibrio parahaemolyticus, Vibrio vulnificus (L+ vibrio) and Vibrio fluvialis (Group F vibrio). During 1980 and the first half of 1981, 17 environmental sites and three sewers were monitored for V. parahaemolyticus and V. vulnificus. Most of the sampling for V. fluvialis was done after October 1980. The sites yielded 1,164 isolates; 613 were identified as V. parahaemolyticus, 245 as V. vulnificus, and 306 as V. fluvialis.

The methodology is essentially that used by the Sea Grant teams of Oregon, Maryland, Florida, and Louisiana. A detailed description of methods is included in another chapter of this publication (Roberts and Seidler, this volume). The parameters for the presumptive identification of these organisms are listed in Table 1.

The V. parahaemolyticus strains follow the pattern listed. Of the strains scored as V. vulnificus, 98.8% were lactose-positive. All strains that were lactose-negative were ONPG-positive. These strains also varied in their ornithine decarboxylase activity with 86% of them positive. Strains

Table 1. Presumptive Parameters for the Identification of Vibrio parahaemolyticus, Vibrio vulnificus, and Vibrio fluvialis

Test	V. parahaemolyticus	V. vulnificus	V. fluvialis
Enrichment	Horie	Horie,BAP,APW	BAP,APW
TCBS	Green	Green	Yellow
TSI	K/A		
KIA		K/A	K/A
Gelatin 0% NaCl	-	-	-
3%	+	+	+
Oxidase	+	+	+
Lysine decarboxylase	+	+	-
Arginine dihydrolase	-	-	+
Ornithine decarboxylase	+	+	-
Indole	+	+	+ or -
ONPG	-	+	+
Sucrose	-	-	+
Arabinose	-	-	+ or -
Growth 0% NaCl	-	-	-
3%	+	+	+
7%	+	-	+
10%	-		
Simmons citrate	+	-	+ or -
0/129 Disk 150 µg			S
10 µg			R
Lactose		+ or -	

resembling V. fluvialis were the most difficult isolates to identify due to their biochemical diversity. Our isolates varied in their indole reaction, arabinose reaction, NaCl growth pattern, and in their sensitivity to the vibriostatic agent 0/129. The percentage of indole-positive strains was 67.3, and 94.3% of the strains were arabinose-positive.

Table 2 shows the variance in 0/129 and NaCl growth patterns. The confirmation or rejection of these deviant strains was determined by agglutination in known Group F antiserum or by having %G+C content consistent with known Group F organisms. Both the serology and genetic studies were performed in Dr. Seidler's laboratory in Oregon (R.J. Seidler, personal communication). Sensitivity to 0/129 separated the Louisiana isolates resembling V. fluvialis into three groups: those consistent with known V. fluvialis strains; those that were more resistant to 0/129; and those that were less resistant. Two of the strains with the typical 0/129 pattern did not agglutinate in known Group F antisera. These were scored as V. fluvialis due to their %G+C content. Strain 407 did not agglutinate in antisera, was only mildly sensitive to 0/129, and was capable of weak growth in 10% NaCl. However, its %G+C content was identical to four strains reported on by Jensen et al. (1980). Strains 317 through 386 were also only midly sensitive to 0/129 but they all agglutinated in known antisera. Again, we have one strain (379) capable of weak growth in the presence of 10% NaCl. Strains 56, 109, 78, and 132 are Oregon isolates included in this table because of their similarity to strains we first isolated in Louisiana waters and called HOG strains for halophilic, oxidase-positive, and gelatinase-positive. The Louisiana isolates resembling these were not scored as V. fluvialis due to base composition analysis of the Oregon strains.

Figure 1 shows the MPN range distribution of isolates presumptively identified as V. fluvialis in Louisiana. The upper figure is the lowest MPN for that station and the bottom figure is the highest MPN from that station. An "NI" indicates that no isolates were detected during the timespan of the study. Vibrio fluvialis was isolated across the state with the highest MPN coming from the Lafayette sewer. Of the 20 stations, 14 yielded isolates.

Table 2. Genetic and/or Serological Identity with Vibrio fluvialis

Strain	Max % NaCl[a]	O/129[b]			%G+C[c]	Agglutination[c]	Identified as V. fluvialis
		10 µg	50	150			
283	7	R	S	S	51.5	–	Yes
288	7	R	S	S	50.6	+	Yes
304	7	R	ND[d]	S	50.0	–	Yes
407	10	R	R	S	50.5	–	Yes
317	7	R	R	S	ND	+	Yes
370	7	R	R	S	ND	+	Yes
378	7	R	R	S	ND	+	Yes
379	10	R	R	S	ND	+	Yes
386	7	R	R	S	ND	+	Yes
56[e]	7	S	S	S	45.0	ND	No
109[e]	7	S	S	S	45.6	ND	No
78[e]	5	S	S	S	43.9	ND	No
132[e]	5	S	S	S	44.0	ND	NO

[a]Growth in maximum %NaCl.

[b]Sensitivity to O/129: S = sensitive, WS = weakly sensitive, R = resistant.

[c]Performed at Oregon State University.

[d]ND = not done.

[e]Oregon State University strains resembling Louisiana HOG (halophilic oxidase-positive, gelatinase-positive) strains.

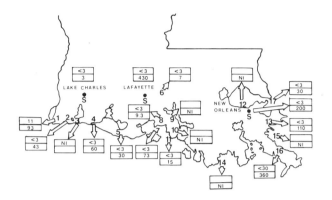

Figure 1. Presumptive Vibrio fluvialis distribution, Louisiana, 1980–1981. Collection stations are designated by number or the letter S for sewer. Arrows point to boxes containing the minimum and maximum most probable number per liter of water. NI indicates no isolates.

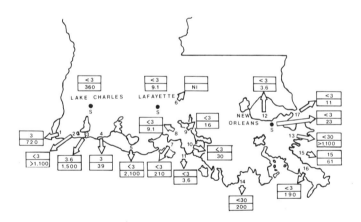

Figure 2. Vibrio parahaemolyticus distribution, Louisiana, 1980–1981. Collection stations are designated by number or the letter S for sewer. Values stated are minimal and maximum most probable numbers per liter of water. NI indicates no isolates.

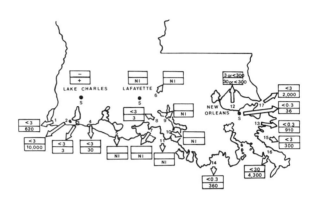

Figure 3. Presumptive Vibrio vulnificus distribution, Louisiana, 1980-1981. Collection stations are designated by number or the letter S for sewer. Values stated are minimum/maximum most probable number per liter of water. NI indicates no isolates.

Vibrio parahaemolyticus is the most widely distributed of the halophiles, being isolated from every station except Station 6 (Figure 2). Station 6 is a freshwater pond used for cultivation of crayfish. Water is supplied primarily from a bayou. Stations 1, 3, 4, and 15 were positive at all samplings. These 4 stations generally have high salinities except following extremely heavy rains and consequent fresh water runoff (Table 3). Stations 1, 2, 3, 5, and 13 had high MPN values.

Figure 3 shows the MPN distribution of isolates presumptively identified as V. vulnificus. This organism is readily detected in the western and eastern portions of the state but low or absent in the central portion. Of the 20 stations, 7 yielded no isolates and most of these cluster around the central coastal area. Salinities are low in the central area due to influx of fresh water from the Atachafalaya Basin (Table 3).

Table 4 depicts our findings on examining 56 market level seafood samples and 16 unprocessed seafood samples

Table 3. Physical Chemical Parameter Ranges for Louisiana Collection Stations

Station	Temperature C° Min.	Max.	Salinity ppt Min.	Max.	Dissolved Oxygen Min.	Max.	pH Min.	Max.
1	6	38	0.91	17.0	8.0	9.9	7.0	8.1
2	9	29	0.57	17.5	3.0	9.6	7.3	8.7
3	7	32	6.9	28.9	7.9	10.2	7.3	8.3
4	10	30	0.27	27.0	7.8	17.6	7.1	8.4
5	12	32	0.18	17.0	4.4	8.6	7.0	7.8
6	14	30	0.005	2.5	3.1	10.8	6.9	7.8
7	10	31	0.63	8.7	6.7	9.1	7.2	7.8
8	16	30	0.54	6.5	4.7	10.1	7.0	7.9
9	15	25	0.004	0.235	6.1	8.2	7.2	8.0
10	6.5	31	0.004	0.072	7.1	8.9	7.2	8.0
11	7	31	0.12	0.44	6.2	9.9	7.1	7.9
12	14	32	0.38	7.84	2.4	5.8	7.1	7.7
13	7	32	7.2	17.7	1.3	6.8	7.2	7.7
14	12	25	0.27	15.0	ND[a]	ND	7.3	8.0
15	ND	31	5.2	15.0	ND	ND	7.5	8.1
16	ND	ND	11.7	17.0	ND	ND	7.4	7.8
17	15	30	4.7	11.0	ND	ND	7.3	7.8

[a]ND = Not done

Table 4. Occurrence in Seafood of Vibrio parahaemolyticus, Vibrio vulnificus, and Vibrio fluvialis

Seafood Sampled	V. parahaemolyticus		V. vulnificus		V. fluvialis	
	Positive	Total	Positive	Total	Positive	Total
Market Level Products						
Crayfish	1	28	0	28	1	28
Crab	1	16	0	16	1	16
Shrimp	0	1	0	1	0	1
Oysters	4	11	4	11	1	11
Collected On Site						
Crab	5	9	3	10	1	9
Oyster	1	7	2	10		

from our collection site. Meat from not less than three crabs and/or oysters captured on site was aseptically removed from the exoskeleton and or shell of the animal, then pooled, blended, and examined. Market level samples were collected from wholesale processing plants as packed for distribution. Vibrio parahaemolyticus was found in 10.7% of the market level products, V. vulnificus in 7.7%, and V. fluvialis found in 5.4% of the market level products. The incidence of all three organisms was higher in the seafood collected on site, with 37.5% positive for V. parahaemolyticus, 25.0% positive for V. vulnificus, and 11.1% positive for V. fluvialis.

SUMMARY AND CONCLUSIONS

Vibrio parahaemolyticus, V. fluvialis, and V. vulnificus have been isolated from Louisiana coastal waters, seafood nurtured by these waters, and also rarely from market level seafood products. The distribution patterns of these halophilic vibrios indicate that these organisms are indigenous to Louisiana coastal waters. Further testing will be required to determine if these environmental vibrios are capable of causing the same diseases as the clinical isolates they resemble.

ACKNOWLEDGMENTS

We gratefully acknowledge the expert technical assistance of Connie Guillory, Kathy Johnson, Joyce Landor, Billie Monsour, Williard Mahfouz, Opal Hair, Susan Searl, Allen Hebert, Mike Purpera, James Gillispie, and Betty Planchard. A special thanks is also extended to Dr. Ramon Seidler, Dr. David Tison, and Mitsuaki Nishibuchi. This work was supported in part by National Oceanic and Atmospheric Administration Office of Sea Grant, Department of Commerce, under Grant NA79AA-D-00128.

REFERENCE

Jensen, J.J., P. Baumann, M. Mandel, and J.V. Lee. 1980. Characterization of facultatively anaerobic marine bacteria belonging to Group F of Lee, Donovan, and Furniss. Curr. Microbiol. 3:373-376.

Chapter 31

THE ROLE OF PLANKTONIC COPEPODS IN THE SURVIVAL AND MULTIPLICATION OF VIBRIO CHOLERAE IN THE AQUATIC ENVIRONMENT

Anwarul Huq, Eugene B. Small, Paul A. West
and Rita R. Colwell

Increasingly, evidence is accumulating that establishes pathogenic Vibrio species, including V. cholerae and V. parahaemolyticus, as naturally occurring members of the aquatic environment (Kaneko and Colwell 1978; Kaper et al. 1979; Blake et al. 1980b; Colwell et al. 1981).

Previous studies have demonstrated an association in aquatic environments between Vibrio spp. and a group of chitinous zooplankton, that is, copepods. The intimate link between zooplankton blooms and the seasonal cycle of V. parahaemolyticus in a tributary of Chesapeake Bay has been elucidated by Kaneko and Colwell (1975; 1978). In addition, Vibrio species are present in the gut of copepods and reflect the bacterial flora of the aquatic milieu in which the plankton live (Simidu et al. 1971; Sochard et al. 1979).

Cholera epidemics in Bangladesh occur at approximately the same time each year, especially when a significant change occurs affecting the aquatic environment. For example, when the monsoon ceases, increases in zooplankton, including copepods, have been recorded in the aquatic environments (A. Huq, unpublished data). Based on these records and observations and current study results, we hypothesized that there is a correlation between the

521

incidence of planktonic copepods and the distribution of $\underline{V}$. cholerae in the aquatic environment. We here report on experimental results to support the hypothesis.

MATERIALS AND METHODS

Experiments have been carried out using Chesapeake Bay water and copepods, as well as local freshwater and copepods from the Dacca, Bangladesh area.

Adult and immature copepods were collected by hand-trawl with a plankton net (#20, 77-μm mesh size) and washed by gently pouring 3 liters of filter-sterilized (0.22-μm) water, from the same collection site, over copepods retained on a metal filter in order to remove surface bacteria. A series of test flasks containing 500 ml of filter-sterilized water were prepared with: (1) live copepods, live bacteria, and live algae; (2) dead copepods and live bacteria; (3) live copepods and dead bacteria; (4) dead copepods and dead bacteria; (5) live algae and live bacteria; (6) live bacteria only. Flasks were incubated at ambient (22-27°C) temperature under static conditions. For experiments using $\underline{V}$. parahaemolyticus, the salinity of the water was adjusted to 30 ppt by addition of NaCl.

The bacterial strains used are listed in Table 1. Vibrio spp. were grown in bacto-peptone (Difco) 1% (w/v) and NaCl 1% (w/v) at pH 8.5. Other strains were cultured in trypticase (BBL) 1% (w/v) and NaCl 1% (w/v) at pH 7.2. For use, strains were grown statically for 12 hours at 30°C, washed twice in phosphate-buffered saline, and added to flasks to a final concentration of ca. 10^4 colony-forming units (cfu)/ml. Dead bacteria were obtained by placing washed cells in a water bath, set at 54°C, for 15 minutes. Death was indicated by the loss of cell motility in hanging drop preparations observed by light microscopy and the loss of ability to grow on Gelatin agar.

Copepods were killed by exposure for 30 minutes at -60°C. Death was indicated by a loss of motility and failure to regain motility during the incubation period of the experiment. The nonaxenic alga culture used to feed the

Table 1. Designation and Source of Bacterial Strains

Species	Strain Number	Source of Isolation
V. cholerae O1 Classical Inaba	CA 401	Clinical isolate from Calcutta, India (1953)
V. cholerae O1 El Tor Ogawa	D-18050	Environmental isolate from riverwater collected at Dacca, Bangladesh (1980)
V. cholerae non-O1	OSU 116	Environmental isolate from algae collected in Tillamook Bay, Oregon (1980)
V. parahaemolyticus	TK 18136	Environmental isolate from river water collected at Teknaf, Bangladesh (1980)
E. coli	E/C744	Environmental isolate from river water collected at Dacca, Bangladesh (1980)
Pseudomonas sp.	PS 11361	Clinical isolate obtained from the ICDDR, B hospital, Dacca, Bangladesh (1981)

copepods was Pseudoisocrysis sp. Copepods were added to flasks to a concentration of ca. 1 copepod/ml water.

For enumeration of each strain, 5 copepods in 2 ml of flask water were homogenized in a tissue grinder. This method counted the bacteria adhering to copepods as well as the bacteria free-living in the flask water. After appropriate decimal dilutions in phosphate-buffered saline, 0.1-ml aliquots were spread onto duplicate agar plates.

Thiosulphate citrate bile salts sucrose (TCBS) agar (BBL) was used to enumerate V. cholerae and V. parahaemolyticus. MacConkey agar (Difco) and Mueller-Hinton agar (Oxoid) were used for E. coli and Pseudomonas sp., respectively.

Representative specimens of intact copepods were randomly selected, removed from the flask, and fixed with Bouin's solution (Baker 1958). Samples were prepared for scanning electron microscopy by the osmium tetroxide-mercuric chloride staining procedure, described by Maugel et al. (1980), and examined under the microscope at an accelerating voltage of 20KV or 30KV.

RESULTS AND DISCUSSION

Strains of V. cholerae in Chesapeake Bay water (salinities 2 ppt, 15 ppt, and 22 ppt), as well as Bangladesh water (salinity 0.2 ppt), demonstrated multiplication to higher numbers when grown in association with live, rather than dead, copepods (Table 2). In addition, V. cholerae survived significantly longer in flasks containing live copepods, compared with V. cholerae inoculated into flasks containing dead copepods. Figure 1 illustrates this phenomenon, showing results for V. cholerae CA 401 in water collected from the Patuxent River, Chesapeake Bay (salinity 2 ppt). The initial count of V. cholerae in all flasks was ca. 10^4 cells per ml, increasing over a 36-hour period to ca. 10^8 cells/ml, in the presence of live copepods, but only to ca. 10^6 cells/ml in flasks containing dead copepods.

Cells were recovered on TCBS agar, that is, survived, up to 14 days when grown in association with live copepods, compared to 6 days in flasks with dead copepods. Among flasks containing viable copepods at the start of the experiment, all of the copepods were dead at 14 days. An interesting observation was that copepods began to die off after incubation for 36 hours, that is, at approximately the same time at which V. cholerae plate counts also began to decrease. Furthermore, the plate count results indicated that the algae culture itself, which was used to feed the live copepods, could not account for the extended survival

Table 2. Influence of the Presence of Live Copepods on the Multiplication of *Vibrio cholerae* in Waters from Chesapeake Bay and Dacca, Bangladesh

Site	Salinity (ppt)	Test Strain	Copepods Present	cfu/ml Initial Count	cfu/ml Maximum Count
Patuxent River	15.0	OSU 116	live	5.70×10^3	9.61×10^6
			dead	5.60×10^3	1.90×10^5
Patuxent River	22.0	CA 401	live	1.15×10^5	3.10×10^7
			dead	9.00×10^4	3.15×10^6
Buriganga River	0.2	D-18050	live	2.39×10^3	7.91×10^5
			dead	6.30×10^3	2.81×10^4

525

of V. cholerae in these systems (Figure 1). Thus, a striking relationship exists between extended survival of V. cholerae in natural water samples and the presence of live copepods.

Other strains tested for incubation periods up to 36 hours did not show a similar trend. V. parahaemolyticus demonstrated approximately one log increase in number in the presence of live copepods alone. The Pseudomonas sp. increased in population size in the presence of both live and dead copepods. However, results obtained for control, with and without copepods, indicated that these increases were not copepod-associated. Counts of E. coli were higher in the presence of dead copepods compared with live copepods.

Examination by scanning electron microscopy revealed that washing freshly caught, live copepods with filter-sterilized water effectively removed virtually all bacteria attached to the copepod surface. Exhaustive examination of copepod surfaces, especially carapace, oral region, and egg sac, failed to reveal the presence of bacteria after washing. On rare occasions, single cells or small clusters of cells were observed around clefts between copepod body parts and these were not considered significant.

All strains of V. cholerae showed extensive attachment to the external surface of live copepods, in addition to a rapid rate of multiplication when grown in association with live copepods contained in Bangladesh and Chesapeake Bay waters. Figures 2 to 4 illustrate this phenomenon with the attachment of live test strain V. cholerae CA 401 when exposed to copepods in water samples collected from the Patuxent River for 36 hours at ambient temperature. Cells were found to concentrate on live copepod surfaces at and around the oral region (Figure 2) as well as on the egg sac surface (Figure 3). At higher magnification, some of the cells covering the egg sac were observed to be undergoing division (Figure 4).

Live copepods incubated with E. coli remained free of attached cells. Very few cells were observed to be attached to the copepod surface when Pseudomonas sp. was used. Many V. parahaemolyticus cells were attached to the

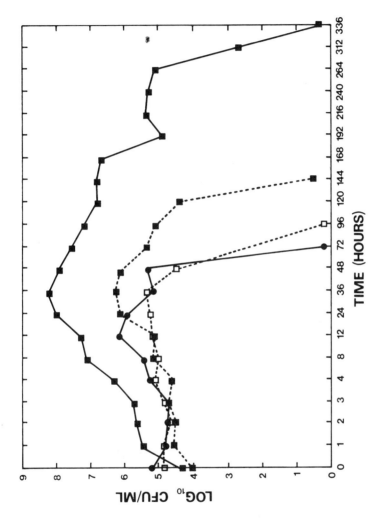

Figure 1. Growth of Vibrio cholerae CA 401 in flasks of Patuxent River water (□---□), and in the presence of live copepods and algae (■——■), dead copepods (■---■), and algae only (●——●).

527

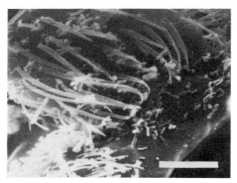

Figure 2. Colonization of a copepod oral region after incubation for 36 hours in Patuxent River water and Vibrio cholerae CA 401. Bar = 10μm.

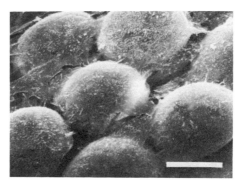

Figure 3. Colonization of a copepod egg sac after incubation for 36 hours in Patuxent River water and Vibrio cholerae CA 401. Bar = 50μm.

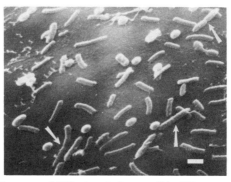

Figure 4. Attachment of Vibrio cholerae CA 401 to a copepod egg sac surface and the presence of dividing cells (arrows). Bar = 1μm.

copepod surface, but not selectively, since the surface appeared evenly covered with bacteria.

Results of survival experiments carried out using flasks of natural water samples, as well as of scanning electron microscopy observations, clearly established a significant association between V. cholerae and copepods, a major component of the zooplankton population in natural waters. The association thus provides further insight into the ecological relationships of V. cholerae in aquatic environment, as well as the epidemiology of cholera.

The specific sites of attachment of V. cholerae on the copepod surface are the oral region and egg sac. Attachment to surfaces at and around the oral region is probably best explained as associated with ingestion of the vibrios as a food source. The study of Sochard et al. (1979) demonstrated that the likely source of vibrios in the copepod gut was the external aquatic environment. Taken into the gut, V. cholerae may be capable of multiplication, subsequently being released into the aquatic environment via fecal pellets and thereby allowing an excellent opportunity for redistribution in the environment (Turner 1979). The specificity of attachment of V. cholerae to the female copepod egg sac may also be important since most planktonic copepods spawn fertilized eggs freely into the water (Sverdrup et al. 1947), thus providing a suitable vehicle for dissemination of V. cholerae. It is not clear why bacteria, other than vibrios, do not concentrate in association with live copepods, under the same experimental conditions. The electrical charge on the waxy layer, the epicuticle, covering copepod surfaces has been suggested previously as a factor limiting attachment (Kaneko and Colwell 1975).

Some implications of these experimental data for the epidemiology of cholera in endemic and nonendemic global areas can now be hypothesized. Every year in Bangladesh there is an epidemic of cholera, commencing around September or October. According to Oppenheimer et al. (1978), zooplankton populations decrease during the monsoon season because of low nutrient conditions; then increase significantly during August and September once the post-monsoon phytoplankton blooms have occurred. The increase in zooplankton populations in the aquatic environment is invariably followed by the appearance of epidemic cholera in Bangladesh. If colonization of copepods with V. cholerae is an important mechanism for distribution of the organism and spreading of the disease, then it is likely that when copepods become abundant, V. cholerae will also become abundant in the environment. The environmental factors and cultural habits of the human population which may effect transfer of V. cholerae from natural waters to the human intestine--and subsequent initiation of epidemic cholera--are not known.

An important question still remains, and that is why V. cholerae serovar O1 is not readily isolated from the aquatic environment during the inter-epidemic periods in Bangladesh. A possible answer may derive from the findings of Singleton et al. (1982), who have demonstrated a nonculturable state into which V. cholerae can enter, yet remain viable and capable of growth, as determined by the nalidixic acid-yeast extract method of Kogure et al. (1979). That is, viable and metabolizing cells were observed by epifluorescence microscopy, but were not culturable on Tryptic Soy Agar (Difco).

Thus, it is possible that V. cholerae cells are present, even during the inter-epidemic monsoon season, when there is significant alteration of the nutritional conditions in the aquatic environment. At such times, the cells themselves may also be altered, that is, under stress and being rendered nonculturable by existing bacteriological plating and/or enrichment methods. During this period, copepods may serve as a reservoir for V. cholerae, allowing multiplication at a later time, when more favorable conditions for growth of the organism occurs in the environment.

Experimentation to illustrate attachment of V. cholerae to copepods, as well as demonstration of the nonculturable state of V. cholerae, have been performed in flask experiments carried out in the laboratory. Although the composition of the aquatic environment can be controlled in such experiments, natural variations in temperature, salinity, oxygen, and nutrient concentrations in the water cannot be considered to be completely replicated in these closed systems. A method suitable for confirming observations made in vitro would be to examine copepods for

V. cholerae immediately after removal from the natural
aquatic environment. Field studies using fluorescent-
antibody detection methods for V. cholerae serovar Ol are
in progress (H.-S. Xu, N.C. Roberts, and R.R. Colwell,
unpublished data).

The epidemic type of cholera has been absent from the
United States for several decades. A recent outbreak,
confined to 11 victims, was reported in Louisiana in 1978
and followed the consumption of improperly cooked crabs,
which had been caught locally (Blake et al. 1980a). Crabs
do not feed directly on zooplankton, but ingestion can
occur as water or the intestinal contents of copepod-feeding
small fish passes through the crab gut. The possibility
that V. cholerae can attach to, and multiply in, the crab
gut requires investigation, since the ecological data suggest
a strong association between the presence of V. cholerae in
the water column and in crab gut contents (Roberts et al.,
this volume). An association between V. cholerae and
copepods, therefore, may assume significance in American
as well as Bangladesh waters.

In contrast, oysters are filter-feeding molluscs which
consume copepods (Churchill 1919). If live copepods are
colonized extensively with V. cholerae in the natural aquatic
environment, then oysters will concentrate V. cholerae in
their tissues. The isolation of V. cholerae serovar Ol from
oysters harvested in a Florida estuary has been previously
reported (Hood et al. 1981).

The counts of free-living V. cholerae in the water
column are typically at least three or four logs less in
number than required to induce cholera in normochloro-
hydric humans (Cash et al. 1974), implying that the
numbers of V. cholerae must increase sufficiently to become
an infective dose before contact with a susceptible human
host occurs. Often, the improper handling of seafood,
contaminated with V. cholerae, provides the opportunity for
multiplication leading to the required infective dose, a
feature of the Louisiana cholera outbreak (Blake et al.
1980a). It is feasible that such increases in number may
also occur in the aquatic environment. The initial concentration of the organism may occur on the copepod and
zooplankton surface and, subsequently, in either crabs or

oysters. Data from studies reported in this volume indicate that counts of V. cholerae in crab and oyster material are generally higher than would be predicted by counts of the organism in the water column. Thus, a concentration process is suggested.

CONCLUSIONS

We conclude that adhesion of cells of V. cholerae onto the surfaces of live copepods may contribute significantly to the survival and distribution of V. cholerae in the aquatic environment. Furthermore, colonization of copepods with V. cholerae may represent the first stage in concentration of cells toward the population size needed to constitute an infective dose to initiate the disease in a human population. It is also suggested that zooplankton samples, as well as water samples, be cultured during an ecological survey for V. cholerae in the aquatic environment.

ACKNOWLEDGMENTS

This work was sponsored, in part, by World Health Organization grant C6/181/70, NIH grant 5R22AI 14242, NSF grant DEB-77-14646, NOAA grant NA81AA-D-00040. We thank Mr. T. Maugel, Mr. D. Brownlee, and Dr. D. Bonar for their advice and assistance during this study.

REFERENCES

Baker, J.R. 1958. Principles of biological micro-techniques. John Wiley, New York.

Blake, P.A., D.T. Allegra, J.D. Snyder, T.J. Barrett, L. McFarland, C.T. Caraway, J.C. Feeley, J.P. Craig, J.V. Lee, N.D. Puhr, and R.A. Feldman. 1980a. Cholera--a possible endemic focus in the United States. N. Engl. J. Med. 302:305-309.

Blake, P.A., R.E. Weaver and D.C. Hollis. 1980b. Diseases of humans (other than cholera) caused by vibrios. Ann. Rev. Microbiol. 34:341-367.

Cash, R.A., S.I. Music, J.P. Libonati, M.J. Snyder, R.P. Wenzel, and R.B. Hornick. 1974. Response of man to infection with Vibrio cholerae. I. Clinical, serologic and bacteriologic responses to a known inoculum. J. Infect. Dis. 129:45-52.

Churchill, E.P. 1919. The oysters and the oyster industry of the Atlantic and Gulf coasts. U.S. Department of Commerce. Bureau of Fisheries Document No. 890, Washington, D.C.

Colwell, R.R., R.J. Seidler, J. Kaper, S.W. Joseph, S. Garges, H. Lockman, D. Maneval, H.B. Bradford, N. Roberts, E. Remmers, I. Huq, and A. Huq. 1981. Occurrence of Vibrio cholerae serotype O1 in Maryland and Louisiana estuaries. Appl. Environ. Microbiol. 41:555-558.

Hood, M.A., G.F. Ness, and G.E. Rodrick. 1981. Isolation of Vibrio cholerae serotype O1 from the eastern oyster Crassostrea virginica. Appl. Environ. Microbiol. 41:559-560.

Kaneko, T., and R.R. Colwell. 1975. Adsorption of Vibrio parahaemolyticus onto chitin and copepods. Appl. Microbiol. 29:269-274.

Kaneko, T., and R.R. Colwell. 1978. The annual cycle of Vibrio parahaemolyticus in Chesapeake Bay. Microb. Ecol. 4:135-155.

Kaper, J., H. Lockman, R.R. Colwell, and S.W. Joseph. 1979. Ecology, serology and enterotoxin production of Vibrio cholerae in Chesapeake Bay. Appl. Environ. Microbiol. 37:91-103.

Kogure, K., U. Simidu, and N. Taga. 1979. A tentative direct microscopic method for counting living marine bacteria. Can. J. Micro. 25:415-420.

Maugel, T.K., D.B. Bonar, W.J. Creegan, and E.B. Small. 1980. Specimen preparation techniques for aquatic organisms. Pages 57-78. Scan. Elect. Microscop. II, SEM, Inc., AMF O-Hare, Chicago, IL.

Oppenheimer, J.R., M.G. Ahmad, A. Huq, K.A. Haque, A.K.M.A. Alam, K.M.S. Aziz, S. Ali, and A.S.M. Haque. 1978. Limnological studies of three ponds in Dacca, Bangladesh. Bangladesh J. of Fisheries 1:1-28.

Simidu, U., K. Ashino, and E. Kaneko. 1971. Bacterial flora of phyto- and zooplankton in the inshore water of Japan. Can. J. Micro. 17:1157-1160.

Singleton, F.L., R.W. Attwell, M.S. Jangi, and R.R. Colwell. 1982. Influence of salinity and nutrient concentration on survival and growth of Vibrio cholerae in aquatic microcosms. Appl. Environ. Microbiol. 43:1080-1085.

Sochard, M.R., D.F. Wilson, B. Austin and R.R. Colwell. 1979. Bacteria associated with the surface and the gut of marine copepods. Appl. Environ. Microbiol. 37:750-759.

Sverdrup, H.V., M.W. Johnson and R.H. Fleming. 1947. The oceans. Prentice-Hall Inc., Englewood Cliffs, NJ.

Turner, J.T. 1979. Microbial attachment to copepod fecal pellets and its possible ecological significance. Trans. Am. Microscop. Soc. 98:131-135.

Chapter 32

EFFECTS OF SURFACE ASSOCIATION AND OSMOLARITY ON SEAWATER MICROCOSM POPULATIONS OF AN ENVIRONMENTAL ISOLATE OF VIBRIO CHOLERAE

M.T. MacDonell, R.M. Baker, F.L. Singleton
and M.A. Hood

Vibrio cholerae has been isolated from a number of diverse aquatic systems, including the brackish waters of the Mississippi River delta and estuaries along the coast of the Gulf of Mexico and the Atlantic Coast (Kaper et al. 1979; Colwell et al. 1981; Hood et al. 1981; Roberts et al., this volume). In order to account for its apparently ubiquitous distribution in brackish and estuarine waters and the apparent lack of correlation between V. cholerae and fecal indicators, it was hypothesized that V. cholerae is a member of the autochthonous estuarine bacterial community (Kaper et al. 1979). Recent studies on the effects of varying environmental parameters on the growth and survival of V. cholerae have supported this hypothesis.

V. cholerae has been shown to survive for extended periods of time in natural estuarine waters (Hood and Ness 1982), brackish water ditches (West and Lee, this volume), and artificial marine salts solutions (Singleton et al. 1982a; b). In the studies by Hood and Ness (1982) and by Singleton et al. (1982a; b), the growth and survival of V. cholerae strains were examined using closed microcosms, as difficulties exist with the study of a specific population of microorganisms in situ, especially in a tidal estuary where organisms encounter constantly changing environmental conditions.

Enhanced survival of some microorganisms in an aquatic environment may be a function of association with surfaces due to the establishment of a more favorable microenvironment (Marshall 1976). Therefore, associations with various artificial surfaces in studies using natural seawater microcosms may indicate affinities for association of microorganisms with surfaces in the natural environment.

Since these closed systems have certain limitations, it was also the purpose of our study to examine some of the factors inherent within the methodology which may influence recovery of V. cholerae from laboratory microcosms. These include the effects of osmotic pressure as well as association with the glass walls of the microcosm.

The Microcosms

Microcosms consisted of 50 ml of natural seawater (salinity = 24 ppt) collected from Pensacola Bay and added to acid-cleaned 125-ml Erlenmeyer flasks. In some experiments the seawater was filtered through 0.2-μm filters (Nucleopore Corp., Pleasanton, CA) to remove any particulate materials prior to autoclaving. Autoclaving was carried out for 15 minutes at 121°C. The microcosms were allowed to adapt to ambient conditions for 24 hours, inoculated with selected cell concentrations of V. cholerae, and incubated for the appropriate periods at ambient temperature, ca. 22°C.

V. cholerae strain WF 110, an environmental isolate (LSU serovar BB) in two physiological states, was employed. Nutrient-enriched cells consisted of a preparation in which the cells were harvested by centrifugation from an 18-hour Brain Heart Infusion broth culture (Difco Laboratories, Detroit, MI) and washed three times in artificial marine salts (Instant Ocean; Aquarium Systems, Mentor, OH). The cells were resuspended in a marine salts solution and this suspension was used as the inoculum. Nutrient-deprived cells were prepared by maintaining cells for a

period of 35 days in an unsupplemented marine salts solution (salinity = 20 ppt), and this solution was used directly
as the inoculum.

Enumeration of V. cholerae from the microcosms was
performed using the spread plate method. All culture
plates were incubated for 24 hours prior to counting total
colony-forming units (cfu).

Effect of Osmolarity

The effect of osmotic pressure of the dilution blanks
and plating media was first examined. Culturable counts
from the microcosms inoculated with both nutrient-enriched
and nutrient-deprived cells were determined using three
methods. The first, representing the standard procedure,
consisted of osmotically imbalanced dilution blanks (0.9%
NaCl; osmolarity = 220 mOsm/l) and culture medium (Brain
Heart Infusion agar, Difco; osmolarity = 330 mOsm/l). The
other two enumeration procedures employed dilution blanks
and plating medium adjusted electrolytically and non-
electrolytically to the osmolarity of the microcosms (525
mOsm/l). These consisted of dilution blanks of marine
salts (electrolyte) and a sucrose solution (nonelectrolyte).
The plating medium was likewise adjusted with marine salts
or sucrose to 525 mOsm/l.

When nutrient-enriched cells were examined, no significant effect ($p < 0.05$) was observed in culturable counts
from either the osmotically balanced or imbalanced protocols
(Table 1). However, there was a marked effect, attributable to osmotic pressure changes, on nutrient-deprived V.
cholerae cells (Table 2). Culturable counts at 1, 2, and 3
hours after inoculation were significantly smaller ($p < 0.05$)
using the unbalanced protocol than with either of the
osmotically balanced protocols. This effect was not detected
beyond the 3-hour sampling, which probably corresponds to
onset of the growth phase. These results suggest that V.
cholerae cells which are subjected to long-term nutrient
deprivation are more sensitive to osmotic pressure changes
than are nonstressed cells.

Table 1. Plating Medium and Diluent Osmolarity Effects on Culturable Counts of <u>Vibrio</u> <u>cholerae</u>[a]

Hours After Inoculation	Balanced Osmotically[b] (marine salts)	Balanced Osmotically[b] (sucrose)	Imbalanced Osmotically[c]
0	1.96×10^4	2.10×10^4 ($\Delta\% = 7.1$)	1.92×10^4 ($\Delta\% = -2.0$)
1	1.9×10^4	1.87×10^4 ($\Delta\% = -2.1$)	1.84×10^4 ($\Delta\% = -3.7$)
2	2.09×10^4	2.03×10^4 ($\Delta\% = -2.9$)	2.06×10^4 ($\Delta\% = -1.4$)
3	3.10×10^4	2.97×10^4 ($\Delta\% = -4.2$)	3.03×10^4 ($\Delta\% = -2.3$)
6	1.21×10^5	1.30×10^5 ($\Delta\% = 7.4$)	1.25×10^5 ($\Delta\% = 3.3$)
12	1.76×10^5	1.72×10^5 ($\Delta\% = -2.3$)	1.81×10^5 ($\Delta\% = 2.8$)
24	1.64×10^6	1.68×10^6 ($\Delta\% = 2.4$)	1.56×10^6 ($\Delta\% = -4.9$)

[a]Strain WF 110, 18 hour growth in BHI broth prior to inoculation.
[b]525 mOsm/liter.
[c]Diluent: 220 mOsm/liter; medium: 330 mOsm/liter.

Table 2. Plating Medium and Diluent Osmolarity Effects on Culturable Counts of Vibrio cholerae[a]

Hours After Inoculation	Balanced Osmotically[b] (marine salts)	Balanced Osmotically[b] (sucrose)	Imbalanced Osmotically[c]
0	1.38×10^4	1.34×10^4 ($\Delta\% = -2.9$)	1.42×10^4 ($\Delta\% = 2.9$)
1	1.79×10^4	1.90×10^4 ($\Delta\% = 6.1$)	1.40×10^4 ($\Delta\% = -21.8$)
2	2.44×10^4	2.25×10^4 ($\Delta\% = -7.8$)	1.31×10^4 ($\Delta\% = -46.3$)
3	2.62×10^4	2.42×10^4 ($\Delta\% = -7.6$)	1.51×10^4 ($\Delta\% = -42.4$)
6	5.30×10^4	5.60×10^4 ($\Delta\% = 5.7$)	5.45×10^4 ($\Delta\% = 2.8$)
12	2.71×10^5	2.73×10^5 ($\Delta\% = <1.0$)	2.83×10^5 ($\Delta\% = 4.4$)
24	2.36×10^6	2.58×10^6 ($\Delta\% = 9.3$)	2.45×10^6 ($\Delta\% = 3.8$)

[a]Strain WF 110 maintained in 20 ppt marine salts for 35 days.
[b]525 mOsm/liter.
[c]Diluent: 220 mOsm/liter; medium: 330 mOsm/liter.

Surface Associations

Particulate Materials. In preliminary experiments it was noted that in microcosms prepared with unfiltered seawater the maximum population size obtained by V. cholerae was consistently twofold less than that obtained in 0.2-µ-filtered seawater microcosms (unpublished results). This was interpreted to reflect the association of organisms with particulate materials and would, therefore, increase the spatial heterogeneity of the population, since different numbers of cells could be expected to be associated with the particles, which affected the observed bacterial counts, that is, one colony ≠ one cell.

Association with $CaCO_3$. The interaction of V. cholerae and inert surfaces was first examined using $CaCO_3$. Nutrient-deprived cells were added to microcosms, incubated for 24 hours at 22°C, and the number of recoverable cells determined before and 10 minutes after the addition of 10 g sterile $CaCO_3$. The results listed in Table 3 show that the addition of $CaCO_3$ resulted in a decrease (of approximately 50%) in cell numbers; that is, 50% of the cells became particle-associated and 50% remained in the planktonic fraction. Samples of both the planktonic cells and those adhering to the $CaCO_3$ were removed and inoculated into new microcosms. The $CaCO_3$ particles containing the associated V. cholerae cells were mechanically vortexed three times in an autoclaved marine salts solution (salinity = 20 ppt) prior to their addition to a new microcosm. The new microcosms were incubated for 24 hours at 22°C and culturable counts were determined before and after the addition of $CaCO_3$. In the microcosms containing the original planktonic cells, a decrease of approximately 50% in counts was observed. However, in microcosms inoculated with particle-associated cells no decrease in counts was noted. These results indicate that two subpopulations of V. cholerae arose in the microcosms: one with the ability to associate with $CaCO_3$ and one without this ability. Furthermore, the results demonstrate that cells without the ability to associate give rise to two populations: cells which can associate and cells which cannot. Cells capable of association also give rise to cells with and without that ability. Those cells which associate with $CaCO_3$ apparently remain associated, while those which do not associate enter the planktonic population.

Table 3. Comparison of $CaCO_3$-Association Effects Between Surface-bound and Planktonic Inocula

Inoculum Source[a]	Population Size			
	Before $CaCO_3$ Addition	After $CaCO_3$ Addition	$\Delta\%$	Corrected $\Delta\%$[b]
Particle-Associated	2.6×10^4	2.8×10^4	8%	-3.4%
Planktonic	8.7×10^2	5.5×10^2	-37%	-48%
Control[c]	9.0×10^1	1×10^2	11%	NA

[a]Microcosms were initially prepared with unfiltered seawater and V. cholerae. After incubation for 24 hours, addition of $CaCO_3$ resulted in a 52% decrease in the planktonic population. Samples of each (planktonic and particle-bound) were removed and used to inoculate new microcosms. After an additional 24 hour incubation, $CaCO_3$ particles were added (see text).
[b]$\Delta\%$sample $-\Delta\%$control.
[c]No particulates added. $\Delta\%$ taken to reflect increase in cell numbers during time interval between assays.

Effect of Nutrient Deprivation on Association. The effects of nutrient deprivation on the ability of V. cholerae cells to associate with $CaCO_3$ were determined using multiple sets of microcosms. Culturable counts were determined before and 10 minutes after the addition of 10 g $CaCO_3$ to the first set of microcosms. From the next set of micro-cosms (incubated for 12 hours) culturable counts were determined before and 10 minutes after the addition of $CaCO_3$. Using each new set of microcosms, incubated for

24, 48, and 72 hours, the procedure was repeated. Figure 1 shows that the proportion of the population able to associate with $CaCO_3$ decreased with increasing time. Initially, 54% of the culturable population was able to associate with $CaCO_3$ particles, but after 72 hours incubation in nutrient-free seawater, only 4% of the culturable planktonic population was capable of surface association.

Association with Silicate (Glass). To determine the portion of the population that would be "lost" from the planktonic fraction due to association of cells to the glass surface of the microcosm, a series of experiments was performed in which microcosms containing glass beads of calculated total surface area were inoculated with nutrient-deprived cells. The percent decrease in culturable counts due to association with the glass beads was similar to that observed with $CaCO_3$ particles, that is, 50%. Extrapolation along a least squares line to a hypothetical "wall-less" microcosm indicated that approximately 17% of the inoculum might be expected to disappear from the culturable count assay due to loss from the planktonic fraction through association with the glass walls of the microcosm (Figure 2).

Association with Chitin. In addition to $CaCO_3$ and glass, the association of nutrient-deprived $\underline{V}$. cholerae cells with chitin was examined. Microcosms were prepared as before using 0.2-μ-filtered and autoclaved natural seawater. These were inoculated with nutrient-deprived cells and culturable counts were determined before and 10 minutes after addition to 1 g of chitin. The results presented in Table 4 show that no decrease in culturable counts was observed after amendment with chitin, suggesting a lack of affinity for this substrate. When sterile $CaCO_3$ was subsequently added to this microcosm, a decrease in the planktonic population of approximately 50% was detected. However, in the reverse experiment--$CaCO_3$ added followed by chitin--$CaCO_3$ removed approximately 50% of the planktonic population, and the cells remaining in the liquid phase did not associate with the chitin particles. Similar results were obtained for all grades and kinds of chitin employed (ball milled--Sigma Chemical Co., St. Louis, MO; grade B

Table 4. Surface Association Effects of Chitin and $CaCO_3$ on Nutrient-Deprived V. cholerae in Seawater Microcosms.

Condition	Log Culturable Count	Δ% Culturable Count
I. Initial inoculum size	6.72	--
After addition of chitin	6.72	0%
After subsequent addition of $CaCO_3$	6.38	-55%
II. Initial inoculum size	6.83	--
After addition of chitin	6.41	-62%
After subsequent addition of chitin	6.41	0%

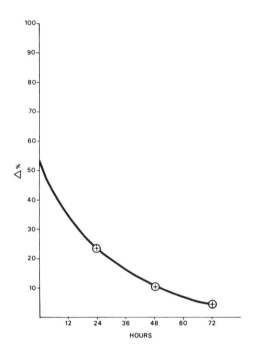

Figure 1. Temporal effect of nutrient deprivation on CaCO₃-association by microcosm populations of V. cholerae.

purified--Eastman Kodak Inc., Rochester, NY; and unpurified crude chitin fragments). This experiment was repeated including nutrient-enriched V. cholerae cells to determine if the physiological condition of the cells influenced surface association. The initial addition of either chitin or CaCO₃ resulted in a decrease of approximately 50% in the planktonic population with no detectable decrease occurring upon addition of the second substrate (Table 5).

DISCUSSION

It is well documented that bacterial associations with various substrates involve many diverse mechanisms,

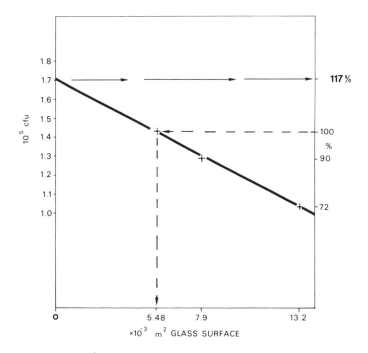

Figure 2. Effect of silicate (glass) microcosm surface on observed population size of microcosm populations of V. cholerae. Least squares line (solid line) generated to indicate expected population size in a hypothetical "surface-less" microcosm.

including those mediated by flagella, pili, fimbrae, slime layers, capsules, and exopolymers. From the results of these studies, it appears that there are, indeed, different mechanisms involved in the association of V. cholerae with chitin, $CaCO_3$, and silicates (glass).

If, in estuarine systems, the V. cholerae population does, in part, exist associated with crustaceans, cells which, for whatever reason, become unattached and enter the water column would seemingly face two alternatives: (1) continue to grow unassociated, or (2) reattach to a host organism. The results of Singleton et al. (1982a) indicate that, in the presence of a proper regime of nutrients and

Table 5. Surface Association Affinity as Reflected by Percent Change ($\Delta\%$) in Culturable Counts for both Nutrient-Enriched and Nutrient-Deprived $\underline{V}.$ cholerae in Seawater Microcosms

Condition	Chitin			CaCO$_3$		
	Culturable Counts			Culturable Counts		
	Before	After	$\Delta\%$	Before	After	$\Delta\%$
Nutrient-Deprived	9×10^2	9×10^2	0%	6×10^4	3.2×10^4	-53%
Nutrient-Enriched	3.6×10^3	2.1×10^3	-42%	4×10^3	2×10^3	-50%

salinity, V. cholerae can survive for extended periods and indeed grow in the planktonic state. Under nutrient deprivation or salinity stress, survival of V. cholerae (as indicated by colony-forming counts) is decreased significantly. Furthermore, V. cholerae can assume a physiological state, associated with nutrient deprivation, characterized by morphological changes and decreases in size (MacDonell and Hood 1982) and metabolic activity (Novitsky and Morita 1978). Through selective association with inert particulates, that is, $CaCO_3$ or sand, cells could be transported to the sediment where they would encounter a microenvironment greatly enriched in available nutrients and may, depending on prevailing conditions, undergo reversion to a nonnutrient-deprived state (MacDonell and Hood 1982). Alternatively, once in the sediment, in which V. cholerae has been shown to survive for extended periods (Hood and Ness 1982), the cells may be taken into organisms feeding on or in the sediment thereby providing the opportunity for reassociation of V. cholerae with higher tropic level organisms.

CONCLUSIONS

1. Osmolarity of the diluents and media employed in the culturable count assay clearly influences the recoverability of nutrient-deprived V. cholerae cells as indicated by microcosm studies.

2. Surface association with glass walls of labware must be considered as a source of error in culturable count assays of V. cholerae.

3. The different affinities demonstrated by nutrient-deprived and nutrient-enriched V. cholerae cells toward $CaCO_3$, chitin, and silicate surfaces in closed microcosms suggest effects of physiological state on analogous surfaces available to V. cholerae in the natural marine environment.

ACKNOWLEDGMENT

The authors gratefully acknowledge Professor K. Ranga Rao for his assistance in reviewing and editing this manuscript.

REFERENCES

Colwell, R.R., R.J. Seidler, J. Kaper, S.W. Joseph, S. Garges, H. Lockman, D. Maneval, H. Bradford, N. Roberts, E. Remmers, I. Huq, and A. Huq. 1981. Occurrence of Vibrio cholerae serotype O1 in Maryland and Louisiana estuaries. Appl. Environ. Microbiol. 41:555-558.

Hood, M.A., G.E. Ness, and G.E. Rodrick. 1981. Isolation of Vibrio cholerae serotype O1 from the eastern oyster, Crassostrea virginica. Appl. Environ. Microbiol. 41:559-560.

Hood, M.A., and G.E. Ness. 1982. Survival of Vibrio cholerae and E. coli in estuarine waters and sediments. Appl. Environ. Microbiol. 43:578-584.

Kaper, J., H. Lockman, R.R. Colwell, and S.W. Joseph. 1979. Ecology, serology and enterotoxin production of V. cholerae in Chesapeake Bay. Appl. Environ. Microbiol. 37:92-102.

MacDonell, M.T., and M.A. Hood. 1982. Isolation and characterization of ultramicrobacteria from a Gulf Coast estuary. Appl. Environ. Microbiol. 43:566-571.

Marshall, K.C. 1976. Interfaces in microbial ecology. Cambridge: Harvard University Press.

Novitsky, J.A., and R.Y. Morita. 1978. Possible strategy for the survival of marine bacteria under starvation conditions. Mar. Biol. 48:289-295.

Singleton, F.L., R.W. Attwell, M.S. Jangi, and R.R. Colwell. 1982. Influence of salinity and nutrient concentration on survival and growth of V. cholerae in aquatic microcosms. Appl. Environ. Microbiol. 43:1080-1085.

Singleton, F.L., R.W. Attwell, M.S. Jangi, and R.R. Colwell. 1982. Effects of temperature and salinity on V. cholerae growth . Appl. Environ. Microbiol. 44: 1047-1058.

Chapter 33

ULTRAMICROVIBRIOS IN GULF COAST ESTUARINE WATERS:
ISOLATION, CHARACTERIZATION AND INCIDENCE

M.T. MacDonell and Mary A. Hood

Due to the recent interest in the problem of overwintering
in the estuary, as well as nutrient scarcity in the open
sea, considerable attention is now being focused on the
filterable bacteria and ultramicrobacteria.

Ultramicrobacteria were first defined by Torrella and
Morita (1981) as bacteria less than 0.3 μ in diameter which
had a very slow growth rate when inoculated onto a
nutrient-rich agar surface and which did not increase
significantly in cell size on this medium. Since filterable
bacteria (Anderson et al. 1965) are generally regarded as
those capable of traversing a 0.45-μ membrane filter, it is
logical to assume that the filterable bacteria would include
the class defined as the ultramicrobacteria.

The isolation of membrane-filterable bacteria has pro-
ceeded rather sporadically since the first report of their
existence by Oppenheimer (1952). Apparently, much of the
difficulty encountered in the isolation of these bacteria has
been caused by use of media inappropriate (Carlucci 1974;
Carlucci and Shimp 1974) to the growth of these organisms.
A significant advance was made toward the solution of this
problem by Torrella and Morita (1981), who employed a less
nutrient-rich solid medium containing a low concentration of
peptone and yeast extract (0.175%). They were able to
obtain growth from some of their isolates, but others either

551

failed to respond or grew for several cell divisions and ceased further division.

Tabor et al. (1981), using polycarbonate membrane filters, demonstrated that bacteria capable of passing through a 0.45-μ pore were ubiquitous in the open sea. As a result of their study, some important observations were presented. They proposed that marine bacteria confronted with conditions of low solutes undergo certain changes, among which are a decrease in volume and a change in morphology. They further suggested that these changes, initiated at the onset of nutrient stress, are associated with the depletion of cellular reserves and that the nature of the marked decrease in volume is a function of the processes of scavenging nonessential cellular components and material.

Numerous investigators have suggested that the little-studied filterable bacteria may represent the true autochthonous bacteria of the sea. Characterization of these microorganisms, however, had remained elusive until Tabor et al. (1981) classified a group of 0.45-μ filterable bacteria taken from the Atlantic Ocean. In contrast to the filterable bacteria, isolation of the ultramicrobacteria has been sufficiently problematic that until recently no published account of their characterization was available.

The purpose of our study was to examine the warmer waters of a relatively unimpacted Gulf Coast estuary for the presence of ultramicrobacteria, to attempt to isolate these organisms, and to phenotypically characterize them.

Isolation

Water samples were taken from five sites located in Perdido Bay, Alabama during the period from April to September 1981. The sites were selected in such a way as to establish a range of pH, flow rates, salinities, and human impact. These samples were passed through 0.2-μ pore nuclepore polycarbonate filters, cultured, and bacteria was characterized by the methods of MacDonell and Hood (1982). Viable ultramicrobacteria were recovered from water samples taken from four out of the five Perdido Bay sites after filtration through 0.2-μ pore diameter poly-carbonate filters.

Characterization

Of 29 isolates, 86% were initially incapable of growth in any of several full-strength nutrient-rich broths, including trypticase soy broth plus marine salts, brain heart infusion broth plus marine salts, and marine 2216 broth, or any full-strength carbohydrate test medium, such as phenol red broth base, decarboxylase base, MRVP media and so on, even when marine salts were present. In order to deter-mine if a lower concentration of nutrients would provide the proper conditions for growth, several seawater dilutions of various media were prepared. The optimum concentration was observed to be an eight-fold dilution of full-strength (Table 1). This dilution permitted the organism to grow while providing enough indicator to allow classical color reactions to be observed in the test media.

The observation that the microorganisms isolated were capable of growth in dilute but not in full-strength broths suggests that the organisms were being inhibited by rich nutrient concentrations. Two of the isolates, UM 106 and UM 403, were examined for their ability to grow at a range of concentrations of trypticase in 15 ppt marine salt water. The growth responses after 36 hours at the various concen-trations are presented in Figure 1. A range of concentra-tions of both yeast extract and proteose peptone produced similar curves. In each case, the optimum concentration for growth of the freshly isolated ultramicrobacteria was 0.04% to 0.05%.

In general, agars were found to be somewhat more inhibitory than broths. Even when using low-nutrient agar media such as BH-ES, it was necessary to condition the organism to the media over a period of several days. This was achieved by heavy inoculation of an area of the BH-ES agar approximately 1 cm in diameter with the enrichment broth, followed by the transfer of the isolate at 48-hour intervals to new media until growth was sufficiently heavy to allow proper isolation for characterization.

Table 1. Response of Five Perdido Bay Ultramicrobacteria (UM 6, UM 7 &, UM 8, UM 9, UM 106) to Various Dilutions of Selected Media[a]

Type of Medium	Dilution of Medium			
	Full-Strength	1/2	1/4	1/8
Phenol Red Broth Base + Glucose	0[b]	0	G[c]	A[d]
Phenol Red Broth Base + Lactose	0	0	G	-[e]
Phenol Red Broth Base + Sucrose	0	0	G	A
Phenol Red Broth Base + Mannose	0	0	G	A
Decarboxylase Base	0	0	G	R[f]
Trypticase Soy Broth	0	0	G	G
Methyl Red Voges-Proskauer Medium	0	0	G	R
OF Medium + Glucose	0	0	0	r[g]

[a] Reprinted, by permission, from M.T. MacDonnell and M.A. Hood. 1982. Appl. Environ. Microbiol. 43:566-571.
[b] 0 = No growth.
[c] G = Growth.
[d] A = Acid production.
[e] - = No reaction.
[f] R = Positive reaction.
[g] r = Weak positive reaction.

554

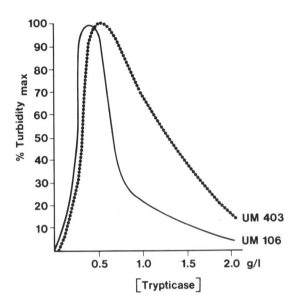

Figure 1. Growth response of isolate UM 106 and UM 403 to nutrient loading. Reprinted, by permission, from M.T. MacDonnell and M.A. Hood. 1982. Appl. Environ. Microbiol. 43:566-571.

Isolate UM 106, after undergoing nutrient conditioning on BH-ES agar for a period of six weeks, was reexamined for its ability to grow at different nutrient levels. Growth responses to various concentrations of trypticase were again determined and compared with those obtained shortly after its collection. The results of adaptation to nutrient-rich media are reflected in the pronounced shift in the isolate's response to low nutrient concentrations (Figure 2).

Adaptation to nutrient media was accompanied by a marked increase in size. Phase contrast microscopic examination of those broth inocula giving rise to visible turbidity within 48 hours indicated microorganisms of a size range of about 0.3-0.4 µ by 1.0-1.5 µ. Those microorganisms, typical of broth inocula not showing visible turbidity until after a period of a week or more, generally appeared as very slender rods only scarcely wide enough to be resolved by the microscope (R.P. = .17 µ) with a length of 0.5-

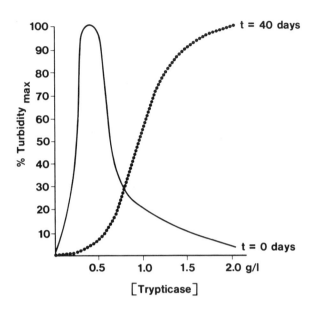

Figure 2. Growth response of UM 106 shortly after isolation (May 15) and after 40 days conditioning to culture media (June 24). Reprinted, by permission, from M.T. MacDonnell and M.A. Hood. 1982. Appl. Environ. Microbiol. 43:566-571.

0.8 μ. Regardless of the initial response to broth media, conditioning sufficient to produce discrete colonies of approximately 1-mm diameter on reduced-nutrient solid media (BH-ES) was accompanied by the development of microorganisms of a "normal" size, 0.5 by 2.0-2.5 μ.

As can be seen from the generic profile (Table 2), 22 (76%) of the isolates were members of the family Vibrionaceae; 18 (62%) belong to the genus Vibrio, of which three (10%) were lactose-positive (L+). Four (14%) were members of the genus Aeromonas; Pseudomonas and Alcaligenes both contributed two (7%) of the isolates, while three (10%) remain unidentified.

Table 2. Generic and Limited Phenotypic Profile of 0.2-µ Filterable Bacteria

Site	Isolate	Oxidase	CAT	LDC	ODC	VP	Citrate	Glucose	Mannose	Sucrose	Hugh-Leifson Lactose	H_2S	MOT	String Test	Sensitivity to 0/129 150 µg	Probable Genus
A	um6	$-^a$	$+^b$	+	+	-	-	+	+	+	-	-	+	+	-	Vibrio
A	um8	+	+	-	+	+	+	+	+	+	-	+	+	+	+	Vibrio
A	um9	+	+	+	+	-	+	+	+	+	-	-	+	+	-	Vibrio
A	um10	+	+	-	+	-	-	+	+	+	-	-	+	+	-	Vibrio
A	um11	-	w^c	+	+	-	-	w	-	-	-	-	+	+	+	Vibrio
A	um13	+	+	+	+	0^d	+	-	-	-	-	-	+	-	+	Alcaligenes
A	um14	+	+	+	+	-	-	-	-	-	-	-	+	+	+	Vibrio
A	um15	+	+	+	+	0	-	-	-	-	-	-	+	+	+	Vibrio
A	um16	+	+	+	+	0	-	-	-	-	-	-	+	+	+	Vibrio
A	um17	+	+	+	+	-	-	-	-	-	-	-	+	-	-	Alcaligenes
A	um18	+	+	+	+	0	-	-	-	-	-	-	+	+	+	Vibrio
B	um106	-	-	+	+	-	+	+	+	+	-	-	-	+	-	unknown
B	um108	+	+	-	-	+	-	+	-	+	-	+	+	+	+	Vibrio
B	um110	+	+	-	+	-	-	+	+	-	-	-	+	-	-	Pseudomonas
B	um111	+	w	-	+	-	+	+	+	-	-	-	+	+	-	Vibrio
B	um112	+	+	-	+	-	+	+	+	-	-	-	+	+	-	Vibrio
B	um113	+	+	-	-	-	-	+	+	-	-	-	+	+	-	Vibrio
B	um114	+	w	+	+	-	+	+	-	-	-	-	-	+	-	Pseudomonas
B	um115	+	+	+	+	-	+	+	+	-	+	-	+	+	+	Vibrio (L+)
B	um116	+	+	+	+	-	+	+	+	+	+	-	+	+	-	Vibrio (L+)
B	um117	+	+	+	+	+	+	+	-	+	-	+	+	+	+	Vibrio (L+)
B	um118	+	+	-	-	-	+	-	-	-	-	-	+	-	-	unknown
B	um119	+	+	-	-	-	-	+	+	+	-	-	+	+	-	Aeromonas
D	um301	+	+	+	+	-	-	+	+	+	-	-	+	+	-	Aeromonas
D	um302	+	+	-	+	-	-	+	+	+	-	-	+	+	-	Vibrio
D	um303	+	+			-	+	+	+	+	-	-	+	-	-	unknown
E	um403	+	w	-	+	-	-	+	-	-	-	-	+	+	-	Vibrio
E	um405	+	+	+	+	-	-	+	w	+	-	+	+	+	-	Aeromonas
E	um406	+	w	+	+	-	+	+	-	-	-	+	+	+	-	Aeromonas

^{a}Negative reaction. ^{b}Positive reaction. ^{c}Weak reaction. ^{d}No growth.

Table 3. Incidence of 0.2-μ Filterable Isolates

Site	Salinity	Character	Average pH	Incidence
A	29–33 ppt.	Fast-flowing Clean Mouth of Perdido Bay	7.8	1 per 5 ml
B	17–21 ppt.	Sationary Extensive shallows Residential	8.3	6 per ml
C	5–7 ppt.	Very slow-flowing Polluted Heavily populated	8.4	None
D	11–13 ppt.	Moderate flow Light marine traffic Rural	8.3	< 1 per 10 ml
E	26–30 ppt.	Slow-flowing Recreational marine traffic Sparsely populated	7.9	1 per 2 ml

Incidence

The incidence of 0.2-μ filterable bacteria per site was determined by a protocol in which replicate tubes containing 1/10 strength Lib-X were inoculated with volumes of filtrate ranging from 50 μℓ to 10 ml. Turbidity produced upon 14 days incubation at 31°C was used as a criterion for assessing presence of bacteria. Table 3 demonstrates a lack of correlation between incidence of ultramicrobacteria and pH, flow rate, or extent of human impact. There was, however, a clear correlation with salinity. The optimum in terms of incidence of 0.2-μ filterable bacteria appeared to center around 17-20 ppt.

DISCUSSION

Because of their size and the environment from which they were collected, the possibility that the Perdido Bay isolates might include host-independent (HI) strains of Bdellovibrio (Burnham and Robinson 1974) was suggested. Although Bdellovibrio are microorganisms about which remarkably little has been documented, they have not been demonstrated to utilize carbohydrates, and many of their phenotypic characteristics remain unidentified. Host-independent (HI) strains are characterized as non-fermentative, nonmotile, catalase-negative curved rods with a tendency to form coils and filaments with an average length of 10 μ (Burnham and Robinson 1974). As this offered little correlation with the Perdido Bay isolates, the possibility that the isolates represented strains of Bdellovibrio was discounted.

It has been suggested by several investigators (Novitsky and Morita 1976, 1977; Tabor et al. 1981; Torrella and Morita 1981) that adaptation to very low solute conditions (starvation) involves a series of processes, including depletion of cellular reserves and degradation of nonessential cellular material, linked to morphological changes in the cell such as rounding up and reduction in volume. Novitsky and Morita (1978) demonstrated, using the marine isolate ANT-300, that after seven days of starvation in seawater, endogenous respiration was reduced by more than 99%. They argued that during evolutionary selection for the ability to maintain viability during nutrient stress, reduction in respiration may have emerged as the means by which macromolecular degradation is controlled. In another study, Novitsky and Morita (1977) showed that certain marine bacteria were able to retain viability for as much as 70 weeks in conditions of starvation with no decrease in numbers. Such results suggest that marine bacteria may retain viability during periods of nutrient stress by maintenance of a state approximating dormancy. We suggest the term "envirotolerant" to describe that state.

CONCLUSION

Considering the characteristics of the ultramicrobacteria, particularly their size and response to nutrients, it seems likely that they represent bacteria in a condition of envirotolerance. The only alternative which readily suggests itself is the possibility that the ultramicrobacteria represent a totally new class of bacteria. Present evidence does not favor such a conclusion. There is sufficient indication that the Perdido Bay isolates, rather than represent a new class of organisms, are marine bacteria of identifiable taxa which have demonstrated the capability of adapting to low nutrient levels. Although it is easy to envision that conditions of relative nutrient stress might occur with some frequency in the deep sea, it is less obvious that an estuarine environment might provide the conditions necessary for nutrient stress adaptation in bacteria. This does not, however, preclude the possibility that the observed ultramicrobacteria are products of the open sea, and that their apparent distribution in the estuary reflects an artifact of the transition from a stressed condition. For these reasons, we feel that estuarine ultramicrobacteria may represent microorganisms not yet recovered from conditions imposed upon them during long-term exposure to deep sea waters. Such a hypothesis suggests a dynamic equilibrium between the microflora of the estuary and that of the open sea.

REFERENCES

Anderson, J.I.W., and W.P. Heffernan. 1965. Isolation and characterization of filterable marine bacteria. J. Bacteriol. 90:1713-1718.

Burnham, J.C., and J. Robinson. 1974. Genus Bdellovibrio. Pages 212-214 in R.E. Buchanan and N.E. Gibbons (Eds.), Bergey's manual of determinative bacteriology, 8th ed. Williams & Wilkins, Baltimore.

Carlucci, A.F. 1974. Nutrients and microbial response to nutrients in seawater. Pages 245-248 in R.R. Colwell and R.Y. Morita (Eds.), Effect of the ocean environment on microbial activities. University Park Press, Baltimore.

Carlucci, A.F., and S.L. Shimp. 1974. Isolation and growth of marine bacterium in low concentrations of substrate. Pages 363-367 in R.R. Colwell and R.Y. Morita (Eds.), Effect of the ocean environment on microbial activities. University Park Press, Baltimore.

Furniss, A.L., J.V. Lee, and T.J. Donovan. 1978. The Vibrios. Public Health Laboratory Services Board Monograph Series II, HMSO, London.

MacDonell, M.T., and M.A. Hood. 1982. Isolation and characterization of ultramicrobacteria from a Gulf Coast estuary. Appl. Environ. Microbiol. 43:556-571.

Novitsky, J.A., and R.Y. Morita. 1976. Morphological characterization of small cells resulting from nutrient starvation of a psychrophilic vibrio. Appl. Environ. Microbiol. 32:617-622.

Novitsky, J.A., and R.Y. Morita. 1977. Survival of a psychrophilic marine vibrio under long-term nutrient starvation. Appl. Environ. Microbiol. 33:635-641.

Novitsky, J.A., and R.Y. Morita. 1978. Possible strategy for the survival of marine bacteria under starvation conditions. Mar. Biol. 48:289-295.

Oppenheimer, C.H. 1952. The membrane filter in marine microbiology. J. Bacteriol. 64:783-786.

Stevenson, L.H. 1978. A case for bacterial dormancy in aquatic systems. Microb. Ecol. 4:127-133.

Tabor, P.S., K. Ohwada, and R.R. Colwell. 1981. Filterable marine bacteria found in the deep sea: Distribution, taxonomy, and response to starvation. Microb. Ecol. 7:67-83.

Torrella, F., and R.Y. Morita. 1981. Microcultural study of bacterial size changes and microcolony and ultra-microcolony formation by heterotrophic bacteria in seawater. Appl. Environ. Microbiol. 41:518-527.

Chapter 34

ISOLATION OF <u>VIBRIO</u> <u>PARAHAEMOLYTICUS</u> FROM
WILD RACCOONS IN FLORIDA

Angelo DePaola and Miles L. Motes

The occurrence of <u>Vibrio</u> infections in humans and the
isolation of <u>Vibrio</u> organisms from environmental sources
have recently received widespread attention (Blake et al.
1980a; Blake et al. 1980b; Bradford and Caraway 1978;
Cameron et al. 1977; DePaola 1981; Kaper et al. 1979).
Vibrios have been isolated in areas remote from sources of
human waste (Kaper et al. 1979). In conjunction with a
primitive weapons hunt for feral swine and white-tailed
deer, the Food and Drug Administration (FDA), in
November 1980, initiated a study to determine whether wild
animals on St. Vincent's Island National Wildlife Refuge in
Apalachicola Bay, Florida harbored <u>Vibrio</u> <u>cholerae</u>. A
concurrent study produced numerous isolates of <u>V</u>. <u>cholerae</u>
O1 and non-O1 from the waters surrounding St. Vincent's
Island.

St. Vincent's Island is 9 miles long and 4 miles wide.
Refuge personnel (one or two persons) are the only human
inhabitants, although at the time of sample collection approximately 100 hunters had camped on the Island for two
nights. Contents from the small intestines of two deer and
two swine were removed during the dressing procedure
(which takes place 1-2 hours after slaughter). Uncoagu-
lated blood collected from the aorta of three deer and three

swine was tested later for the presence of antibodies against O1 and non-O1 strains of V. cholerae.

In a separate refuge project, raccoons were being captured in live traps in an attempt to reduce their numbers. These animals were sacrificed by gunshot to the head. Contents of the small and large intestines were collected and pooled for V. cholerae analysis, and blood was removed from the aorta. V. cholerae MPN analysis was performed by diluting and inoculating 10^{-1} to 10^{-6} g of the intestinal contents of each animal type into alkaline peptone broth and incubating for 6 hours at 35°C. The isolation procedure for V. cholerae is described in the 5th edition of the Bacteriological Analytical Manual (Food and Drug Administration, 1978). Three blood serum samples from each type of animal were tested for the presence of antibodies against V. cholerae by Dr. Harry Smith of the Vibrio Reference Laboratory (VRL) in Philadelphia; however, no antibodies were detected.

Vibrio cholerae was not found in the intestinal contents of the feral swine or white-tailed deer. Samples from the intestinal contents of two raccoons trapped on subsequent nights revealed organisms suspected to be V. cholerae. Dilutions were as high as 1:100,000 in one sample. Biochemical characterization of ten of these isolates yielded the following pattern: acid from aerobic glucose (+); anaerobic glucose (+); mannitol (+); inositol (-); sucrose (-); arabinose (+); decarboxylation of lysine (+); ornithine (+); dihydrolation of arginine (-); string test (+); oxidase (+); catalse (+); Gram stain reaction (-); growth in 1% tryptone without NaCl (-); growth in 1% tryptone with 0.5% NaCl (+). On the basis of sucrose and arabinose fermentation and NaCl requirement, the isolates were identified as Vibrio parahaemolyticus.

Representative isolates from each raccoon were sent to the FDA facility at the Howard A. Taft Center in Cincinnati, where Dr. Robert Twedt assessed their pathogenic potential. Negative Kanagawa phenomenon test results suggested a lack of pathogenicity. Because of the relatively high correlation of human pathogenicity with a positive Kanagawa reaction, rabbit ileal loop tests were not performed.

The role of wild animals in the distribution of vibrios is receiving greater attention, as indicated by other findings presented in this volume. Roberts et al. (this volume) report the finding of $\underline{V.}$ $\underline{parahaemolyticus}$ in seagulls in Louisiana, and Lee et al. (this volume) note the incidence of $\underline{V.}$ $\underline{cholerae}$ non-O1 in seagulls in England.

In previous studies (Dutta et al. 1963) "rabbit-passaged" strains of $\underline{V.}$ $\underline{cholerae}$ non-O1 were shown to increase in pathogenicity; the serotypes of $\underline{V.}$ $\underline{cholerae}$ O1 were found to change when the organisms were passed through the gastrointestinal tract of germ-free mice (Sack and Miller 1969). These observations suggest that wildlife may contribute to the occurrence of certain vibrios by providing a mechanism for their concentration. Further study is needed to determine the effect of wild animals on the incidence of pathogenic vibrios in the environment.

REFERENCES

Blake, P.A., R.E. Weaver, and D.G. Hollis. 1980a. Diseases of humans (other than cholera) caused by vibrios. Ann. Rev. Microbiol. 34:341-367.

Blake, P.A., D.T. Allegra, J.D. Snyder, T.J. Barrett, L. McFarland, C.T. Caraway, J.C. Feeley, J.P. Craig, J.V. Lee, N.D. Puhr, and R.A. Feldman. 1980b. Cholera--a possible endemic focus in the United States. N. Engl. J. Med. 302:305-309.

Bradford, H.B., and C.T. Caraway. 1978. Follow-up on Vibrio cholerae serotype Inaba infection--Louisiana. CDC Morbid. Mortal. Wkly Rep. 27:388-389.

Cameron, J.M., K. Hester, W.L. Smith, E. Caviness, T. Hosty, and F.S. Wolf. 1977. Vibrio cholerae-- Alabama. CDC Morbid. Mortal. Wkly Rep. 26:159-160.

DePaola, A. 1981. Vibrio cholerae in marine foods and environmental waters: A literature review. J. Food Sci. 46:66-70.

Dutta, N.K., M.V. Panse, and H.I. Jhala. 1963. Choleragenic property of certain strains of El Tor, nonagglutinable, and water vibrios confirmed experimentally. Br. Med. J. 1:1200-1203.

Food and Drug Administration. 1978. Vibrio cholerae. In Bacteriological Analytical Manual, 5th ed. Association of Official Analytical Chemists, Arlington, VA.

Kaper, J., H. Lockman, R.R. Colwell, and S.W. Joseph. 1979. Ecology, serology, and enterotoxin production of Vibrio cholerae in Chesapeake Bay. Appl. Environ. Microbiol. 37:91-102.

Sack, R.B., and Miller, C.E. 1969. Progressive changes of vibrio serotypes in germ-free mice infected with Vibrio choelrae. J. Bateriol. 99:688.

Chapter 35

THE RELATIONSHIP BETWEEN FECAL COLIFORM
LEVELS AND THE OCCURRENCE OF
VIBRIOS IN APALACHICOLA BAY, FLORIDA

G.E. Rodrick, N.J. Blake, M. Tamplin,
J.E. Cornette, T. Cuba and M.A. Hood

Currently in the state of Florida, over 2.2 million acres have been classified for shellfish harvesting. Some 22% or 512,577 acres have been classified as approved; 5% or 110,281 acres as conditionally approved; 13% or 292,484 as prohibited; and 60% or 1,352,635 acres remain unclassified (Florida Department of Natural Resources 1980). Over 88% of all Florida oysters are harvested from Franklin County which includes Apalachicola Bay.

The classification of seawater for shellfish harvesting is based upon bacteriological standards relying primarily on the fecal coliform test. Specifically, shellfish harvesting waters are approved if the fecal coliform most probable number (MPN) does not exceed 14/100 ml seawater in more than 10% of the samples tested. In addition, fresh and frozen shellfish meats are considered to be satisfactory if the fecal coliform MPN does not exceed 2.3/g and the 35°C aerobic plate count is not more than 500,000/g (Hunt et al. 1976).

Recent reports however, indicate that potentially pathogenic vibrios may be part of the normal estuarine ecosystem and not of human fecal origin (Colwell et al. 1977; Blake 1980). It seems likely, therefore, that fecal coliform standards can not be used alone to rule out infectious hazards from vibrios in shellfish. This study examines the relationship between fecal coliform standards and the levels of Vibrio parahaemolyticus, V. cholerae, V. vulnificus, and V. alginolyticus in seawater and oysters from both approved and unapproved shellfish harvesting areas in Apalachicola Bay, Florida.

Determination and Enumeration
of Fecal Coliforms and Vibrios

Seawater and oyster (Crassostrea virginica) samples were collected from eight different stations in Apalachicola Bay which were located in approved, conditionally approved, and prohibited shellfish harvesting areas (see Figure 1). All samples were collected, handled, transported, and prepared for bacteriological analysis according to established techniques (American Public Health Association 1970).

The enumeration of fecal coliforms in seawater and oyster samples followed the methods of Hunt and Springer (1978) using A-1 broth. The isolation and enumeration of V. parahaemolyticus, V. cholerae, V. vulnificus, and V. alginolyticus in seawater and oyster samples followed a modification of the Food and Drug Administration method (1978). Aliquots of oyster homogenates were serially diluted tenfold from 10^{-1} to 10^{-6} using 1% peptone water, pH 7. One-ml aliquots were then inoculated into alkaline peptone broth, pH 8.4, and incubated 8-12 hours at 35°C. Culture tubes showing turbid growth were then streaked onto thiosulfate citrate bile salt sucrose agar (TCBS, Difco Laboratories, Detroit, MI) and incubated for approximately 20 hours at 35°C. Both green and yellow colonies were selected and screened for the presence of cytochrome oxidase. All colonies giving a positive cytochrome oxidase test were then tested biochemically using an API 20E system (Analytab Products, Plainview, NY). Coliform MPN analyses were performed on all samples positive or negative for vibrios using a 3-tube series reference table.

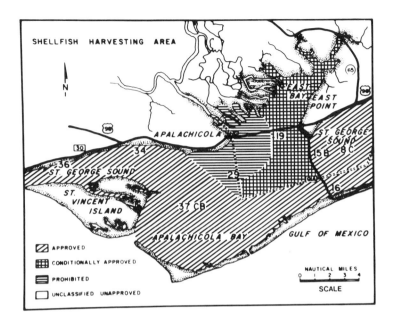

Figure 1.   Collection stations in Apalachicola Bay, Florida.

Seawater Fecal Coliform MPN and the Occurrence of Vibrios

The percentage of seawater samples containing vibrios collected from approved stations when the seawater fecal coliform MPN was $\leq$ 14/100 ml and > 14/100 ml with an aerobic plate count of less than 500,000 colonies is shown in Table 1.   When the seawater fecal coliform MPN was $\leq$ 14, V. cholerae occurred in 8.6% of the samples while V. parahaemolyticus, V. alginolyticus, and V. vulnificus occurred in 51.4%, 25.7%, and 37.1% of the seawater samples, respectively.   Overall, 75% of the seawater samples collected from approved stations contained at least one Vibrio species.   In contrast, the occurrence of V. cholerae was threefold higher (23.5% vs. 8.6%) when the seawater fecal coliform MPN was > 14, while the occurrence of other vibrios was markedly less.

Table 1.   Percent of Seawater Samples Containing Vibrios when Seawater Fecal Coliform MPN ≤ 14 and > 14

	Approved Site		Unapproved Site	
Species	MPN ≤ 14	MPN > 14	MPN ≤ 14	MPN > 14
V. cholerae	8.6	23.5	0	29.4
V. parahaemolyticus	51.4	17.6	8.6	41.2
V. alginolyticus	25.7	5.9	2.9	17.6
V. vulnificus	37.1	17.6	2.9	17.6

The same analysis was performed for unapproved shellfish harvesting sites. The data in Table 1 show that when the seawater fecal coliform MPN was ≤ 14 V. cholerae was not present and V. parahaemolyticus, V. alginolyticus, and V. vulnificus were present at low levels ranging from 8.6% to 2.9% (see Table 1). When the percentage of vibrios was calculated for a fecal coliform MPN > 14, V. parahaemolyticus was found in 41.2% of the seawater samples, while V. cholerae was found in 29.4%, and both V. alginolyticus and V. vulnificus were present in 17.6% of the seawater samples (see Table 1).

Seawater Fecal Coliform MPN and
the Occurrence of Vibrios in Oysters

The percentage of oyster samples containing vibrios when the fecal coliform MPN was ≤ 14/100 ml and > 14/100 ml seawater at both approved and unapproved stations was also determined (see Table 2).

Vibrios were found in more than 50% of the oyster samples analyzed when the seawater fecal coliform MPN was ≤ 14 at approved stations. The percentage of oyster

Table 2. Percent of Oyster Samples Containing Vibrios when Seawater Fecal Coliform MPN ≤ 14 and > 14

Species	Approved Site		Unapproved Site	
	MPN ≤ 14	MPN > 14	MPN ≤ 14	MPN > 14
V. cholerae	16.3	28.6	10.0	14.2
V. parahaemolyticus	37.5	57.1	8.6	57.1
V. alginolyticus	21.9	0	12.9	28.6
V. vulnificus	40.9	42.8	12.9	28.6

samples analyzed which contained vibrios was 16.3 for V. cholerae; 37.5 for V. parahaemolyticus; 21.9 for V. alginolyticus, and 40.9 for V. vulnificus. When the seawater fecal coliform MPN exceeded 14, 28.6% contained V. cholerae, 57.1% had V. parahaemolyticus, 42.8% possessed V. vulnificus; V. alginolyticus was not found.

In unapproved sites, when the seawater fecal coliform MPN was < 14, a low percentage of occurrence of V. cholerae (10%), V. parahaemolyticus (8.6%), V. alginolyticus (12.9%), and V. vulnificus (12.9%) were found. In addition, the percent occurrence of all four vibrios was markedly higher when the seawater fecal coliform MPN was > 14.

Oyster Meat Fecal Coliform Levels
and the Occurrence of Vibrios

When the oyster fecal coliform MPN was ≤ 2.3/g wet weight of oyster meats, over one-third of the oyster meats contained V. parahaemolyticus, V. alginolyticus, and V. vulnificus. Vibrio cholerae was found in 12.8% of the oyster samples (see Table 3). When the fecal coliform MPN was > 2.3/g wet weight of oyster meat taken from approved

Table 3. Percent of Oyster Samples Containing Vibrios when Oyster Meat Fecal Coliform MPN $\leq$ 2.3/g[a] and > 2.3/g

	Approved Site		Unapproved Site	
Species	MPN $\leq$ 2.3	MPN > 2.3	MPN $\leq$ 2.3	MPN > 2.3
V. cholerae	12.8	22.2	0	22.0
V. parahaemolyticus	38.5	33.3	0	56.0
V. alginolyticus	37.7	11.1	0	44.0
V. vulnificus	33.3	22.2	0	22.0

[a]Wet weight.

sites, the occurrence of V. cholerae increased 1.7-fold while the other vibrios decreased.

Analysis of oysters from unapproved shellfish harvesting water yielded no vibrios when the oyster meat MPN was $\leq$ 2.3. A high percentage occurrence was found, however, when the MPN was greater than 2.3. Interestingly, when the seawater taken from approved sites had an acceptable fecal coliform MPN standard of 14, it was found that 45.7% of the oyster meats exceeded the 2.3 fecal coliform MPN per gram wet weight standard (see Table 4).

When both the seawater MPN fecal coliform ($\leq$ 14/100 ml) and oyster meat MPN fecal coliform standards ($\leq$ 2.3/g wet weight of meat) are taken together, less than 6% of all oyster samples contained vibrios and then at very low levels (an MPN < 10).

SUMMARY AND CONCLUSIONS

Results presented indicate little relationship between the presence of Vibrio parahaemolyticus, V. cholerae, V. alginolyticus, and V. vulnificus and the standard fecal

Table 4. Percent Occurrence of Vibrios in Oyster Meats when Oyster Fecal Coliform MPN $\leq 2.3/g$[a] and $> 2.3/g$ and the Seawater Fecal Coliform MPN was ≤ 14[b]

Fecal Coliform MPN		Percent Occurrence of Vibrios in Oyster Meat
Seawater	Oyster Meat	
≤ 14	≤ 2.3	5.0
≤ 14	> 2.3	95.0

[a]Wet weight.
[b]From approved harvesting sites.

coliform MPN value (14/100 ml) for seawater and oyster meats (2.3/g). In addition, when seawater fecal coliform levels were acceptable (≤ 14 MPN), only 54.3% of the oysters sampled met the acceptable fecal coliform levels. This difference may be due to the oyster's ability to filter foreign material.

However, when both seawater and oyster meats met the acceptable fecal coliform levels, less than 5% of oyster tested contained vibrios, and then at low levels. It is possible, when both seawater and oyster fecal coliform standards are met, to predict a low occurrence of vibrios.

In summary, it is clear that both seawater and raw or improperly cooked oysters can serve as a vehicle for the transmission of vibrio infections even when considered safe by existing government and state standards.

Current federal and state guidelines use fecal coliform levels in an attempt to prevent the consumption of shellfish subjected to fecal contamination. Although such guidelines seem to be adequate in the prevention of diseases associated with contamination of human feces, these guidelines may be ineffective in predicting the presence of certain potentially pathogenic vibrios, which seem to be part of the normal estuarine microflora and not completely of human fecal origin. Given the lack of correlation between fecal coliform MPN and the presence of vibrios, a combination of criteria seems to be called for in evaluating shellfish quality.

ACKNOWLEDGMENTS

This work was supported by Florida Sea Grant, National Oceanic and Atmospheric Administration Office of Sea Grant, Department of Commerce, under Grant 125720073/257*V73.

REFERENCES

American Public Health Association. 1970. Recommended procedures for the examination of seawater and shellfish. 4th Ed. American Public Health Association, New York.

Blake, P.A., R.E. Weaver, and D.G. Hollis. 1980. Diseases of humans (other than cholera) caused by vibrios. Ann. Rev. Microbiol. 34:341-367.

Colwell, R.R., and J. Kaper. 1977. Vibrio species as bacterial indicators of potential health hazards associated with water. Pages 115-125 in A.W. Hoadley and B.J. Dutka (Eds.), Bacterial indicators/health hazards associated with water. ASTM STP635. American Society for Testing and Materials, Philadelphia.

Department of Natural Resources. 1980. National Register for the State of Florida. History of Changes.

Food and Drug Administration. 1978. Bacteriological Analytical Manual. Association of Official Analytical Chemists, Washington, D.C.

Hunt, D.A., J. Miescier, J. Redman, and A. Salinger. 1976. Molluscan shellfish, fresh frozen oyster, mussels, or clams. Pages 530-552 in M.L. Speck (Ed.),

Compendium of methods for the microbiological examination of foods. A.P.H. Intersociety/Agency Committee on Microbiological Methods of Foods.

Hunt, D.A., and J. Springer. 1978. Comparison of two rapid test procedures with the standard EC test for recovery of fecal coliform bacteria from shellfish-growing waters. J. Assoc. Off. Anal. Chem. 61:1318-1323.

Implications for the
Seafood Industry

Chapter 36

PREVENTION OF FOOD-BORNE DISEASE CAUSED BY VIBRIO SPECIES

Paul A. Blake

Prevention of food-borne disease caused by Vibrio species cannot be achieved by reliance on a single control measure such as prevention of sewage contamination. It requires knowing which Vibrio species cause food-borne disease, the foods that are their vehicles of transmission, the food-handling errors that increase the risk of infection, the reservoirs and ecology of these Vibrio species, and the host factors that place humans at increased risk of infection.

Prevention of food-borne disease caused by Vibrio species is a difficult topic because there are at least as many questions as there are answers. Nine Vibrio species have been associated with disease in man (Table 1). I have divided the species Vibrio cholerae into two groups: those that are O group 1 and those that are of other O groups. Each of these groups is further subdivided by whether the strains are toxigenic. By toxigenic, I mean capable of producing cholera toxin or a very similar toxin. Vibrio damsela and Vibrio hollisae are the proposed names for two Vibrio species that we have known at the Centers for Disease Control (CDC) as EF 5 and EF 13. Vibrio mimicus is similar to V. cholerae and some strains can produce cholera toxin. Vibrio vulnificus is the name currently given to an organism that has been referred to in the past

Table 1. Vibrio Species Associated with Disease in Man

V. alginolyticus
V. cholerae O1 (tox$^{+,-}$)^a; non-O1 (tox$^{+,-}$)
V. damsela (EF 5)
V. fluvialis (Group F, EF 6)
V. hollisae (EF 13)
V. metschnikovii (enteric group 16)
V. mimicus (tox$^{+,-}$)
V. parahaemolyticus
V. vulnificus

---

^{a}tox$^+$ = toxigenic; tox$^-$ = nontoxigenic.

by a variety of names including Beneckea vulnifica and lactose-positive vibrio.

The diseases that have been associated with these nine Vibrio species (Blake et al. 1980) are shown in Table 2. The disease categories are self-explanatory except for primary septicemia and secondary septicemia. While these are not optimal terms, no better ones have been suggested. By primary septicemia, I mean the onset of systemic infection without any apparent primary focus of infection-- such as an infected wound or a gastrointestinal illness. By secondary septicemia, I mean systemic infection occurring after a primary focus of infection has appeared--usually a wound infection but sometimes a gastrointestinal illness.

Toxigenic V. cholerae O1 is the cause of true cholera while the other V. cholerae can cause a variety of diseases. Nontoxigenic strains of V. cholerae O1 appear to be of trivial importance as a cause of human disease, although they have been isolated from diarrheal stool and from a severe wound infection. Gastrointestinal illness is the most common disease caused by non-O1 Vibrio cholerae, and both toxigenic and nontoxigenic strains have been isolated from people with diarrheal disease. In this country, the vast majority of strains from humans are nontoxigenic. Non-O1 V. cholerae diarrhea can range in severity from very mild

Table 2. Diseases Associated with Vibrio Species

Species	Gastrointestinal	Wound Infection	Ear Infection	Primary Septicemia[a]	Secondary Septicemia[b]
V. alginolyticus		X	X		X
V. cholerae O1	(tox$^+$, ? tox$^-$)[c]	(tox$^-$)			
V. cholerae non-O1	(tox$^{+,-}$)	(tox$^-$)	?	(tox$^-$)	(tox$^-$)
V. damsela		X			
V. fluvialis	?				
V. hollisae	X				
V. metschnikovii	?				
V. mimicus	(tox$^{+,-}$)	?		?	?
V. parahaemolyticus	X	X	X		X
V. vulnificus		X		X	X

[a]Occuring without apparent primary focus of infection.
[b]Occurring after a wound infection.
[c]tox$^+$ = toxigenic; tox$^-$ = nontoxigenic.

to a disease as severe as the more severe forms of true cholera. Non-O1 V. cholerae have also been associated with wound infections and with primary and secondary septicemias and, as far as I know, these organisms have always been nontoxigenic.

Vibrio damsela is a newly described organism, and we have just reviewed a series of six cases reported to CDC from the United States over the last ten years; all had wound infections without a diarrheal illness. Vibrio fluvialis has been isolated from diarrheal stools in many countries, but as far as I know it has not been isolated from stool in the United States. Vibrio hollisae is another newly described Vibrio species; we have just reviewed a series of ten cases reported to CDC from the United States over the last ten years and have found that all but one were gastrointestinal illnesses. Although not, as far as I know, in this country, Vibrio metschnikovii has occasionally been isolated from stool.

For public health purposes, Vibrio mimicus can probably be approached in the same way as non-O1 V. cholerae. However, we are just starting to study the diseases associated with isolation of this organism. In 1980, there was a large outbreak of diarrheal disease caused by nontoxigenic V. mimicus in Louisiana. Easily the most common disease caused by Vibrio parahaemolyticus is gastrointestinal illness, but V. parahaemolyticus has also caused wound infections, ear infections, and, rarely, secondary septicemia. Vibrio vulnificus has caused the most severe extra-intestinal infections associated with Vibrio species. V. vulnificus wound infections and primary septicemias are not uncommon in the United States, and many of the wound infections lead to secondary septicemias. There have been rare isolations from diarrheal stools, but it is not clear that these organisms were the cause of the diarrhea.

When we consider only food-borne disease, we can eliminate wound infections, ear infections, and almost all of the secondary septicemias, leaving a simple table with only five Vibrio species and two diseases (Table 3). These are the Vibrio species that we currently have to worry about when we try to prevent food-borne disease in the United States. All of these species except for Vibrio vulnificus

Table 3. Food-borne Disease Associated with Vibrio Species in the United States

	Disease	
Species	Gastro-intestinal	Primary Septicemia
V. cholerae O1 (tox$^+$)^a	X	
V. cholerae non-O1 (tox$^{+,-}$)	X	X
V. hollisae	X	
V. mimicus (tox$^+$, tox$^-$)	X	?
V. parahaemolyticus	X	
V. vulnificus		X

^{a}tox$^+$ = toxigenic; tox$^-$ = nontoxigenic.

are associated with gastrointestinal disease. Vibrio vulnificus is by far the most common cause of primary septicemia among the Vibrio species. Almost half of the reported cases are fatal. Non-O1 V. cholerae is an unusual cause of primary septicemia, and Vibrio mimicus has not yet been thoroughly investigated.

Vehicles of Transmission

Table 4 shows the foods that have been strongly impli-cated as vehicles of transmission of these Vibrio species in the United States, or that have been suspected but not proven. All of these foods come from water, and with the exception of a turtle and boiled crayfish, all are seafoods that would come from brackish or seawater. I do not think that we should necessarily focus upon these specific foods as being the primary vehicles of transmission of these specific organisms. Only with continued epidemiologic and

Table 4. Food-borne Disease Associated with Vibrio Species by Type of Food, United States

Species	Food
V. cholerae 01	Boiled crabs, shrimp ?, turtle ?
V. cholerae non-01	Raw oysters
V. hollisae	Raw oysters, cooked seafood ?
V. mimicus	Boiled crawfish, raw oysters ?
V. parahaemolyticus	Cooked crabs, shrimp, lobster
V. vulnificus	Raw oysters, raw fish ?

ecologic investigations will we be able to determine if some types of seafood are much more likely than others to transmit specific Vibrio species. For now, it might be prudent to think of all seafoods as being potential vehicles of transmission for all of these Vibrio species.

There are a few things related to this table that are worthy of note. One is that Vibrio parahaemolyticus, the most common cause of disease among these Vibrio species, in this country is almost invariably associated with eating cooked seafood which has been mishandled after cooking, allowing the organism to multiply. Food-borne Vibrio vulnificus and non-01 V. cholerae have thus far been associated almost exclusively with raw seafoods, especially oysters (Blake et al. 1979; Morris et al. 1981). The boiled crabs that caused cases of cholera were usually eaten less than half an hour after cooking, so multiplication after cooking was usually not an important factor (Blake et al. 1980b). However, in one instance the crabs were allowed to incubate for almost 6 hours after cooking, and four out of the five persons who ate them became ill. This suggests that multiplication may have occurred and that handling after cooking is a concern in preventing cholera.

Reservoirs for Vibrio Species

Another important factor in trying to prevent food-borne Vibrio disease is the reservoir for each of these species-- specifically, is the organism free-living (autochthonous), or does it come from human feces, or is it both free-living and sewage-associated (Table 5)?

Until recently toxigenic V. cholerae O1 was thought to persist exclusively in man, and its extra-human existence was thought of as survival in food or water after it left the human intestine. However, recent events in Australia and the United States have suggested that toxigenic V. cholerae O1 can persist for years in an area with few or no known human infections. Now it appears that these organisms can persist and multiply, perhaps indefinitely, in fresh water in Australia and in brackish coastal water in the United States (Blake et al. 1980b; World Health Organization 1980). Certainly infection of man can greatly amplify the threat posed by toxigenic Vibrio cholerae O1, since a person with severe cholera discharges enormous numbers of the organisms in his stool. However, we should probably be thinking of prevention and control of the disease in the United States rather than of eradication of the organism, which may be impossible.

The reservoir for non-O1 V. cholerae, both toxigenic and nontoxigenic, is unclear to me. While we cannot totally rule out the possibility that all pathogenic strains ultimately come from man, it is much more likely that toxigenic and nontoxigenic non-O1 V. cholerae causing disease in man sometimes come from sewage and sometimes are free-living organisms (Blake et al. 1980a). Thus, protection of raw oysters from sewage contamination may greatly decrease the risk to the consumer, but I doubt that it can eliminate all risk of a non-O1 V. cholerae infection.

We do not know if Vibrio hollisae and Vibrio mimicus are sewage-associated. The ecology of Vibrio parahaemolyticus has been studied extensively in the United States and in other countries, and there is no doubt that it is a free-living organism and is not sewage-associated. It is conceivable that the Kanagawa-positive strains that produce gastrointestinal disease in man are of sewage origin, but

Table 5. Principal Reservoirs for Vibrio Species Associated with Food-borne Disease in the United States

Species	Reservoir	Sewage Association
V. cholerae O1	Man--transient infection-- chronic carrier (rare) fresh water (Australia) ? coastal water (U.S.) ?	Yes May also be free-living
V. cholerae non-O1 (tox[+],[−])	Unclear--probably coastal water, fresh water, man, and animals	Yes Probably also free-living
V. hollisae	Probably coastal water	Unknown
V. mimicus	Probably coastal water, perhaps fresh water	Unknown
V. parahaemolyticus	Estuarine and coastal water	Free-living Possibly Kanagawa[+] strains
V. vulnificus	Coastal water Brackish water	Free-living

[a]tox[+] = toxigenic; tox[−] = nontoxigenic.

this is sheer speculation. As far as I know, <u>Vibrio vulnificus</u> is not sewage-associated. It is found in coastal waters, and one wound infection occurred after exposure to a brackish river in New Mexico, hundreds of miles from the sea.

Host Risk Factors

Another factor to be considered in disease prevention is whether the disease occurs in apparently "normal" people and whether there are factors that place some persons at greatly increased risk (Table 6). All of these food-borne <u>Vibrio</u> species apparently can cause disease in normal people except for <u>Vibrio vulnificus</u>. There have been rare instances in which food-borne <u>Vibrio vulnificus</u> infections have occurred in apparently normal people, but we cannot be certain that their defenses were not compromised. Among the host risk factors, lack of gastric acid has been repeatedly shown to be a risk factor for cholera. It may prove to be a risk factor for all of these organisms when we know more about them.

The other important risk factor is liver disease, especially cirrhosis of the liver. This is most dramatic in primary septicemia caused by <u>Vibrio vulnificus</u>, in which about 75% of the cases have liver disease (Blake et al. 1979). Pre-existing liver disease is also prominent among persons with septicemia caused by non-O1 <u>V. cholerae</u> (Blake et al. 1980a). In the one case I know of in which septicemia occurred after <u>Vibrio parahaemolyticus</u> gastrointestinal disease, the patient had cirrhosis (Tay and Yu 1978).

CONCLUSION

Table 7 summarizes some of the measures that may help control disease caused by <u>Vibrio</u> species. The first potential control measure is the control of fecal contamination. This is listed first because it is the foundation of the shellfish sanitation program that we rely on to make

Table 6. Host Risk Factors in Food-borne Disease Associated with Vibrio Species in the United States

Species	Occurrence in "normal" people	Host Risk Factors
V. cholerae O1	Yes	Lack of gastric acid
V. cholerae non-O1	Yes	Cirrhosis of liver
V. hollisae	Yes	None well-established
V. mimicus	Yes	None well-established
V. parahaemolyticus	Yes	None well-established Cirrhosis of liver
V. vulnificus	Rare	Cirrhosis and other liver disease, diabetes ?

shellfish that are eaten raw as safe as possible. Control of fecal contamination will certainly prevent hepatitis A, typhoid, and other diseases. Control of fecal contamination should decrease the risk of toxigenic V. cholerae O1 infections and decrease the risk of both toxigenic and non-toxigenic V. cholerae non-O1 infections, because it should decrease the number of these organisms in seafoods. However, since both of these organisms can apparently be free-living, I doubt that control of fecal contamination can eliminate the risk of infection with these organisms. Control of fecal contamination will probably have no effect on Vibrio vulnificus or on Vibrio parahaemolyticus, with the possible exception of any contribution that sewage may make to the Kanagawa-positive Vibrio parahaemolyticus population.

The next control measure is cooking. Obviously, thorough cooking will kill all vibrios and eliminate them as a health hazard. However, seafood is not always cooked thoroughly. Cooked seafood ranges from clams that are just steamed until they open, achieving an internal temperature of about 115°F (45°C); through crabs boiled for eight

Table 7. Prevention of Disease Caused by _Vibrio_ Species in Seafoods

Species	Control Fecal Con- tamination	Adequate Cooking	Time & Temperature	Season	High Risk Persons Avoid Raw Seafood
V. cholerae Ol (tox⁺)[a]	±Yes	Yes	Yes	±Yes	Yes
V. cholerae non-Ol (tox⁺,⁻)	±Yes	Yes	Yes	±Yes	?
V. hollisae	?	Yes	?	?	?
V. mimicus	?	Yes	?	?	?
V. parahaemolyticus	No (? for K⁺)	Yes	Yes	±Yes	?
V. vulnificus	No	Yes	?	±Yes	Yes

a tox⁺ = toxigenic; tox⁻ = nontoxigenic.

589

minutes that are red and have firm, apparently well-cooked meat but still have live Vibrio cholerae in them; to seafood that is so well cooked that it is sterile.

One must also consider the handling of food after cooking; even if food is sterilized by cooking, there is often ample opportunity for contamination after cooking by other raw seafood or by contaminated hands or surfaces. Time and temperature are other considerations. If the cooked seafood is not eaten immediately or kept at a temperature of below 40°F (4°C) or above 140°F (60°C), multiplication of the vibrios may occur, increasing the probability that the consumer will be infected. Time and temperature are also important when seafood is eaten raw: if the seafood is handled inappropriately, the vibrios present could multiply or they could die off, and different species may act differently.

Another possible control measure is the season when the seafood is harvested. The four Vibrio spp. listed in Table 7 with reasonable information on seasonality have a seasonal fluctuation in the incidence of disease which probably reflects, among other things, seasonal fluctuation in the number of each of these species in water. Thus, there is at least the potential for partial control of food-borne Vibrio disease by restricting consumption of raw seafoods to certain months of the year. These months would probably vary depending on the local ecology. Direct measurement of the numbers and types of vibrios in shellfish and shellfish waters, and the temperature, salinity, and other characteristics of the water, may eventually be a useful adjunct to fecal coliform counts in determining when raw shellfish from a growing area represent relatively little hazard to consumers. However, much more work on the ecology, epidemiology, and pathogenesis of Vibrio species must be done before such Vibrio counts can be incorporated into shellfish regulations.

A final control measure would be for persons at high risk such as those with low gastric acid to avoid raw sea-food. The Vibrio species that is most likely to kill is Vibrio vulnificus, and people with liver disease and other underlying diseases are at a vastly increased risk of food-borne Vibrio vulnificus infection. It would be prudent for those persons to avoid raw seafood completely.

REFERENCES

Blake, P.A., M.H. Merson, R.E. Weaver, D.G. Hollis, and P.C. Heublein. 1979. Disease caused by a marine vibrio. N. Engl. J. Med. 300:1-5.

Blake, P.A., R.E. Weaver, and D.G. Hollis. 1980. Diseases of humans (other than cholera) caused by vibrios. Ann. Rev. Microbiol. 34:341-367.

Blake, P.A., D.T. Allegra, J.D. Snyder, T.J. Barrett, L. McFarland, C.T. Caraway, J.C. Feeley, J.P. Craig, J.V. Lee, N.D. Puhr, and R.A. Feldman. 1980. Cholera--A possible endemic focus in the United States. N. Engl. J. Med. 302:305-309.

Morris, J.G. Jr., R. Wilson, B.R. Davis, I. K. Wachsmuth, C.F. Riddle, H.G. Wathen, R.A. Pollard, P.A. Blake. 1981. Non-O group 1 Vibrio cholerae gastroenteritis in the United States. Ann. Int. Med. 94:656-658.

Tay, L., M. Yu. 1978. Vibrio parahaemolyticus isolated from blood cultures. Sing. Med. J. 19:89-92.

World Health Organization. 1980. Cholera surveillance. WHO Wkly. Epidemiol. Rec. 14:101-102.

Chapter 37

SANITARY PRECAUTIONS FOR THE SEAFOOD PACKER
IN PREVENTING DISEASE CAUSED BY
VIBRIO SPECIES

Michael W. Paparella

Seafood technologists are concerned with the wholesomeness
and safety of all seafoods--a concern that extends from raw
material to finished product. In Maryland, commercial
harvests concentrate mainly on crabs, oysters, clams, and
some finfish. The quality of Maryland seafood, and seafood
in general, is affected by many factors: the method of
handling the catch, containerization, storage on board, and
transport to and from the dock. Throughout the preparation, pasteurization, canning, and freezing of crab, oyster,
clam meats, and fish fillets, sanitation and the associated
problems of bacteriology are of primary importance to the
processor (Riemann and Bryan 1979).
    Fresh seafoods are highly perishable and will spoil
rapidly if mishandled. Moreover, they serve as an excellent growth medium for food-borne pathogenic bacteria,
which at permissive temperatures, may grow rapidly to
infectious levels. To guard against food poisoning, and to
protect his product from spoilage or impoundment, the
processor relies on the sanitation function of his quality
control program.
    Quality control in the seafood industry encompasses all
steps necessary to protect the integrity of the product.
Its aim is to prevent spoilage, contamination, or other

influences that may render the product unsafe or objection-
able from the standpoint of smell, taste, texture, or
appearance. In the broadest sense, quality control begins
with the waters where the food is harvested (Colwell and
Kaper 1977).

The most serious hazard that the processor faces on a
day to day basis is bacterial contamination of his product.
Although the great majority of seafood packers abide by the
federal and state health rules and regulations, violations do
occur. One such violation resulted in this country's first
food-borne disease outbreak caused by V. parahaemolyticus
(Paparella 1979; Fishbein and Olson 1971; Nelson 1971;
Dadisman et al. 1973). Steamed crabs were the vehicle of
the August 1971 infection. The crabs were cooked and
shipped immediately in a refrigerated truck by a reputable
Eastern Shore processing plant to a retail outlet in Elkton,
Maryland. At Elkton, the steamed crabs were stored for
several hours in close proximity to raw crabs without
adequate refrigeration. Customers representing two separate picnics picked up the crabs from the retail outlet the
following day. About two-thirds of the guests at each
picnic became ill with diarrhea, severe abdominal cramps,
nausea, vomiting, mild fever, headache, and chills.
Cultures of food from the picnics and of stools isolated from
the persons afflicted did not yield enteric pathogens
normally encountered in food poisoning outbreaks.

No causative agent was apparent, yet 350 people had
become ill. Further testing by the State Health Department
Laboratory for V. parahaemolyticus proved positive. Cultures were sent to the Food and Drug Administration, which
then reported the first confirmed outbreak of V. parahaemolyticus gastroenteritis in the western hemisphere.

V. parahaemolyticus was first reported as the etiologic
agent of an outbreak of food poisoning in Osaka, Japan in
1950 (Dadisman et al. 1973). In Japan, where seafood is
consumed raw or partially cooked, more than half of all
cases of bacterial food poisonings reported are due to this
microorganism.

To prevent food-borne disease due to V. parahaemolyticus, health authorities and food technologists emphasize

the need for proper handling practices; that is, thorough cooking, avoidance of cross-contamination between cooked and raw foods, and storage of cooked foods at temperatures either under 4°C or over 60°C (Riemann and Bryan 1979).

Accumulated evidence indicates that Vibrio species, including Vibrio parahaemolyticus, live at large in the Chesapeake Bay (Kaper et al. 1979; Colwell et al. 1977). They have been found in a wide variety of locations--in finfish and shellfish, in mud, sediment, and water samples primarily from coastal water locations. The association of vibrios with zooplankton has been well established, and the vibrios comprise a large part of the total population of plankton in the summer months. These organisms have a seasonal incidence, highest in the warmer weather, paralleling the temperature of the water in which they are found. They are sensitive both to heat (killed at 55°C in 10 minutes) and to cold. When stored in baskets in hot weather, as was the case at the retail outlet in Elkton, the low concentration of vibrios found in healthy blue crabs quickly explode into astronomically large populations.

In the case of V. cholerae, as with V. parahaemolyticus, the importance of proper handling can not be overemphasized. Careful hygiene provides almost complete protection against the disease since it is transmitted through foods and beverages that are contaminated with disease-producing bacteria, usually from the stools of cholera victims. Apparently, ingestion of a large number of bacteria is necessary to produce the disease, and most people who become infected with V. cholerae do not get the severe form of the disease (R. Colwell, personal communication). When elementary sanitary precautions are taken, even the medical workers who care for the cholera patients almost never come down with the disease.

Until 1978, only two cholera cases had been reported in the United States since 1911. In 1978, however, eleven people contracted the disease in Louisiana (Greer 1981; Greer 1979; Centers for Disease Control 1981). All eleven had consumed home-prepared crabs. Health officials quickly recognized and isolated the cause of the outbreak. None of the patients died; two showed no symptoms at all. The public was informed that the situation was under control. In spite of the reassurance, the seafood industry--in Louisiana especially--experienced a loss of confidence. Business slumped dramatically; in parts of the state seafood production was temporarily shut down.

The problem turned out to be an old one: improper handling. Cooked crabs had been stored for several hours without refrigeration in the same baskets they had been held in while still alive. The cholera bacteria had increased at a logarithmic rate until the number of vibrios reached into the millions per gram of crab.

The threat of cholera is always with us. Two cases occurred in 1981 in East Texas (R. Colwell, personal communication). On May 7, a 42-year-old man developed the classical symptoms of cholera and was admitted to the hospital. He improved rapidly with fluid replacement and was discharged 12 days later. On June 21, a 65-year-old man, living 40 miles distant from the first, came down with the same symptoms. On admission to the hospital, he was severely dehydrated. He died two weeks later with complications due to renal and pulmonary failure. In these two cases, precise food histories could not be obtained. The first ate locally caught fish and a turtle during the week before the onset of the illness; the second ate shrimp in a stew one week before his illness.

Sanitation Procedures

Although pathogenic vibrios are present in most, if not all, of the United States coastal marine environment, they do not represent a serious health hazard when proper sanitation procedures are implemented. Just as good sanitation will prevent Salmonella and Shigella from contaminating our chicken salad, so will it prevent vibrios from contaminating our seafood.

Sanitation must be considered in its many forms, starting with surface appearance cleanliness (or "broom cleanliness"), and including personal hygiene, uniforms, work habits, design of equipment, and means and frequency of cleaning equipment. Sanitation extends to the design and location of buildings and their relationship to other nearby operations. Another important aspect of sanitation is the exclusion of foreign materials from the finished product and the exclusion of all kinds of pests (e.g., insects, rodents, dogs, cats, birds, bats) from the areas where processing operations take place. Finally, sanitation also extends to the proper discharge of all waste materials.

Implementation of a sanitation program must be reasonable and practical since the program requires the support of every member of the organization to work. And it must work. Food and Drug Administration (FDA) regulations are written such that food need not necessarily be contaminated to be banned from commerce. Food may be embargoed if it <u>might have been</u>, <u>could have been</u>, <u>may have been</u>, or <u>might become</u> contaminated. Moreover, the FDA has declared its intention to prosecute any organization and its chief executive officer(s) for violation of any sanitary practice if they do not cooperate in eliminating the conditions which brought about the violation and in maintaining a program of strict sanitary control. A first conviction is a misdemeanor, punishable by a fine of up to $1000 and/or one year in prison. A second conviction, which need not be of the same kind, is a felony with attendant loss of citizenship, a fine of up to $10,000, and three years in prison. The nature of the violation, FDA spokesmen emphasize, is relatively unimportant if prosecution was deemed necessary. Those companies with multiple installations or with plants and warehouses in different locations are treated as a single entity regardless of where the violation occurs.

The manager of a seafood processing plant (who may also be its principal executive officer) is ultimately responsible for maintaining a sanitary plant. Generally, he will delegate some of this responsibility and authority--by setting up a quality control department if the plant is large enough to warrant it. In the case of a smaller plant, someone with a basic knowledge of sanitation procedures should be appointed sanitarian to oversee the sanitation program.

The sanitarian should be directly responsible to top management. In addition to implementing a preventive program including regular application of control measures, he must be available daily to investigate reports of faulty procedures.

The sanitarian functions in both regulatory and advisory capacities, and he should have the authority to bring about any necessary changes. Additionally, he must act as liaison with the regulatory agencies. Often he is the best person to accompany a regulatory inspector during a routine inspection. In short, employment of a qualified sanitarian with specific responsibilities will usually result in a more rapid recognition of sanitation problems and in better communication with management concerning the origin and solution of real or potential problems.

The sanitarian's inspections might take one of three forms: (1) Horizontal--following the flow of product material from receiving through processing to storage and shipping; (2) Vertical--observing a single operation in process for a period of time; and (3) "Hazard Analysis and Critical Control Points"--a new name for an old technique based on assigning the hazard of risk at each step in a processing cycle (Riemann and Bryan 1979). A critical control point is a processing step where the material in process undergoes a change of state; that is, a change in particle size, texture, temperature, or character by incorporating another ingredient. Whatever form the inspection takes, the sanitarian should present management with written reports augmented by meetings as necessary.

REFERENCES

Centers for Disease Control. 1978. Morbid. and Mortal. Wkly. Rep. 27(39):367.

Colwell, R.R. and J. Kaper. 1977. Vibrio species as bacterial indicators of potential health hazards associated with water. ASTM STP635, American Society for Testing and Materials, Philadelphia.

Colwell, R.R., J. Kaper, and S.W. Joseph. 1977. Vibrio cholerae, Vibrio parahaemolyticus, and other vibrios:

occurrence and distribution in Chesapeake Bay.
Science 198:394-396.

Dadisman, T.A., Jr., R. Nelson, J.R. Molenda, and H.J.
Garber. 1973. Vibrio parahaemolyticus gastroenteritis
in Maryland. I. Clinical and Epidemiologic Aspects.
Am. J. Epidem. 96(6):414-426.

Fishbein, M., and J.C. Olson, Jr. 1971. Vibrio
parahaemolyticus: A real foodborne disease problem.
FDA Papers, Sept.:16-22.

Greer, A. 1979. Squelching the cholera scare. NOAA
Magazine 9(4):48-49.

Greer, J. 1981. The cholera connection. Maryland Sea
Grant, Maryland Sea Grant Program, University of
Maryland 4(4):10-12.

Kaper, J., H. Lockman, R.R. Colwell, and S.W. Joseph.
1979. Ecology, serology, and enterotoxin production of
Vibrio cholerae in Chesapeake Bay. Appl. Environ.
Microbiol. 37:91-103.

Nelson, R. 1971. Vibrio parahaemolyticus gastroenteritis
report. Presented Interstate Environmental Health
Seminar, Ocean City, MD, September 28, 1971.

Paparella, M.W. 1979. Vibrios--their significance in the
crab industry. Information Tips, Marine Products
Laboratory, Center for Environmental and Estuarine
Studies, University of Maryland 79(4):4 pages.

Riemann, H, and F.L. Bryan (Eds.) 1979. Food-borne
infections and intoxications. 2nd Ed. Academic, New
York.

Chapter 38

FACTORS AFFECTING THE ADHERENCE OF VIBRIO CHOLERAE TO BLUE CRAB (CALLINECTES SAPIDUS) SHELL

M.A. Dietrich, C.R. Hackney and R.M. Grodner

Eleven sporadic incidents of cholera occurred in Louisiana in 1978. The blue crab (Callinectes sapidus) was presumed to be the vehicle for the cholera transmission (Blake et al. 1980). These eleven incidents were the first documented cases of cholera in Louisiana since 1911, although one case of cholera was reported in Texas in 1973. The same bacteriophage type of Vibrio cholerae O1 caused both the Louisiana and Texas incidents and it is possible that the V. cholerae strain that caused these incidents was surviving as a free-living agent during the five-year period. This hypothesis is somewhat contrary to the long-held idea that V. cholerae O1 has only a limited survival ability in the marine environment (Mizaki et al. 1967; Pesigan et al. 1967; Sakazaki 1979). Yet, recent isolations of V. cholerae O1 from the Chesapeake Bay and the Gulf Coast have led many researchers to propose that V. cholerae O1 is actually part of the autochthonous flora of brackish coastal waters (Colwell and Kaper 1977).

V. cholerae O1 is a chitinase-positive bacterium and its survival time in the marine environment may be enhanced by association with the chitin of the shells of marine fauna such as the blue crab. Nalin et al. (1979) reported that V. cholerae will adsorb to chitin and suggested that this association might decrease the infective dose needed to establish infection. However, no one has reported on the adherence of V. cholerae to crab shell fragments. Since the latter consists of 75% calcium carbonate, 5-10% protein and 15-20% chitin, the conditions for V. cholerae adherence to crab shell may be quite different than those for chitin alone (Welinder 1974). The purpose of this study was to examine environmental factors and those shell components which might influence the adsorption of V. cholerae to crab shell fragments, and to determine if scanning electron microscopy could be used to demonstrate V. cholerae's adherence.

MATERIALS AND METHODS

Preparation of the Crab
Shell Fragments

Crabs were obtained from local fish markets, and killed by freezing at -20°C. Subsequently, the dorsal shells were removed, washed of residual tissue, broken into fragments, and the membraneous layer removed. Shells were auto-claved at 121°C for 15 minutes to sterilize the fragments.

Adherence Procedure

V. cholerae O1 cells were grown to the late log phase in trypticase soy broth (TSB) at 35°C, harvested by centrifugation at 4000g, washed once in the medium to be used in the incubation system, and resuspended to an Optical Density (OD) 650nm of 1.0. Approximately 5 ml of the V. cholerae inoculum was added to 1 gram of crab shell fragments and the system was incubated at 35°C for up to 5 hours. Following incubation, the suspending medium was poured off and the shell fragments were repeatedly washed, with gentle shaking, in the suspending menstrum to remove all remaining nonadhering cells (approximately 7 times). Thereafter, the shell fragments were added to 100 ml of dilution water (1% bacto/peptone, Difco), 0.85% NaCl, and 0.01% antifoam B (Sigma) and blended for 20 seconds at high speed to remove the adhering cells. These cells were enumerated on TSB plus 1.5% agar by the spread plate method. TSB plus 1.5% agar (TSBA) was used instead of trypticase soy agar because the colonies were much larger and easier to enumerate.

Suspending media included synthetic seawater (American Public Health Association 1976); distilled water; NaCl concentrations ranging from 0 to 3.5%; 0.1 M phosphate buffer adjusted to pH values of 4, 5, 6, 7, 8, 9; and 0.01 M $MgSO_4$. All incubations were at 35°C unless otherwise noted. In addition to crab shell fragments, glass fragments were similarly tested for V. cholerae adherence.

Separation of Crab Shell
into Component Parts

The crab shell fragments were decalcified and depro-teinated by the method of Welinder (1974a), which includes the addition of large excesses of trichloroacetic acid. They were then incubated at room temperature for 48 hours to decalcify the shell and further treated with an excess of 1.0 M NH_4OH for 4 days at 5°C.

Preparation of Scanning
Electron Microscopy Specimens

Specimens were placed in a fixative of 2.5% glutaral-dehyde in 0.1 M sodium cacodylate (pH 7.2) for 1 hour. Following this, the fixative was removed and specimens were stored in 0.1 M sodium cacodylate for 6 days. Specimens were prepared for scanning electron microscopy (SEM) by washing in distilled water, dehydration in 2,2-dimethoxypropane, and critical point drying. The dry specimens were mounted on aluminum stubs with aluminum paint, sputtercoated with 200 Å gold-palladium, and viewed with a Hitachi S-500 scanning electron microscope operating at 25 Kv.

RESULTS AND DISCUSSION

<u>V</u>. <u>cholerae</u> adhered readily to the shell of the blue crab. This adherence was affected by time, age of culture, temperature of incubation, pH, and components of the suspending medium. When <u>V</u>. <u>cholerae</u> was incubated with crab shells at two different temperatures for 5 hours, there appeared to be a linear to quadratic relationship between the amount of adherence and time. The cells adhered more readily at 35°C than at 25°C.

<u>V</u>. <u>cholerae</u> cells suspended in either distilled water or synthetic seawater were incubated with either sterile or nonsterile shell fragments and glass fragments. No significant difference was noted between the adherence of <u>V</u>. <u>cholerae</u> to sterile and nonsterile shells incubated in distilled water at 35°C (Table 1). Likewise, there was no significant difference in adherence to sterile and nonsterile shells incubated in synthetic seawater at 35°C (Table 2). However, a substantial difference is noted between the number of cells adhering to the shell fragments in the synthetic seawater and distilled water systems. Incubation

Table 1. Adherence of <u>Vibrio</u> <u>cholerae</u> to Sterile and Nonsterile Crab Shells and to Glass Incubated in Distilled Water at 35°C

Time (hours)	Cell Counts per Gram[a]		
	Sterile	Nonsterile	Glass
0	7.0×10^5	8.6×10^5	1.8×10^5
2.5	7.8×10^6	2.0×10^7	1.0×10^4
5	7.0×10^6	2.0×10^6	8.5×10^4

[a]Initial inoculum: 1.5×10^8 cells/g of shell.

Table 2. Adherence of Vibrio cholerae to Sterile and Nonsterile Crab Shells, and Glass Incubated in Synthetic Seawater at 35°C

Time (hours)	Cell Counts per Gram[a]		
	Sterile	Nonsterile	Glass
0	1.4×10^6	1.0×10^6	7.0×10^3
2.5	3.9×10^7	5.7×10^7	1.4×10^4
5	1.4×10^8	1.8×10^8	1.4×10^5

[a]Initial inoculum: 6.1×10^7 cells/g of shell.

for 5 hours in the seawater resulted in an increase of two logs.

Since the synthetic seawater solution enhanced the ability of vibrios to adhere, the solution was separated into its individual components, and these were used separately in combinations as suspending media for further adherence studies. Sodium chloride and magnesium salts both promoted adherence; however, the counts were highest in the synthetic seawater (Table 3).

Since NaCl appeared to influence adherence, studies were performed to determine the percentage of salt which would yield the greatest degree of attachment. The optimum salt concentrating for adherence is approximately 1.5 to 2.0% (Table 4) at the end of a 3-hour incubation at 35°C.

The pH of the suspending medium also affected the ability of V. cholerae to adhere to the shell fragments (Table 5). Adherence was favored by slightly acid to neutral pH values.

Since chitin only accounts for 15-20% of the total crab shell, we investigated the possibility that other components of the crab shell beside chitin influence V. cholerae's

Table 3. Adherence of Vibrio cholerae to Sterile Crab Shell as a Function of the Components of Synthetic Seawater at 35°C

Cell Counts per Gram[a,b]

Time (hours)	Distilled Water	0.4 M NaCl	Magnesium Salts[c]	SSW[d]
0	1.0×10^7	1.5×10^7	1.5×10^7	4.9×10^6
2.5	3.7×10^7	5.8×10^7	7.1×10^7	3.6×10^7
5	2.0×10^7	6.7×10^7	4.4×10^7	2.2×10^8

[a] Initial inoculum: 1.4×10^7 cells/g of shell.
[b] Mean of two trials.
[c] 0.03 M MgCl and 0.01 M MgSO$_4$.
[d] Synthetic seawater.

Table 4. Adherence of _Vibrio cholerae_ to Crab Shells as a Function of Salt Concentration after 3-Hours Incubation at 35°C

Salt Concentration	Cell Counts per Gram of Shell[a,b]
0%	5.0×10^7
0.5%	8.6×10^7
1.0%	1.7×10^8
1.5%	1.9×10^8
2.0%	2.2×10^8
2.5%	1.3×10^8
3.0%	1.1×10^8
3.5%	4.2×10^7

[a]Initial inoculum: 1.4×10^7 cells/g of shell.
[b]Mean of two trials.

Table 5. Adherence of _Vibrio cholerae_ to Crab Shells as a Function of pH after 3-Hours Incubation at 35°C

pH	Cell Counts per Gram of Shell[a,b]
4	2.3×10^6
5	3.8×10^6
6	7.2×10^6
7	9.9×10^6
8	1.6×10^6
9	1.4×10^6

[a]Initial inoculum: 1.4×10^7 cells/g of shell.
[b]Mean of two trials.

adherence. Crude chitin can be extracted from crab shell by first treating the shell with acid and then treating these decalcified fragments with base to remove the protein (Welinder 1974a). The adherence ability of V. cholerae was examined at each stage of treatment. If chitin was the component of the crab shell which most influences adherences, then more cells should adhere to a gram of crude chitin than to a gram of crab shell fragments. We did not observe this (Table 6). Approximately the same number of cells adhered to the gram of crab shell containing only 0.15 to 0.2 g chitin as to 1 g of crude chitin. Furthermore, Nalin et al. (1979) used 4% NaCl in their adherence systems and noted "good" adherence. We noted that adherence to the crude chitin was similar in synthetic seawater containing either 2 or 4% NaCl. Conversely, adherence to the intact shell was inhibited at high NaCl concentrations. This indicates that other components, probably calcium carbonate, may be important for V. cholerae's adherence to crab shell.

Electron microscopy studies were conducted in an attempt to illustrate the mechanism of attachment. The cells

Table 6. Adherence of Vibrio cholerae to Components of the Crab Shell after 3-Hours Incubation at 35°C in Synthetic Seawater

Treatment	Result	Counts per Gram
Untreated	Crab shell fragment	1.4×10^8
Excess Trichloracetic Acid 48 hours	Decalcified fragments	1.0×10^5
Excess/1m NH_4OH 5 days, 5°C	Decalcified and deproteinated fragments (crude chitin)	1.9×10^8

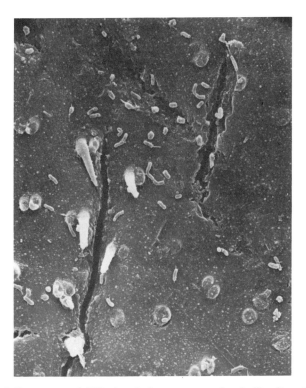

Figure 1. Adherence of Vibrio cholerae to crab shell after 2.5 hours incubation in synthetic sea water at 35°C. Magnification 2750X.

were often clustered near projections protruding from the shell which may indicate possible trapping of cells and prevention of removal by washing procedures (Figure 1).

Cells incubated in distilled water appeared distorted compared to cells incubated in synthetic seawater; however, cells were still able to maintain their ability to adhere to the crab shell fragments.

SUMMARY

The results of this study support the work of Nalin et al. (1979) on the adherence of V. cholerae to chitin.

However, this study also indicated that other components of the crab shell beside chitin influence the adherence of V. cholerae to crab shell. The optimum conditions for adsorption were salt concentration of 1.5 to 2%, pH values of 7, and a temperature of approximately 35°C. It is possible that V. cholerae may associate with crabs and other marine fauna and that this association may prolong its survival in the marine environment. We are currently investigating this possibility.

REFERENCES

American Public Health Association. 1976. Compendium of methods for the microbiological examination of food. APHA, Washington, D.C.

Blake, P.A., D.T. Allegra, J.D. Snyder, T.J. Barrett, L. McFarland, C.T. Caraway, J.C. Feeley, J.P. Craig, J.V. Lee, N.D. Puhr, and R.A. Feldman. 1980. Cholera--a possible endemic focus in the United States. N. Engl. J. Med. 302:305-309.

Colwell, R.R., and J. Kaper. 1977. Vibrio cholerae, Vibrio parahaemolyticus, and other vibrios: occurrence and distribution in Chesapeake Bay. Science. 198:394-396.

Mizaki, K., S. Iwahara, K. Asto, S. Jujimoto, and K. Atbara. 1967. Basic studies on the viability of El Tor vibrios. Bull. W.H.O. 37:773-778.

Nalin, D.R., V.D. Reid, M.M. Levine, and L. Cisneros. 1979. Adsorption and growth of Vibrio cholerae on chitin. Infect. Immun. 25:768-770.

Pesigan, T.P., J. Plantilla, and M. Rolda. 1967. Applied studies on the viability of El Tor vibrios, Bull. W.H.O. 37:779-786.

Sakazaki, R. 1979. Vibrio infections. Pages 189-206 in
H. Riemann and F.L. Bryan (Eds.), Food-borne
infection and intoxication. Academic Press, New York.

Welinder, B.S. 1974a. The crustacean cuticle. I.
Studies on the composition of the cuticle. Comp.
Biochem. Physiol. 47A:779-780.

Welinder, B.S. 1974b. The crustacean cuticle. II.
Composition of the individual layer in Cancer pagurus
cuticle. Comp. Biochem. Physiol.. 52A:659-663.

Chapter 39

THE EFFECTS OF STORAGE ON VIBRIO
CONCENTRATIONS IN SHELLFISH

Mary A. Hood and Gregory E. Ness

Recent outbreaks of cholera and cholera-like gastroenteritis along the Gulf Coast have implicated shellfish as the source of contamination (Weissman et al. 1975; Centers for Disease Control 1978; Blake et al. 1980). In Florida, outbreaks of cholera have been traced to the consumption of raw oysters (Centers for Disease Control 1979; 1980). In addition to cholera, a number of other food-borne diseases have been associated with shellfish and are caused by several Vibrio species as reviewed by Blake (this volume). It was evident from the increasing number of outbreaks that the relationship between these bacteria and shellfish needed to be examined. Therefore, studies were designed to determine the effects of several commonly used storage and handling methods on the levels of Vibrio cholerae, V. parahaemolyticus, and the lactose-positive Vibrios (Lac[+] vibrios or V. vulnificus) in two economically important species of shellfish: oysters, Crassostrea virginica; and clams, Mercenaria campechiensis.

The shellfish examined in our studies were collected from two of the most productive shellfish harvesting areas in Florida, Apalachicola Bay and Tampa Bay, and the sites from which they were collected represented a range of water qualities, including three prohibited shellfish harvesting areas, a conditionally approved harvesting area, and two approved harvesting areas. A procedure developed by Dr. Norman Blake (University of South Florida) in which the samples were transported in portable refrigeration units (Koolatron Industries, Ontario, Canada) ensured that the samples reached the laboratory quickly (within 6 to 8 hours after collection) under well-controlled conditions. With one exception, temperatures were maintained below 12°C during shipment of the samples.

The shellfish samples were prepared for microbiological analysis using standard recommended procedures (American Public Health Association 1970). V. cholerae was enumerated using the methods described by Kaper et al. (1979) and Hood et al. (1981). Numbers of V. parahaemolyticus were determined by an MPN series using glucose salt Teepol enrichment broth followed by streaking onto TCBS (Food and Drug Administration 1978), and confirming colonies by the API 20E system (Analytab Products, Inc., Plainview, NY), oxidase reaction, 0/129 sensitivity, and salt requirement. The Lac$^+$ vibrios were enumerated by reincubating the V. cholerae alkaline peptone broths for an additional 6 hours, streaking onto TCBS, and confirming green colonies using the API 20E system, oxidase reaction, 0/129 sensitivity, lactose fermentation, and salt requirement (R.J. Seidler, personal communications).

Statistical analysis including analysis of variants and linear correlation analysis was conducted using SAS programs at the Institute for Statistical and Mathematical Modeling (University of West Florida). Probability levels were considered significant if they were observed at the 95% level of confidence or above.

Storage Procedures

Oysters are generally stored and shipped in two ways. For local markets, the animals are left in their shells and shipped as shellstock. They are also processed, packaged in tins or plastic containers, and shipped to markets. Oyster houses in Florida generally process the shellfish by shucking and washing the meats. Our experiments were designed to examine both shellstock and processed oysters.

Four temperatures (2°C, 8°C, 20°C, and 35°C) and three time intervals (7, 14, and 21 days) were chosen for the shellstock experiments as they represented real conditions to which oysters might be exposed. In the shucked or processed experiments, a storage temperature of 8°C was selected after a survey of the local supermarkets revealed that this temperature was one under which processed oysters were generally held. Fourteen days was the maximum number of days for storage as the Food and Drug Administration recommends this time limitation to ensure the quality of the meats.

Processing oysters consisted of a treatment designed to simulate the procedure used in most Florida oyster processing houses. The oysters were first sucked into cold (4°C) tap water of drinking quality after which they were removed, placed on a nylon screen (to simulate the scimmer process), and sprayed with cold tap water for 2 minutes. Shell particles and debris were removed by hand, and the meats were then transferred to a container equipped with an air-stone rod (to simulate the blower process). Small air bubbles were blown into the water causing the oyster meats to circulate slowly and the gills to expand so that the meats were thoroughly cleaned. Exposure to this treatment was conducted for 5 minutes after which the meats were transferred to sterile glass jars and stored.

Time and Temperature for Storage

The most dramatic effects of storing oysters as shellshock were observed at 7 days (Figure 1). V. cholerae levels increased significantly by nearly one log at 2°C, while mean levels of V. parahaemolyticus increased at 20°C and the Lac[+] vibrios increased at 20°C and 8°C. However, after 7 days of storage, the levels of vibrios either remained statistically the same as initial levels (as with V. cholerae) or declined (as with V. parahaemolyticus and the Lac[+] vibrios).

Oysters that were shucked but not washed had significantly lower concentrations of vibrios than shellstock (Figure 2), and, with the single exception of the Lac[+]

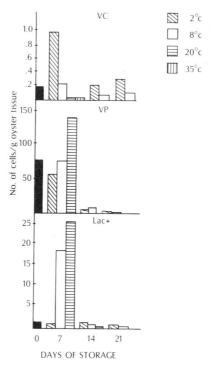

Figure 1. The effect of temperature and time on the levels of V. cholerae (VC), V. parahaemolyticus (VP), and the Lac+ Vibrios (Lac+) in oysters stored as shellstock.

vibrio levels at 7 days, the recoverable numbers of vibrios declined with storage. In the fully processed oysters, mean levels of V. cholerae were higher than in unwashed oyster meats (Figure 3), but statistically these differences were not significant. It was observed that after 7 days of storage, V. cholerae was rarely isolated from either washed or unwashed oyster meats. V. parahaemolyticus and the Lac+ vibrios in shucked oysters showed several responses under storage, but because of large variations among replica samples, the differences were not significant. However, V. parahaemolyticus levels like V. cholerae did significantly decline with storage time.

Site location and the physical/chemical parameters of salinity, dissolved oxygen, and the total and volatile

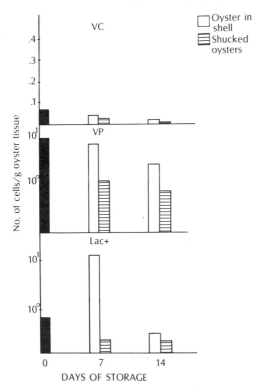

Figure 2. The effect of shucking on the levels of V. cholerae (VC), V. parahaemolyticus (VP), and the Lac[+] Vibrios (Lac[+]) in stored oysters (held at 8°C).

suspended matter of the waters from which the oysters were collected had no significant effect on the concentration of V. cholerae under any storage condition. However, there was a significant interaction among V. cholerae levels in stored shellstock and environmental temperature above 30°C. When water temperatures were above 30°C, levels of V. cholerae in stored oysters were higher. Correlation analysis revealed that at 7 days of storage as shellstock the Lac[+] Vibrio levels strongly correlated to the temperature and salinity of the harvesting waters, and at 14 days, V. parahaemolyticus correlated to temperature and salinity. This suggests that oysters harvested from waters whose temperatures and salinities are high are likely to develop

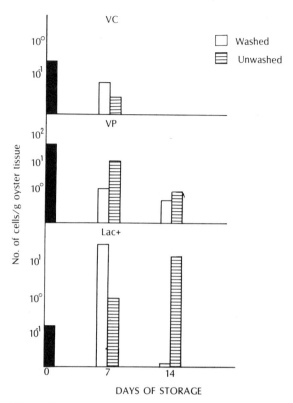

Figure 3. The effect of washing on the levels of V. cholerae (VC), V. parahaemolyticus (VP), and the Lac[+] Vibrios (Lac[+]) in stored oysters (held at 8°C).

higher concentrations of vibrios under storage than oysters harvested from waters of low temperatures and salinities.

In contrast to oysters, clams had relatively lower initial levels of vibrios, and under storage conditions, little changes in the concentration of these bacteria occurred (Figure 4). V. cholerae was isolated from only one clam sample by Dr. G.E. Rodrick (personal communication) while mean levels of V. parahaemolyticus and Lac[+] vibrios were less than 1 cell/g and 0.2 cells/g tissue, respectively. At 2°C storage, vibrios were rarely recovered from clams while at 8°C, mean levels of V. parahaemolyticus and Lac[+] vibrios increased only slightly.

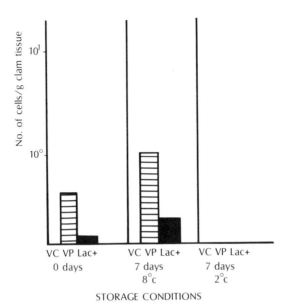

Figure 4. The effect of temperature on the levels of V. cholerae (VC), V. parahaemolyticus (VP), and the Lac$^+$ vibrios (Lac$^+$) in stored clams.

SUMMARY AND CONCLUSIONS

Storage of oysters as shellstock appears to be the treatment that may result in the survival and growth of vibrios, while processing, that is, shucking and washing, appears to result in an overall decline in vibrios. At cold storage temperatures, V. cholerae and the Lac$^+$ vibrios increased in stored shellstock, but in shucked oysters, the levels of V. cholerae and V. parahaemolyticus significantly declined. The reason why such responses occur is probably a function of many complex factors including the composition of the initial microbial load and the physiology of the oyster. However, from a practical standpoint, the safety of oyster meats for consumption depends on the manner in which the shellfish are handled and stored. From the studies discussed here it appears that the processing of oysters is an effective means of preventing increases in the levels of vibrios, especially V. cholerae and V. parahaemolyticus.

The observation that certain types of shellfish are more likely to harbor vibrios than others allows efforts to be directed toward finding solutions to the problem of making those shellfish products safer. For example, clams may be far less likely a source of vibrio-related gastrointestinal illness than oysters because the initial concentrations of vibrios were found to be low and the levels of these bacteria changed little under storage conditions.

REFERENCES

American Public Health Association. 1970. Recommended Procedures for the Examination of Seawater and Shellfish, 4th ed. APHA, Washington, D.C.

Blake, P.A., D.T. Allegra, J.D. Snyder, T.J. Barrett, L. McFarland, C.T. Caraway, J.D. Feeley, J.P. Craig, J.V. Lee, N.D. Puhr, and R.A. Feldman. 1980. Cholera--a possible endemic focus in the United States. N. Engl. J. Med. 302:305-309.

Centers for Disease Control. 1978. Follow-up on Vibrio cholerae serotype Inaba infection--Louisiana. Morbid. Mortal. Wkly. Rpt. 27:388.

Centers for Disease Control. 1979. Non-O1 Vibrio cholerae infections--Florida. Morbid. Mortal. Wkly. Rpt. 28:571-572.

Centers for Disease Control. 1980. Cholera--Florida. Morbid. Mortal. Wkly. Rpt. 29:601.

Food and Drug Administration. 1978. Bacteriological Analytical Manual. Association of Official Analytical Chemists, Washington, D.C.

Hood, M.A., G.E. Ness, and G.E. Rodrick. 1981. Isolation of _Vibrio cholerae_ serotype O1 from the eastern oyster, _Crassostrea virginica_. Appl. Environ. Microbiol. 41:559-560.

Kaper J., H. Lockman, R.R. Colwell, and S.W. Joseph. 1979. Ecology, serology, and enterotoxin production of _Vibrio cholerae_ in Chesapeake Bay. Appl. Environ. Microbiol. 37:91-103.

Weissman, J.B., W.E. DeWitt, J. Thompson, C.N. Muchnick, B.L. Portnoy, J.C. Feeley, and E.J. Gangarosa. 1975. A case of cholera in Texas, 1973. Am. J. Epidemiol. 100:487-498.

INDEX

Page numbers followed by *t* indicate tables; page numbers followed by *f* indicate figures.